The Equine Distal Limb

Atlas of Clinical Anatomy and Comparative Imaging

J.-M. Denoix
CIRALE, Equine Clinical Unit
INRA (Department of Animal Health), Anatomy Department
Ecole Nationale Vétérinaire d'Alfort
Paris, France

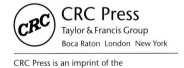

CRC Press
Taylor & Francis Group
Boca Raton London New York

CRC Press is an imprint of the
Taylor & Francis Group, an **informa** business

To Nathalie, my wife,
who shared these years of labour
and is a continuing support
in my achievements.

With my admiration and love.

CRC Press
Taylor & Francis Group
6000 Broken Sound Parkway NW, Suite 300
Boca Raton, FL 33487-2742

© 2000 by Taylor & Francis Group, LLC
CRC Press is an imprint of Taylor & Francis Group, an Informa business

No claim to original U.S. Government works

Visit the Taylor & Francis Web site at
http://www.taylorandfrancis.com

and the CRC Press Web site at
http://www.crcpress.com

Contents

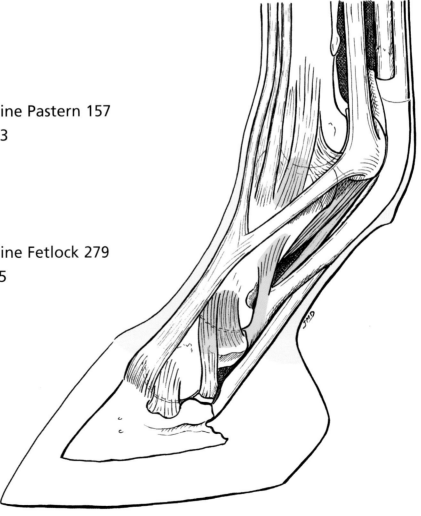

Foreword

Jean-Marie Denoix is the world's foremost equine musculoskeletal system anatomist, and using this anatomical knowledge he has become one of the world's leading equine diagnostic ultrasonographers. No-one is better qualified to compile a reference atlas of clinical anatomy correlated with images obtained by radiography, diagnostic ultrasonography and magnetic resonance imaging.

The diagnosis of lameness depends first and foremost on a detailed clinical evaluation, but it is then necessary to decide on the most appropriate imaging modality (or modalities) to use in order to help in the final diagnosis. Advanced imaging techniques require an in-depth knowledge of anatomy for accurate interpretation; especially when using magnetic resonance imaging this must be a three-dimensional concept of anatomy.

This book is a unique contribution to equine medicine and will be an invaluable reference text. The image quality is extraordinarily high and the multiple views of each area of the distal limb provide an extremely detailed evaluation. The text clearly highlights our current limitations in localizing pain sufficiently accurately to specific anatomical structures. It emphasizes the vital importance of the knowledge of normal anatomy and the need for highly detailed evaluations using a variety of imaging techniques in order to gain maximum information about the normality or otherwise of the structures in the area under investigation.

Magnetic resonance imaging has the potential in the future to enhance greatly our diagnostic capabilities in the distal limb, particularly within the foot. This book provides an excellent database of normal MRI anatomy. This work will therefore be essential for anyone involved in complex lameness evaluations, and those utilizing advanced imaging techniques.

Sue Dyson MA VetMB PhD DEO FRCVS

Preface

In the last ten years, the constant development of imaging modalities has reinforced the need for a better knowledge of anatomy. Diagnostic imaging is now a major part of the clinical examination of lame horses and will be even more important in the future.

Many of the classic books and manuals on the subject provide an anatomical basis for the understanding of the general constitution of the horse's locomotor apparatus and are very useful for a comprehensive, overall knowledge of the anatomy of the equine limbs. But with the growing importance of diagnostic techniques, there is a need for reference anatomical documents providing immediate support for the interpretation of diagnostic images.

The purpose of this book is to feature a direct source of information based on real, fresh anatomical specimens very close to live anatomy. It provides reference images of the foot, pastern and fetlock – the most commonly involved areas in equine locomotor problems. The reference images include dissections, segmental anatomic sections and diagnostic images (radiographs and ultrasound scans as well as magnetic resonance imaging scans). Following the general approach of morphological sciences, based on relationships of anatomical structures and a direct analogy between images, no text is provided, but there is precise and complete labelling for each specimen or cross-section.

The anatomical specimens presented in this book were prepared using various techniques of fine dissection performed on fresh limbs, as well as on limbs injected with coloured latex into the vessels and/or synovial cavities of joints or tendon sheaths. The anatomical cross-sections were made at regular intervals in the three complementary planes of the space, after injection of coloured latex into the vessels and/or synovial cavities. Since the specimens were prepared, and the latex injected, over a considerable period of time, the colour of the latex may differ between specimens.

The clinical importance of each anatomical section is illustrated by correlated diagnostic imaging documents: plain or contrast radiographic studies, ultrasound scans of sound live horses and magnetic resonance imaging scans performed on sound isolated limbs.

The anatomical terms used in this book are close to those recommended in the Fourth Edition of the *Nomina Anatomica Veterinaria* (1994) and the illustrated *Veterinary Anatomical Nomenclature* (Schaller, 1992), but they also take into account usage among English-speaking anatomists and clinicians, which can be found in conventional books. At the end of the book there is an alphabetical index in English, with Latin equivalents for readers in non-English speaking countries.

The objective of this atlas is to provide the clinician with the anatomical basis required for the main steps in the clinical examination of locomotor problems in horses, including:

- Interpretation of local deformity (inspection), based on the topography of subcutaneous structures.
- Regional analgesia (nerve blocks) and intrasynovial analgesia (joint or tendon sheaths blocks), based on precise anatomical landmarks.
- Interpretation of diagnostic analgesia, using nerve and synovial relationships.
- Preparation and interpretation of soft tissue images, especially ultrasound scans.
- Anatomical landmarks for orthopaedic surgery and local injection or treatment.

My priority has been to produce a book that is informative and easy to use; I hope it will be useful in resolving the diagnosis of a large variety of clinical conditions involving the equine distal limb and for the teaching of locomotor diseases in the horse.

Jean-Marie Denoix

Acknowledgements

Many individuals contributed and helped in the production of this book. I would like to thank especially P. Perrot and B. Bousseau for their invaluable help in the preparation of the anatomical sections, in the presentation of the book, as well as in the labelling of the legends.

Many thanks to Professor Mathieu (Hopital Henri Mondor, Creteil-F) for having allowed us to produce the MRI scans in his department, and to Dr J. Tapprest who provided many of them.

Finally, I would like to acknowledge all the equine practitioners and colleagues who regularly encouraged me to complete this book, as they wished to have at their disposal the iconography performed on the anatomy and diagnostic imaging of one of the main parts of the horse's locomotor system.

Grants and assistance in the production of the book

This work has been completed thanks to the financial support of the INRA (National Institute of Agronomic Research – Department of Animal Health), and of the Haras Nationaux (French Horse Breeding Institute).

General Presentation of the Atlas

Objective

The aim of this book is to show the anatomy of the horse's distal limb (foot, pastern and fetlock) exclusively in the form of dissected anatomical specimens, anatomical cross-sections and diagnostic imaging documents – radiographs, ultrasonograms, magnetic resonance imaging (MRI) scans – with explanatory legends.

These illustrations should provide:

- Basic anatomical data, as required for physical examination and for carrying out diagnostic analgesia (nerves and synovial blocks).
- Reference images for interpreting diagnostic imaging (radiographs, ultrasonograms and MRI scans).
- Anatomical guidelines, references and illustrations required for actual treatment (e.g. for surgical approaches or local injections into joint cavities and tendon sheaths, as well as in other anatomical locations).

This atlas is focused on the distal parts of the equine forelimb which is the most frequently involved area when osteoarticular and tendon lesions occur in horses.

Materials and methods

The book contains illustrations of reference anatomical specimens and cross-sections, in conjunction with radiographic and ultrasonographic images. MRI scans are also widely used to demonstrate the correlation between anatomy and imaging techniques. Thus, the diagnostic images can easily be compared to the anatomical cross-sections performed in the transverse, frontal and sagittal planes, in order to accurately identify each joint structure, tendon or vessel.

The legends are presented mainly in English according to the recommendations of the International Committee on Veterinary Anatomical Nomenclature (*Nomina Anatomica Veterinaria*, Fourth Edition, 1994). Because of their worldwide use, some Latin names have also been employed, especially for the hoof and corium.

Anatomical illustrations

Detailed photographs of precise and cleaned anatomical dissections of fresh and injected specimens cover all aspects of the areas considered in the book. For each region they are presented from the most superficial anatomical layers to the deepest. Information on the topography of each anatomical structure is provided with these specimens.

There are also highly detailed anatomical cross-sections, performed on isolated frozen limbs after the injection of coloured latex into the vessels (arteries and veins) and/or synovial cavities of joints and tendon sheaths.

The limbs have been clipped to avoid contamination by hair and the cross-sections have been performed in the three complementary planes of the space (sagittal, transverse and frontal planes) in order to accurately define the identity, size and topography of each joint or tendon structure.

All planes of section are defined and illustrated with line drawings by the author.

General Presentation of the Atlas

In each area selected, casting specimens have also been prepared to illustrate the regional vascular supply or synovial cavities.

Diagnostic images

Based on precise and clear anatomical data, the purpose of this atlas is to present, with each anatomical cross-section, correlated diagnostic images:

- Plain and contrast radiographs of sound horses with no history of lameness, as well as normal isolated limbs.
- Reference ultrasound scans made using sound horses.
- MRI scans of isolated limbs with no lesions of the locomotor system.

The radiographs were produced using high definition single emulsion films (Kodak Min R). An 8 ratio grid with parallel lead sheaths was used for dorsopalmar and lateromedial projections of the foot. The exposure varied from 60 to 70 kV and from 12 to 63 mAs.

Sound adult horses with no history of lameness provided reference transverse and longitudinal (sagittal, parasagittal and frontal) ultrasonographic images of the foot, pastern and fetlock; these images were made with a non-portable machine (Aloka 2000) equipped with 7.5 MHz linear and convex linear probes and a 10 MHz sector probe. The skin of the area was clipped and a standoff pad was placed between the skin and probe in order to improve contact with the limb and enhance visualization of superficial structures. All the longitudinal and transverse ultrasound scans were recorded on 3/4 inch U-Matic videotapes to allow complete retrospective analysis and manipulation.

MRI scans were performed on selected normal freshly isolated limbs. These images were produced with a 1.5 Tesla field machine (Magnetom-Siemens) using a T1 weighted sequence. Some of the MRI scans were performed after injection of 'fat material' or latex into the arteries or veins in order to highlight the position of these structures.

Legends have been placed consistently on ultrasonograms and occasionally on radiographs. In general, legends have not been added to MRI scans, except when some vessels have undergone specific preparation, as their appearance is closely related to the anatomical sections that accompany them.

Presentation

Sections

For each of the anatomical regions shown – foot, pastern and fetlock – four types of images are provided:

1 Anatomical views (dissected specimens).
2 Sagittal cross-sections (anatomical cross-sections, ultrasound scans, MRI scans) as well as lateromedial radiographs.
3 Transverse cross-sections (anatomical cross-sections, radiographs, ultrasound or MRI scans).
4 Frontal cross-sections (anatomical cross-sections, ultrasound scans, MRI scans) and dorsopalmar radiographs.

Design

The material on each anatomical specimen or cross-section is displayed on a double page. All dissected specimens or sagittal sections are presented with the dorsal aspect facing to the left; the corresponding ultrasound scans are presented with the distal aspect on the right. All transverse sections are presented with the dorsal aspect up; the corresponding transverse ultrasonograms are presented as they are displayed on the monitor, with the superficial structures on the top and the dorsal or medial aspect on the left.

The Equine Foot

Dissections of the Equine Foot

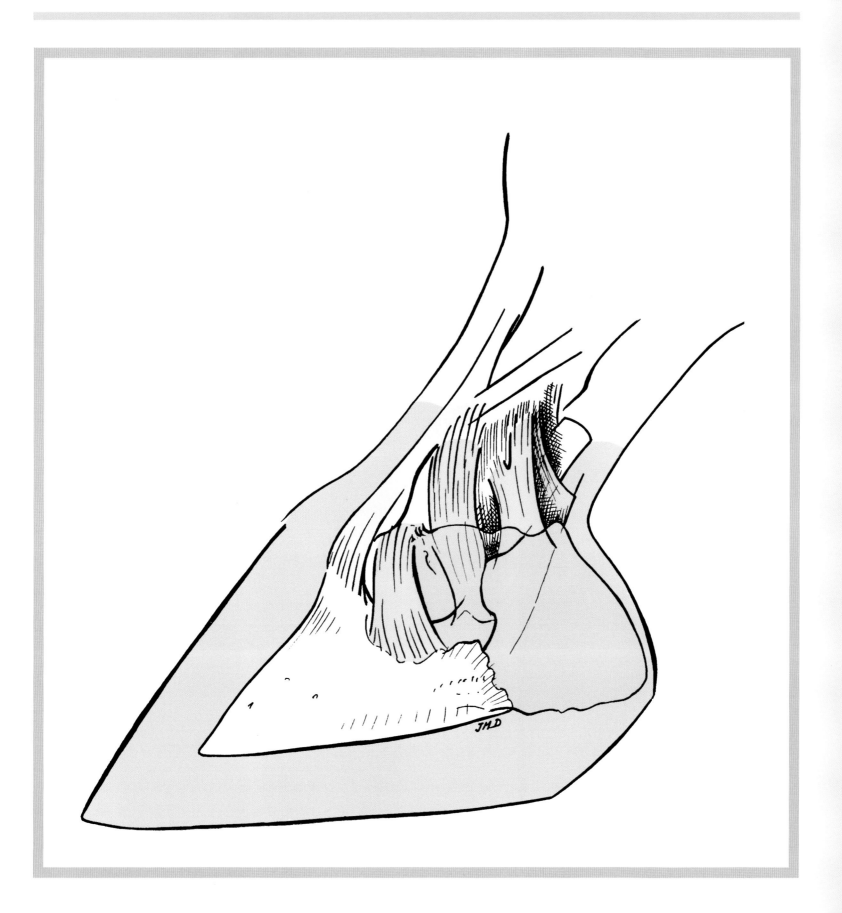

Dissection 1: Corium and Hoof – Dorsal Part

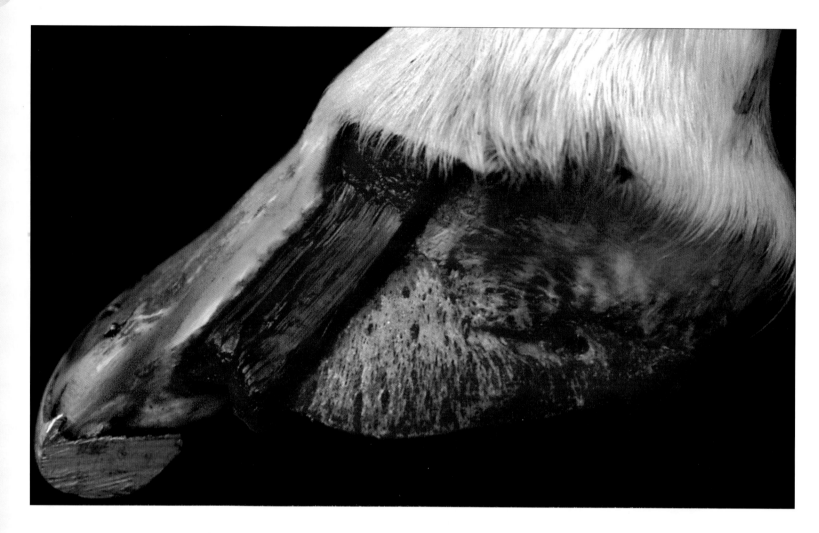

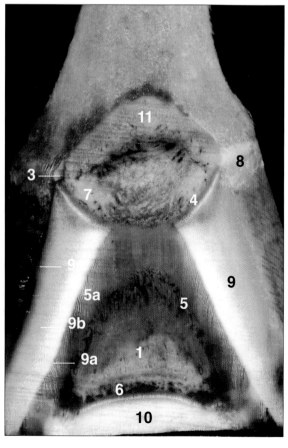

Frontal anatomical section of the foot.

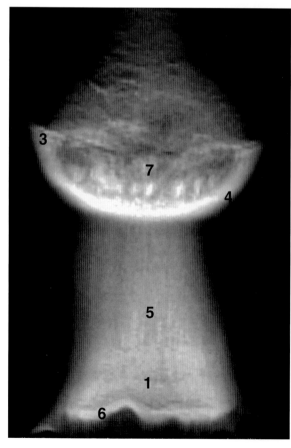

Frontal MRI scan of the foot.

Dissection 1: Corium and Hoof – Dorsal Part

1 Distal phalanx
  1a Foramen of the palmar process
  1b Parietal sulcus
2 Ungular cartilage
3 Corium limbi
4 Corium coronae
5 Corium parietis
  5a Dermal lamellae
6 Corium soleae
7 Pulvinus coronae
8 Periople
9 Hoof wall
  9a Stratum internum
  9b Stratum medium
  9c Stratum externum
10 Sole
11 Skin
12 Shoe

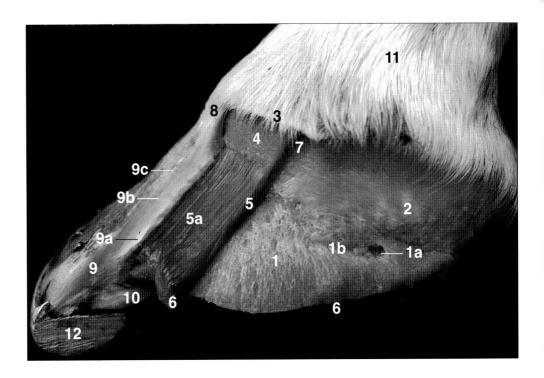

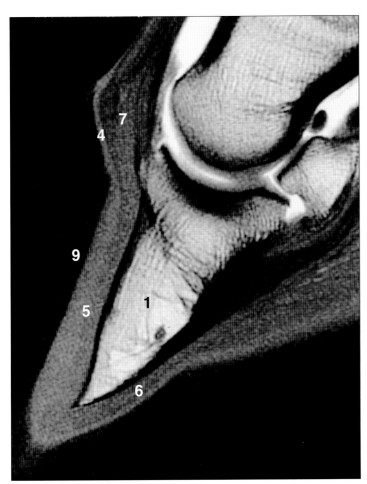

Sagittal MRI scan of the foot after injection of contrast material in the distal interphalangeal joint.

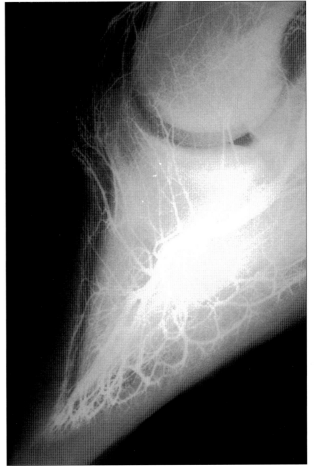

Contrast radiographic study of the arteries (arteriography) of the corium, lateromedial view.

Dissection 2: Corium (After Removal of the Hoof) – Collateral Part

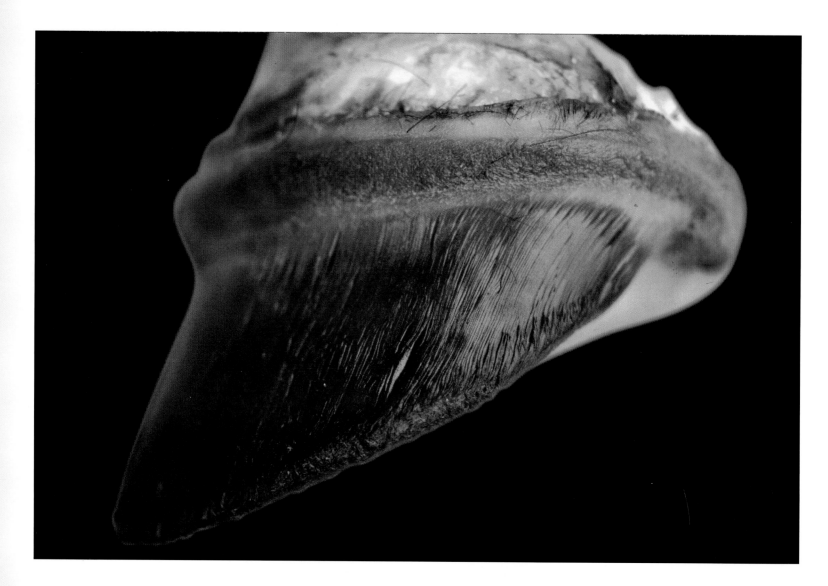

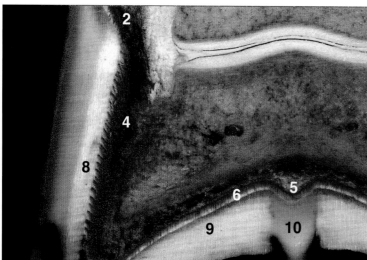

Frontal section of the equine foot after injection of latex in the synovial cavities and vessels.

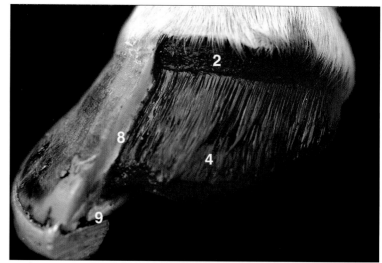

Dorsomedial aspect of the foot after removal of the medial part of the hoof.

Dissection 2: Corium (After Removal of the Hoof) – Collateral Part

1 Ungular cartilage
2 Corium coronae
   2a Dermal papillae
3 Corium limbi
4 Corium parietis
   4a Dermal lamellae
5 Corium cunei
6 Corium soleae
   6a Dermal papillae
7 Heel
8 Hoof wall
9 Sole
10 Frog (apex)

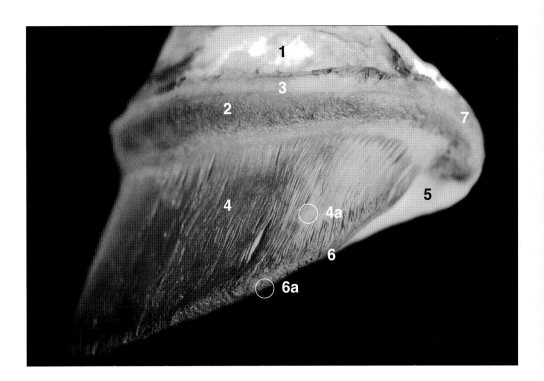

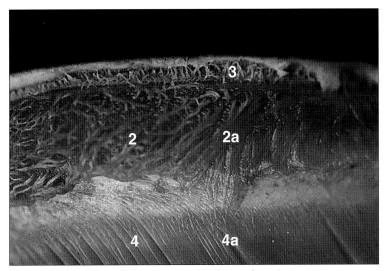

Dermal papillae of the corium limbi and corium coronae.

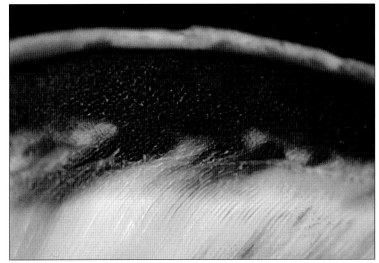

Coronal sulcus: conical depressions of the epidermis coronae that fit with the dermal papillae of the corium coronae.

Dissection 3: Corium Soleae and Corium Cunei – Distal View

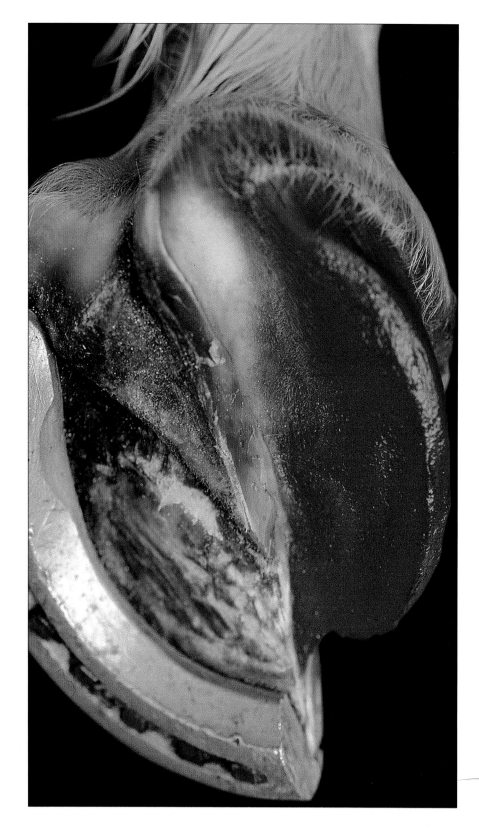

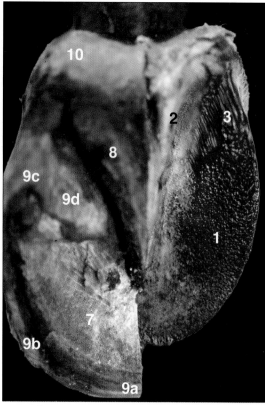

Distal aspect of the foot after removal of the lateral part of the hoof.

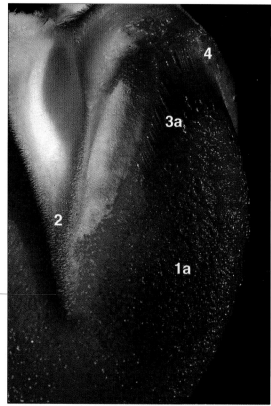

Distal aspect of the corium (after removal of the hoof).

1 Corium soleae
   1a Dermal papillae
2 Corium cunei
3 Corium parietis
   3a Dermal lamellae
4 Corium coronae
5 Corium limbi
6 Skin
7 Sole
   7a Body
   7b Branch
   7c Angle
8 Frog
   8a Apex
   8b Body
   8c Branch
   8d Central cuneal sulcus
   8e Paracuneal sulcus
9 Hoof wall
   9a Dorsal part
   9b Collateral part
   9c Heel
   9d Bar (inflex part)
10 Bulb of the heel
11 Shoe

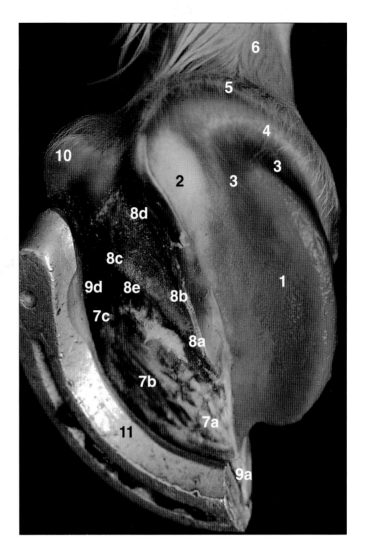

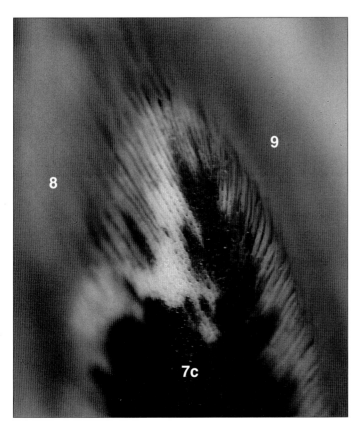

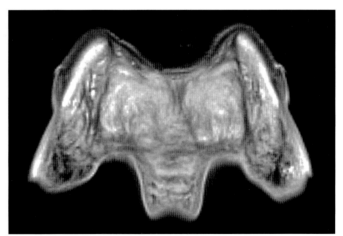

Frontal MRI scan of the foot showing the different parts of the corium.

Proximal aspect of the sole angle showing conical depressions for the dermal papillae of the corium soleae.

Dissection 4: Vessels and Nerves of the Digit – Medial View

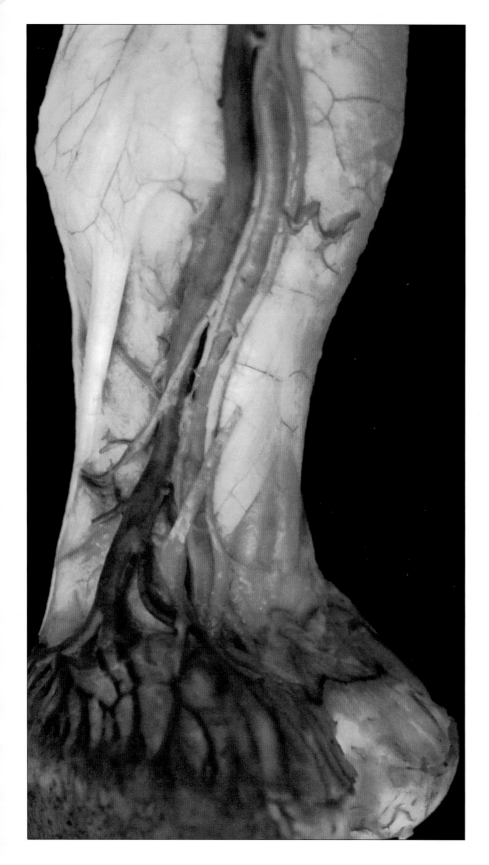

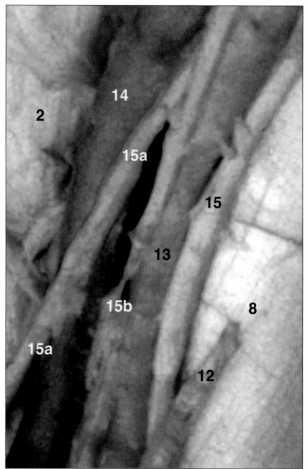

Close up view of the digital vessels and nerves (see dotted area in illustration on opposite page).

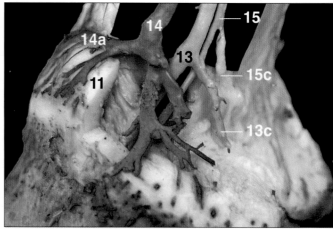

Dissected specimen showing the proper digital vessels and nerve after partial removal of the ungular cartilage.

1 Fetlock region
2 Proximal phalanx (P1)
3 Dorsal digital extensor tendon
4 Extensor branch of the third interosseous muscle
5 Palmar annular ligament
6 Proximal digital annular ligament
7 Distal digital annular ligament
8 Superficial digital flexor tendon (distal branch)
9 Deep digital flexor tendon
10 Digital cushion
11 Ungular cartilage
12 Ergot ligament
13 Proper palmar digital artery
    13a Ergot ramus
    13b Dorsal ramus of P1
    13c Ramus of the digital torus
14 Proper palmar digital vein
    14a Coronal vein
    14b Superficial ungular plexus
    14c Parietal plexus
    14d Lateromedial palmar anastomosis
    14e Dorsal ramus of P1
15 Proper palmar digital nerve
    15a Dorsal ramus
    15b Intermediate ramus
    15c Ramus of the digital torus (see also page 8)

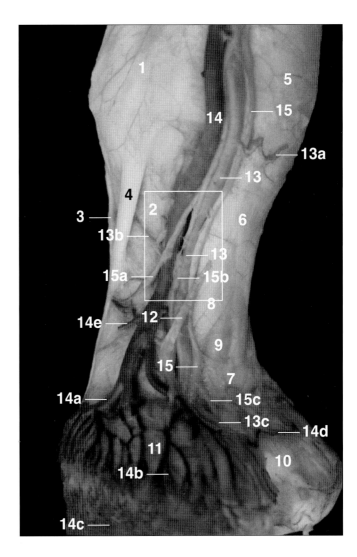

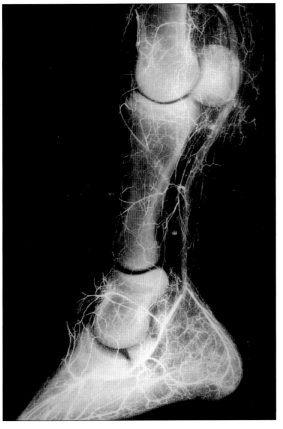

Arterial supply of the digit (only half is shown after a sagittal section).

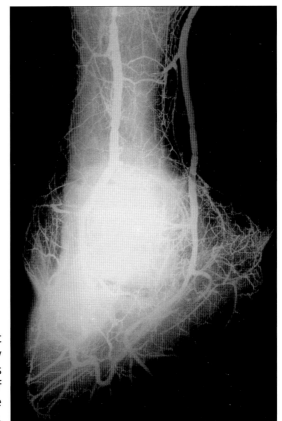

Contrast radiographic study of the arteries (arteriography) of the digit, oblique view.

Dissection 5: Veins of the Foot – Medial View
(Hoof Wall and Corium Removed)

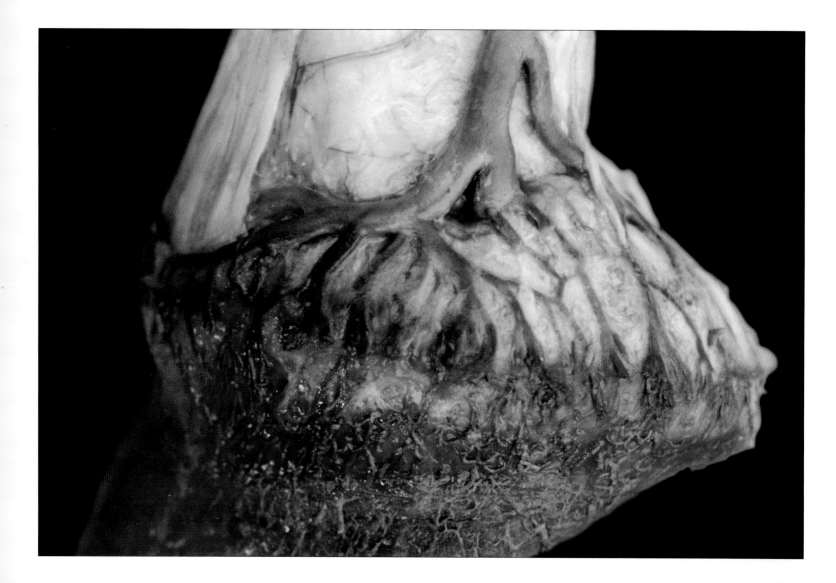

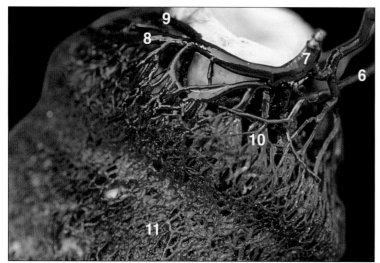

Casting preparation of the veins and arteries of the foot.

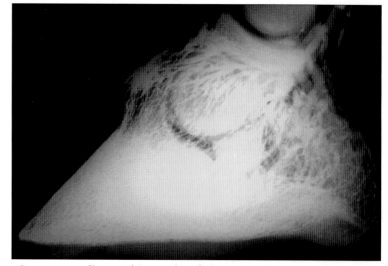

Contrast radiographic study of the veins (venography) and plexi of the foot, lateromedial view.

Dissection 5: Veins of the Foot – Medial View
(Hoof Wall and Corium Removed)

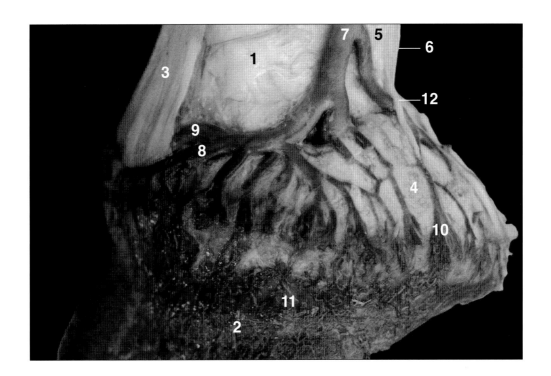

1 Middle phalanx
2 Distal phalanx
3 Dorsal digital extensor tendon
4 Ungular cartilage
5 Ergot ligament
6 Proper palmar digital artery
7 Proper palmar digital vein

8 Coronal vein
9 Dorsal ramus (vein) of the middle phalanx
10 Superficial ungular plexus
11 Parietal plexus
12 Intermediate ramus of the proper palmer digital nerve

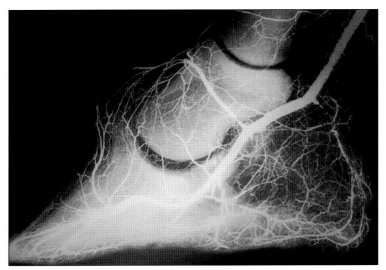

Contrast radiographic study of the arteries (arteriography) of the foot, lateromedial view.

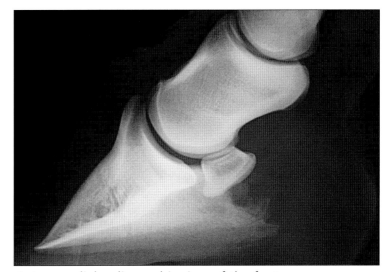

Lateromedial radiographic view of the foot.

Dissection 6: Vessels and Nerves – Palmarolateral View

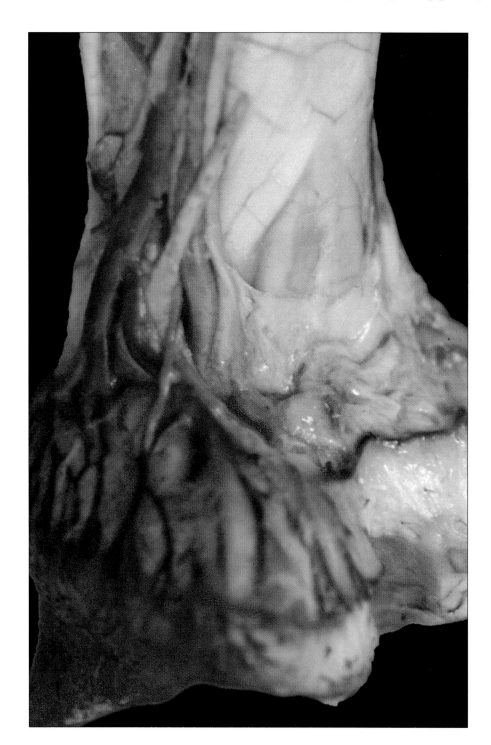

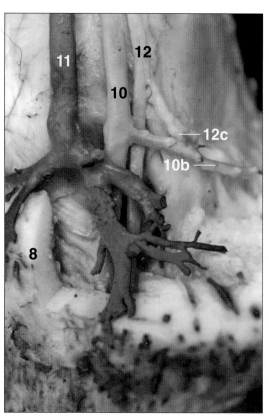

Dissected specimen with incomplete removal of the ungular cartilage.

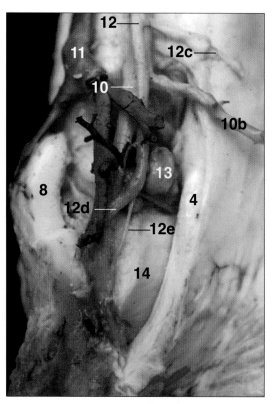

Dissected specimen with incomplete removal of the ungular cartilage and deep digital flexor tendon.

1 Proximal phalanx (P1)
2 Extensor branch of the third interosseous muscle
3 Superficial digital flexor tendon (distal branch)
4 Deep digital flexor tendon
5 Palmar wall of the palmar distal recess of the digital sheath
  5a Mesotendon
6 Distal digital annular ligament
7 Digital cushion
8 Ungular cartilage
9 Ergot ligament
10 Proper palmar digital artery
  10a Dorsal ramus of P1
  10b Ramus of the digital torus
11 Proper palmar digital vein
  11a Coronal vein
  11b Superficial ungular plexus
  11c Parietal plexus
  11d Lateromedial palmar anastomosis
12 Proper palmar digital nerve
  12a Dorsal ramus
  12b Intermediate ramus
  12c Ramus of the digital torus
  12d Ramus for the corium and distal phalanx (page 12)
  12e Ramus for the distal sesamoid bone (page 12)
13 Distal interphalangeal joint cavity (page 12)
14 Distal sesamoid bone (page 12)

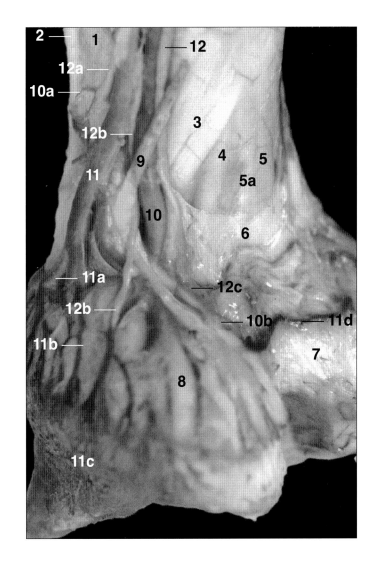

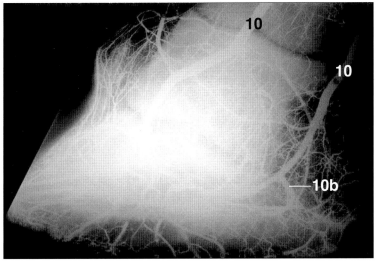

Contrast radiographic study of the arteries (arteriography) of the foot, oblique view.

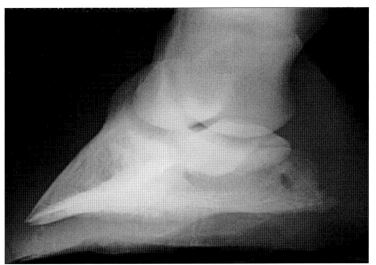

Dorsomedial-palmarolateral oblique radiographic view of the foot.

Preparation 7a: Venography of the Foot

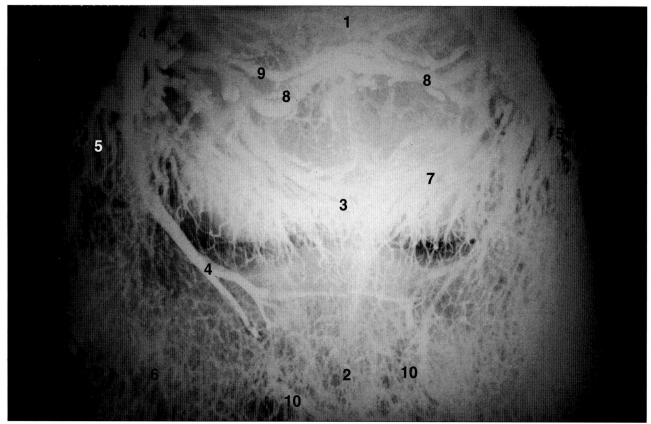

Contrast radiographic study of the veins (venography) of the foot, dorsopalmar view.

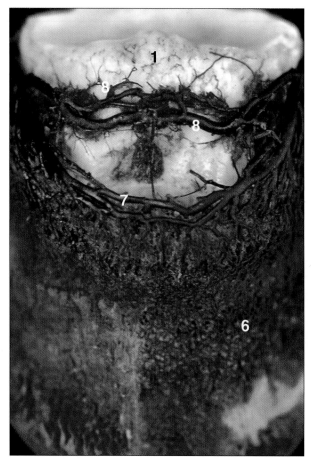

Casting preparation of the veins and arteries of the foot, dorsal view.

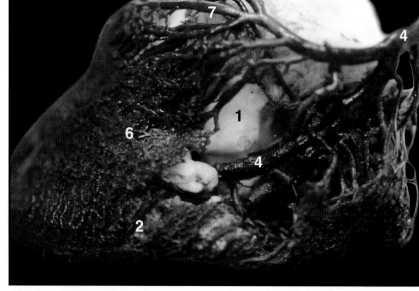

Casting preparation of the veins and arteries of the foot, lateral view.

1 Middle phalanx (P2)	**7** Coronal vein
2 Distal phalanx	**8** Dorsal ramus (vein)
3 Distal sesamoid bone	of P2
4 Proper palmar digital	**9** Palmar ramus (vein)
vein	of P2
5 Ungular plexus	**10** Terminal arch
6 Parietal plexus	

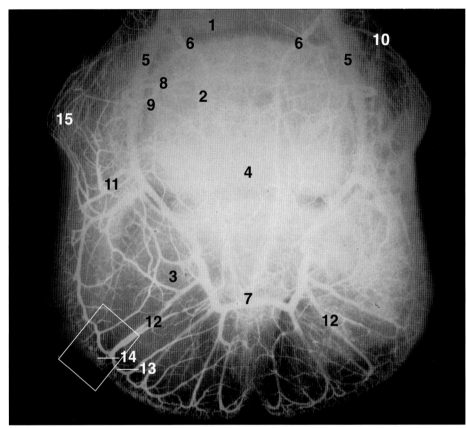

1 Proximal phalanx
2 Middle phalanx (P2)
3 Distal phalanx (P3)
4 Distal sesamoid bone
5 Proper palmar digital artery
6 Ramus of the digital torus
7 Terminal arch
8 Palmar ramus of P2
9 Dorsal ramus of P2
10 Coronal artery
11 Dorsal ramus of P3
12 Perforating rami
13 Solar marginis artery
   (circumflex artery)
14 Arteries of the corium
   parietis
15 Arteries of the corium
   coronae
16 Distal artery and vein of the
   distal sesamoid bone (close-up
   view shown below)

Contrast radiographic study of the arteries (arteriography) of the foot, dorsopalmar view.

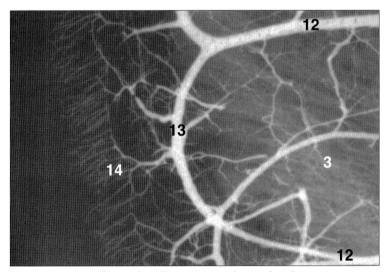

Close-up view from the illustration above (within dotted area).

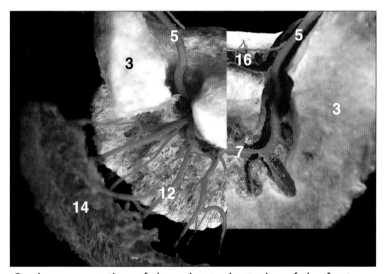

Casting preparation of the veins and arteries of the foot, distal view.

Dissection 8: Digital Cushion and Ungular Cartilage – Palmaromedial View

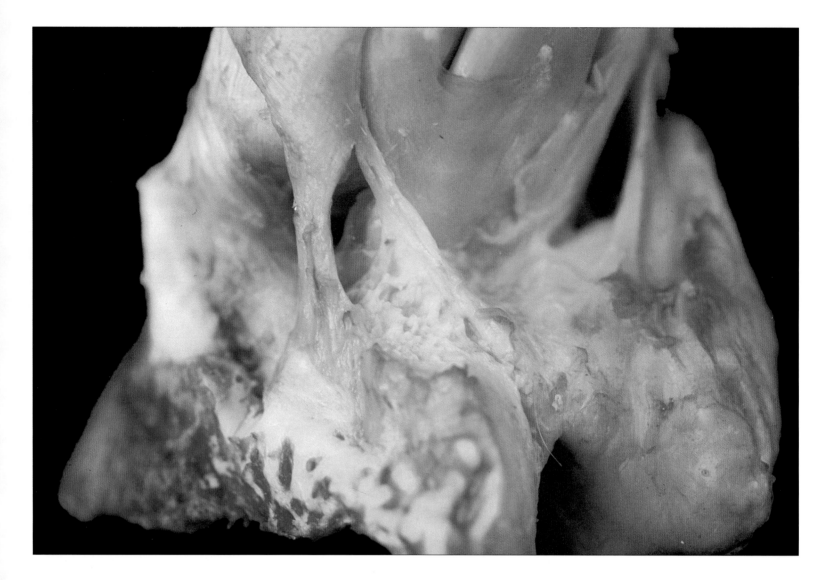

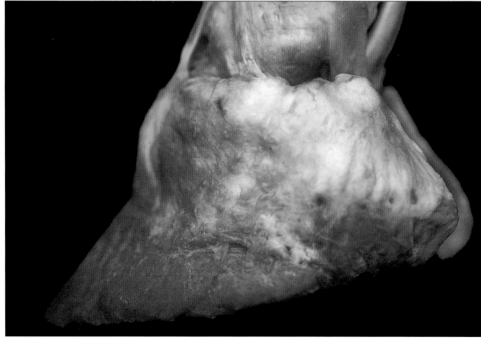

Medial view.

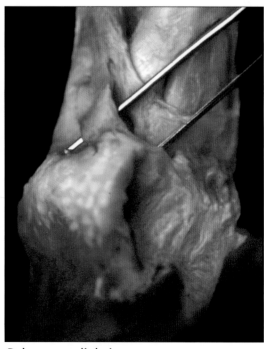

Palmaromedial view.

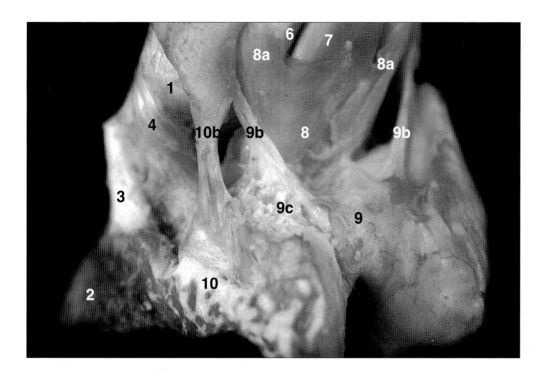

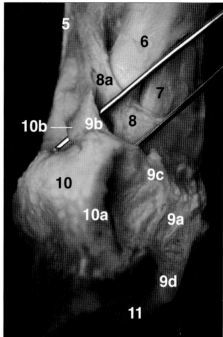

Palmaromedial view.

1 Middle phalanx
2 Distal phalanx
3 Collateral ligament of the distal interphalangeal joint
4 Collateral sesamoidean ligament
5 Dorsal digital extensor tendon
6 Superficial digital flexor tendon (distal branch)
7 Deep digital flexor tendon
8 Distal digital annular ligament
   8a Proximal attachment
9 Digital cushion
   9a Section plane
   9b Proximal attachment
   9c Toric part
   9d Cuneal part
10 Ungular cartilage
   10a Section plane
   10b Chondrocompedal ligament
11 Corium cunei

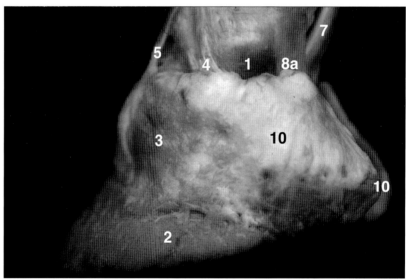

Medial view.

Dissection 9: Interphalangeal Joints – Collateral (Lateral or Medial) View

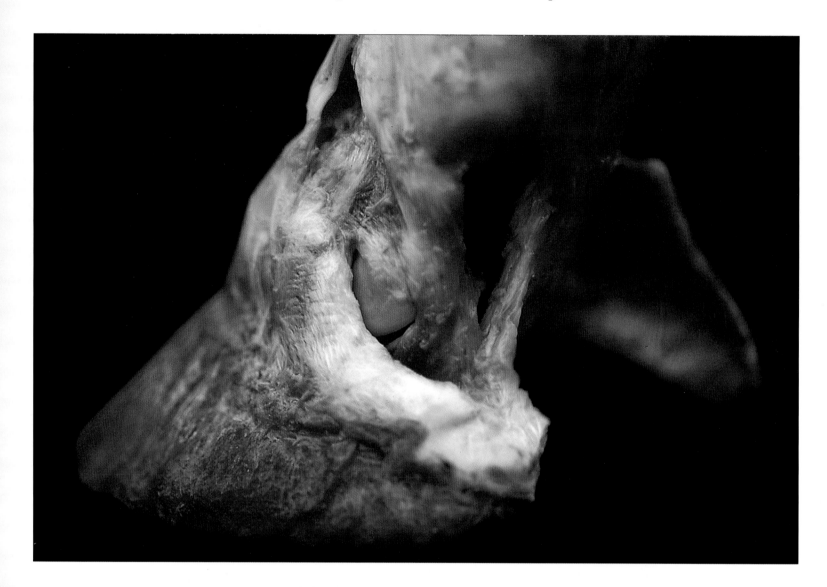

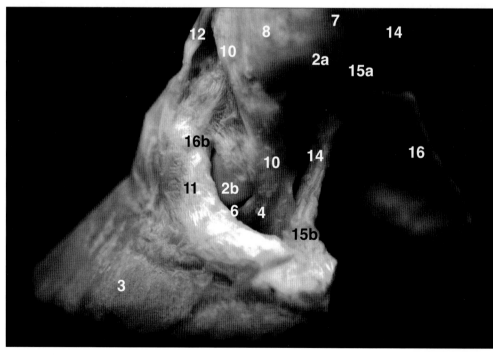

Dissection 9: Interphalangeal Joints –
Collateral (Lateral or Medial) View

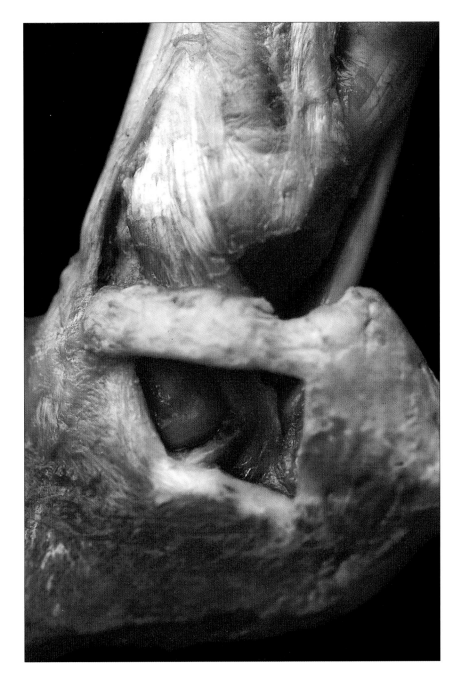

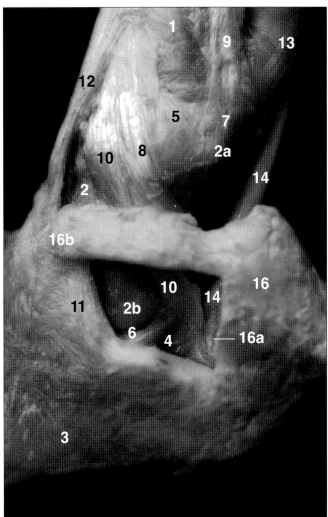

1 Proximal phalanx
2 Middle phalanx
  2a Flexor tuberosity
  2b Distal condyle
3 Distal phalanx
4 Distal sesamoid bone
5 Proximal interphalangeal (PIP) joint
6 Distal interphalangeal (DIP) joint
7 Middle scutum
8 Collateral ligament of the PIP joint
9 Abaxial palmar ligament of the PIP joint

10 Collateral sesamoidean ligament
11 Collateral ligament of the DIP joint
12 Dorsal digital extensor tendon
13 Superficial digital flexor tendon (distal branch)
14 Deep digital flexor tendon
15 Distal digital annular ligament
  15a Proximal attachment
  15b Distal attachment
16 Ungular cartilage
  16a Window cut in it
  16b Chondrocoronal ligament

Dissection 10: Distal Interphalangeal Joint and Podotrochlear Apparatus – Collateral View

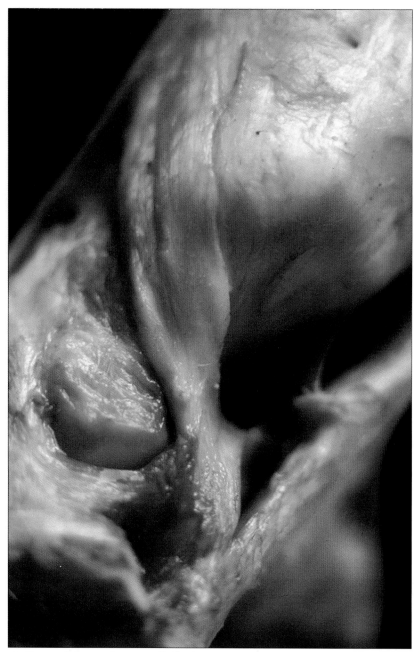

Collateral (lateral or medial) view.

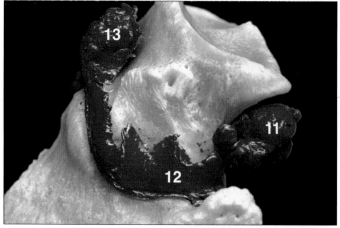

Casting preparation of the DIP joint cavity, lateral view.

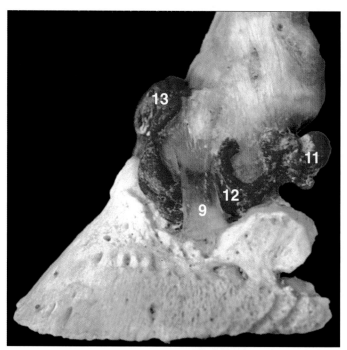

Casting preparation of the DIP joint cavity, lateral view.

Dissection 10: Distal Interphalangeal Joint and Podotrochlear Apparatus – Collateral View

1 Proximal phalanx
2 Middle phalanx
   2a Flexor tuberosity
   2b Distal condyle
3 Distal phalanx
4 Distal sesamoid bone
5 Proximal interphalangeal (PIP) joint
6 Distal interphalangeal (DIP) joint
7 Middle scutum
8 Collateral ligament of the PIP joint
9 Collateral ligament of the DIP joint
10 Collateral sesamoidean ligament
11 Proximopalmar recess of the DIP joint
12 Collateral recess of the DIP joint
13 Dorsal recess of the DIP joint
14 Dorsal digital extensor tendon
15 Deep digital flexor tendon
16 Dorsal distal recess of the digital sheath
17 Proximal recess of the podotrochlear bursa
18 Separation between the synovial recesses
19 Needle

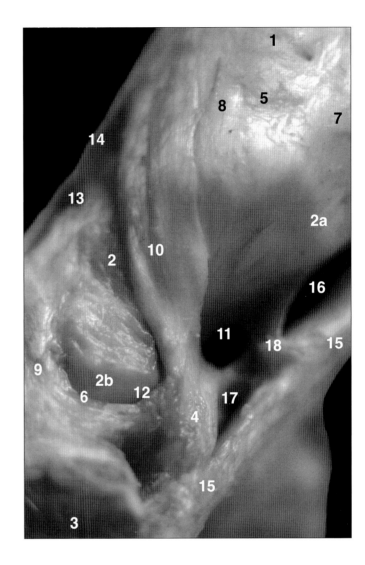

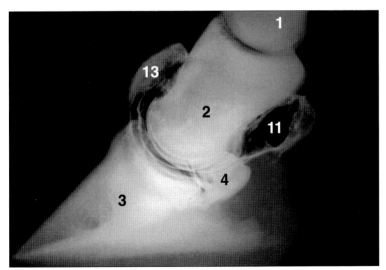

Double contrast radiographic study of the DIP joint cavity (arthrography), lateromedial projection.

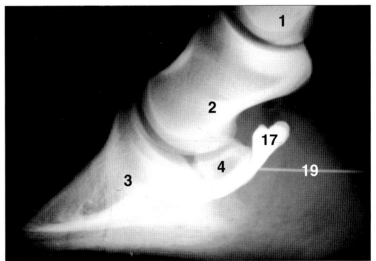

Contrast radiographic study of the podotrochlear bursa (bursography), lateromedial projection.

Dissection 11: Palmar Structures of the Foot and Distal Pastern – Palmar View

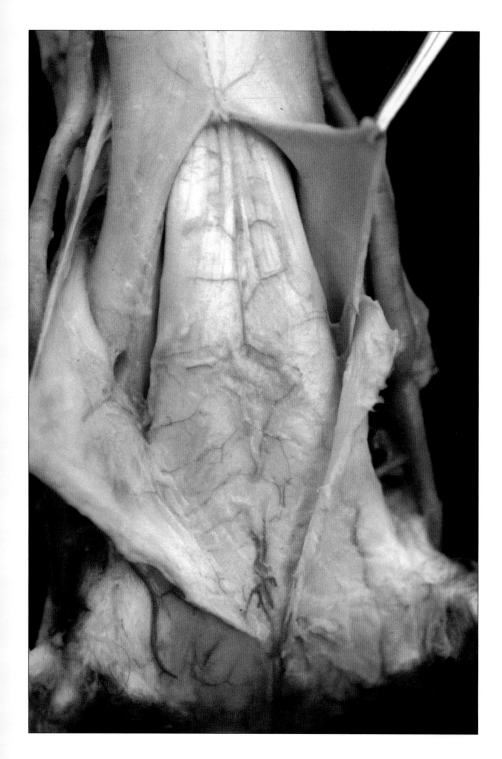

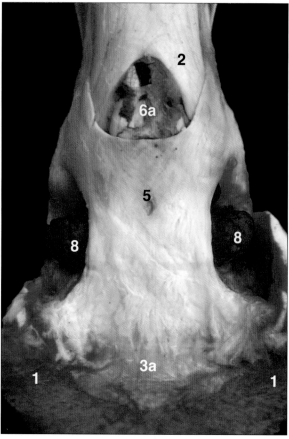

Dissection after coloured latex injection within the digital sheath and DIP joint cavities.

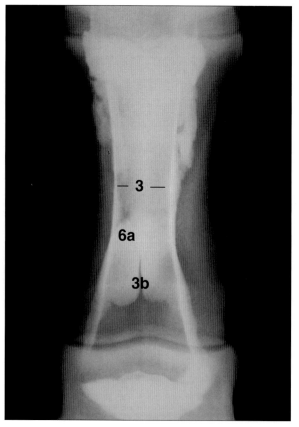

Contrast radiographic study of the digital sheath (tendinography), dorsopalmar view.

1 Distal phalanx (palmar process)
2 Superficial digital flexor tendon
  (distal branch)
3 Deep digital flexor tendon
  3a Distal attachment
  3b Mesotendon
4 Proximal digital annular ligament
5 Distal digital annular ligament (reclined)
  5a Proximal attachment
  5b Distal attachment
6 Palmar wall of the digital sheath
  (reflected)
  6a Palmar distal recess of the digital
  sheath
7 Proper palmar digital artery
  7a Palmar ramus of the middle
  phalanx
8 Proximopalmar recess of the distal
  interphalangeal joint cavity
  (top right, page 22)

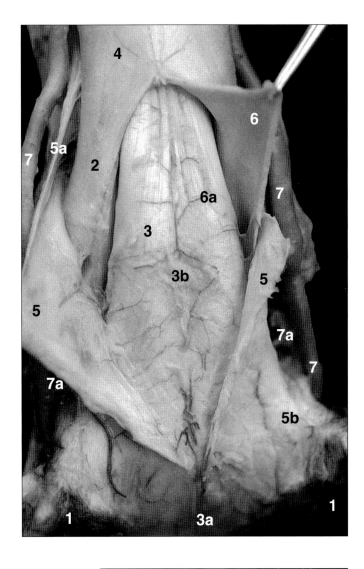

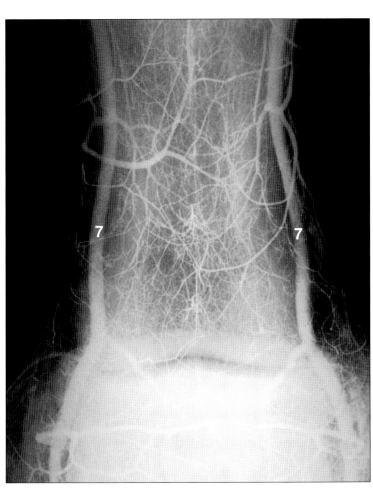

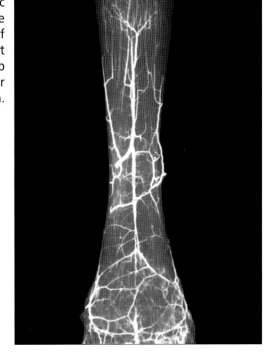

Contrast
radiographic
study of the
arterial supply of
the digital part
of the deep
digital flexor
tendon.

Contrast
radiographic
study of the
arteries
(arteriography)
of the digit,
dorsopalmar
view.

Dissection 12: Palmar Structures of the Foot – Palmar View

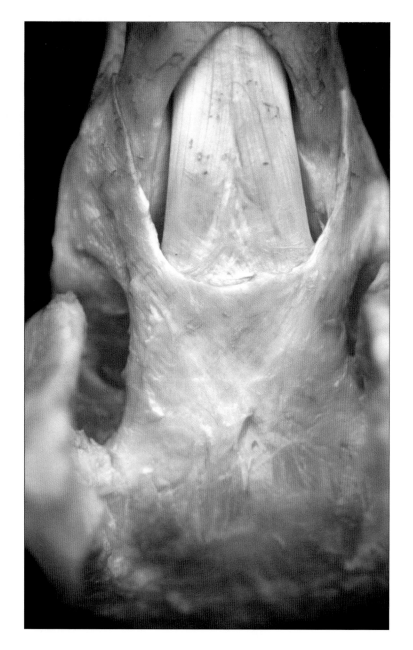

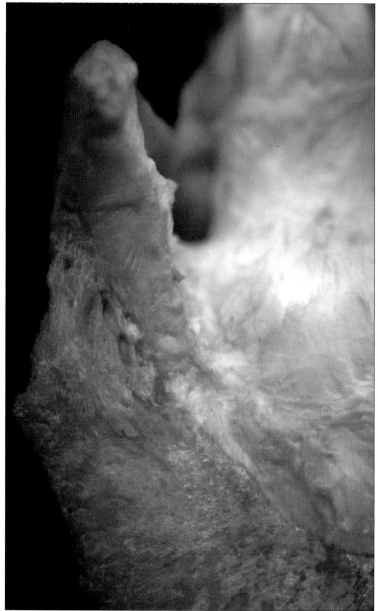

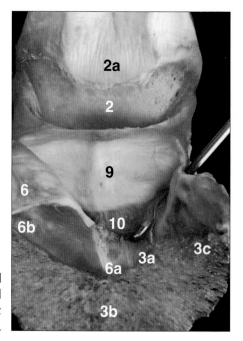

Palmar view of the dissected foot. Half of the deep digital flexor tendon was removed; the other part is reflected.

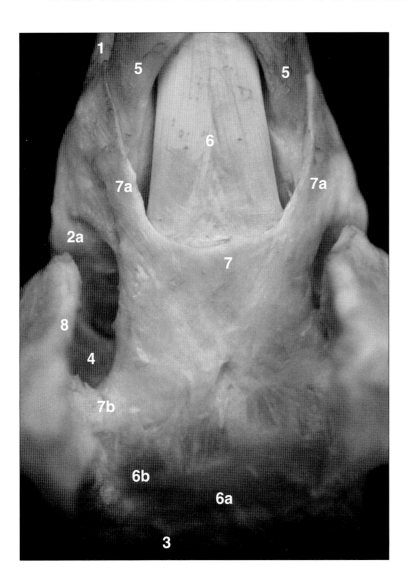

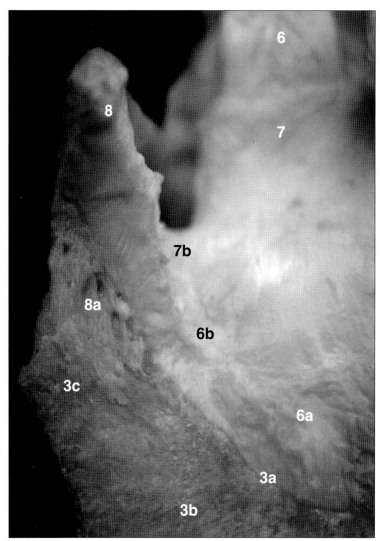

1 Proximal phalanx
2 Middle phalanx
   2a Flexor tuberosity
3 Distal phalanx
   3a Semilunar line
   3b Planum cutaneum
   3c Palmar process
4 Collateral sesamoidean ligament
5 Superficial digital flexor tendon
   (distal branches)
6 Deep digital flexor tendon
   6a Sagittal distal insertion
   6b Collateral distal insertion
7 Distal digital annular ligament
   7a Proximal attachment
   7b Distal attachment
8 Ungular cartilage
   8a Chondroungular ligament
9 Distal sesamoid bone (page 24)
10 Impar distal sesamoidean ligament (page 24)

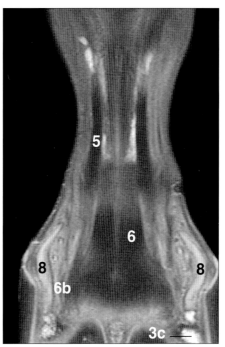

Frontal MRI scan of the palmar
structures of the digit after
injection of latex in the arteries
and veins.

Dissection 13: Distal Interphalangeal Joint and Podotrochlear Apparatus – Palmar View

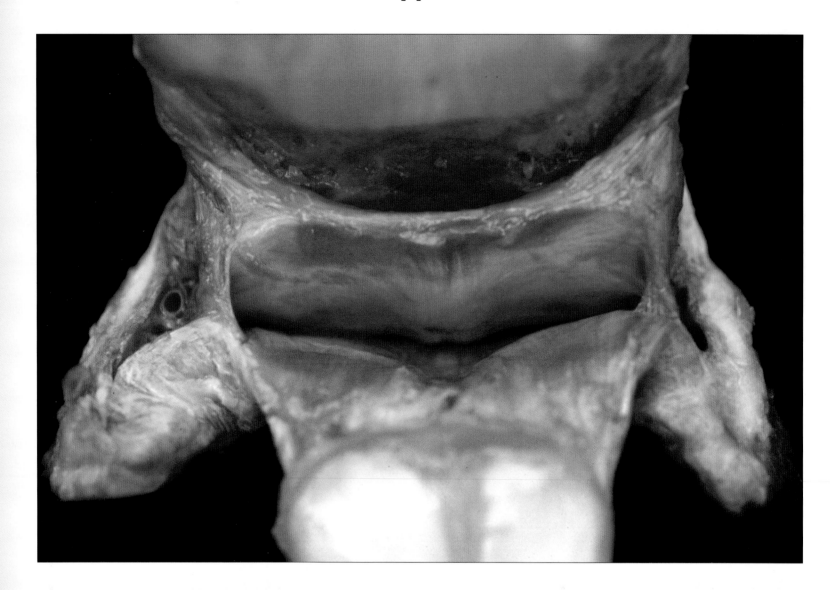

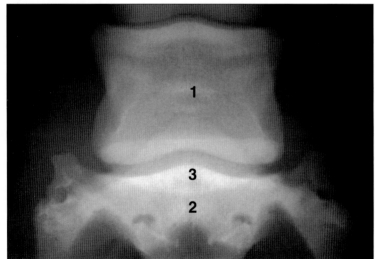

Dorsopalmar (horizontal) radiographic view of the foot.

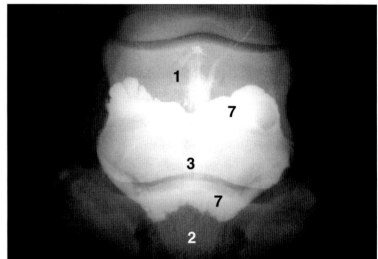

Contrast radiographic study of the podotrochlear bursa (bursography), dorsopalmar view.

Dissection 13: Distal Interphalangeal Joint and Podotrochlear Apparatus – Palmar View

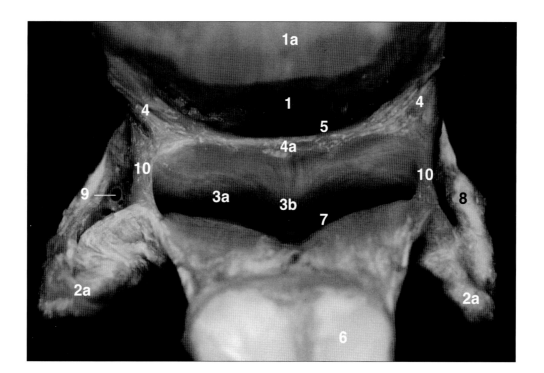

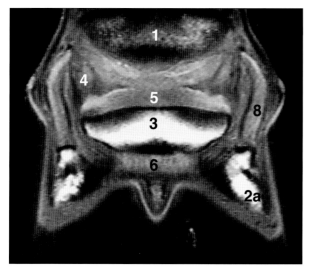

Frontal MRI scan of the podotrochlear apparatus after injections of latex in the arteries and veins.

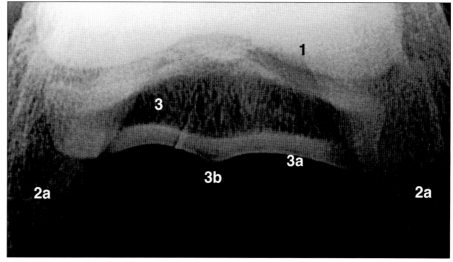

Palmaroproximal-palmarodistal oblique (sky-line) radiographic view of the palmar structures of the foot.

1 Middle phalanx
  1a Flexor tuberosity
2 Distal phalanx (P3)
  2a Palmar process
3 Distal sesamoid bone
  3a Flexor surface
  3b Sagittal ridge
4 Collateral sesamoidean ligament
  4a Sagittal union

5 Proximopalmar recess of the distal interphalangeal joint
6 Deep digital flexor tendon (DDFT) (reclined)
7 Podotrochlear bursa
8 Ungular cartilage (most of it was removed)
9 Proper palmar digital artery
10 Collateral attachment between the distal sesamoid bone, the DDFT and P3

Dissection 14: Podotrochlear Apparatus

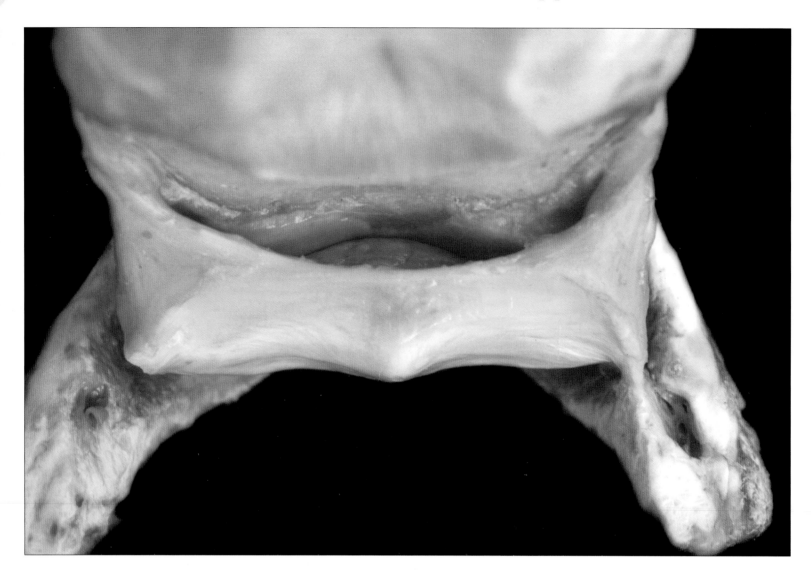

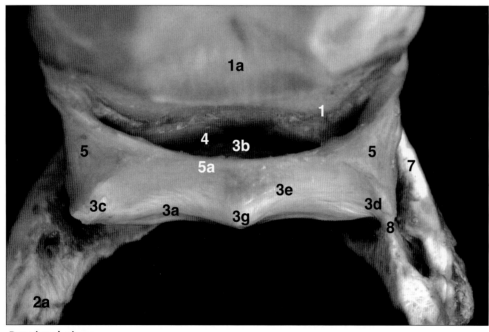

Proximal view.

1 Middle phalanx
  1a Flexor tuberosity
2 Distal phalanx
  2a Palmar process
  2b Flexor surface
  2c Semilunar line
  2d Planum cutaneum
  2e Solar sulcus
  2f Solar foramen
3 Distal sesamoid bone
  3a Flexor surface
  3b Proximal articular
      border
  3c Lateral angle

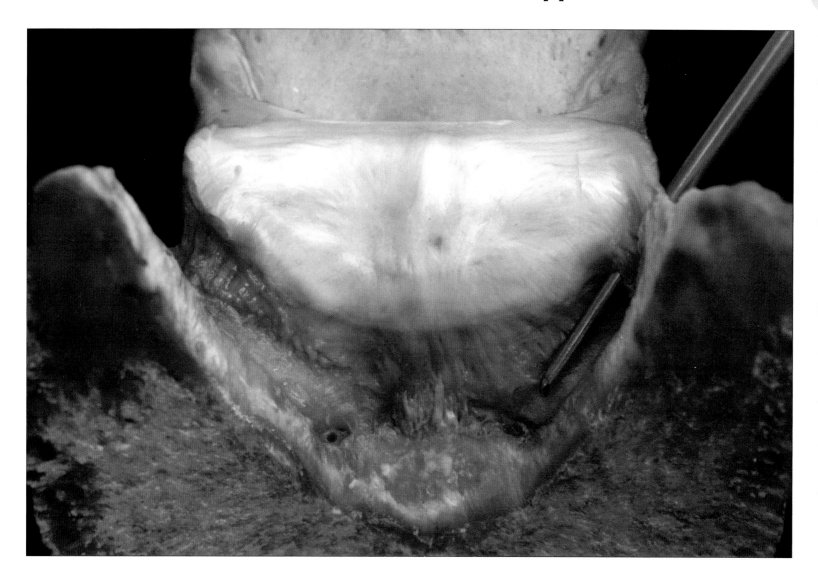

3d Medial angle
3e Proximal border
3f Distal border
3g Sagittal ridge
4 Distal interphalangeal joint
5 Collateral sesamoidean ligament
  5a Sagittal union
6 Impar distal sesamoidean ligament
7 Ungular cartilage
8 Chondrosesamoidean ligament

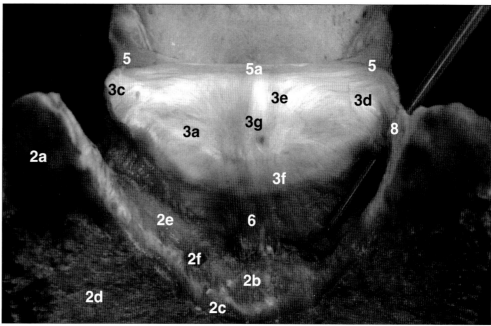

Palmar view.

Dissection 15: Distal Interphalangeal Joint

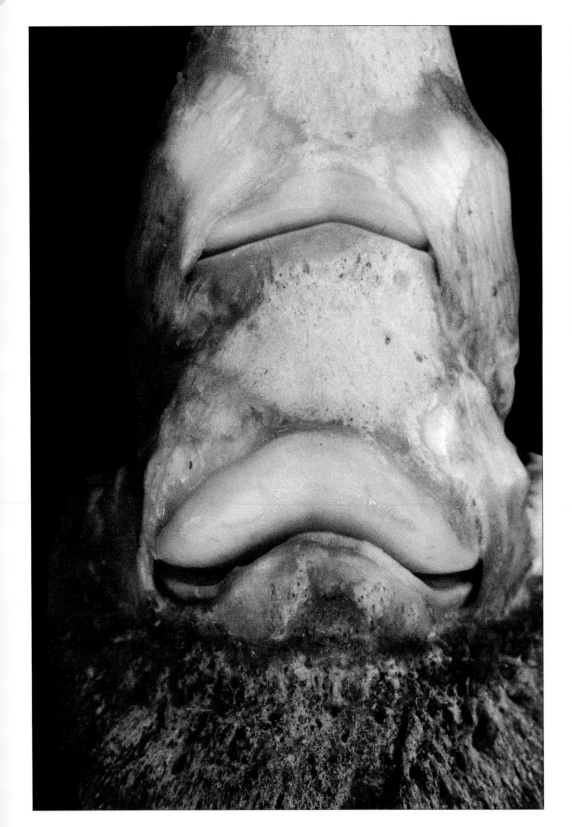

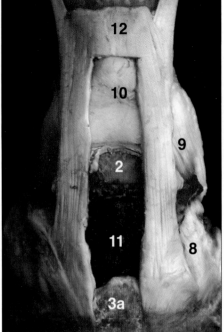

Dissection after coloured latex injection in the joint cavities, dorsal view.

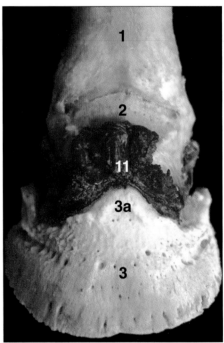

Casting preparation of the DIP joint cavity, dorsal view.

1 Proximal phalanx
2 Middle phalanx
  2a Extensor process
3 Distal phalanx
  3a Extensor process
  3b Parietal surface
  3c Articular surface
  3d Palmar process
4 Distal sesamoid bone
  4a Articular surface
  4b Proximal border
5 Proximal interphalangeal (PIP) joint
6 Distal interphalangeal (DIP) joint
7 Collateral ligament of the PIP joint
8 Collateral ligament of the DIP joint
9 Collateral sesamoidean ligament
  9a Sagittal reunion
10 Dorsal recess of the PIP joint cavity
   (page 30)
11 Dorsal recess of the DIP joint cavity
   (page 30)
12 Dorsal digital extensor tendon
   (page 30)

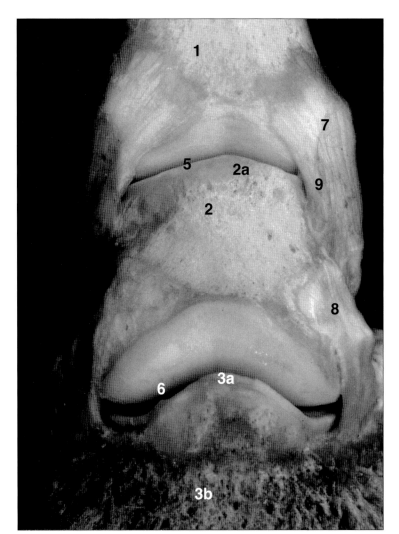

Dorsal view.

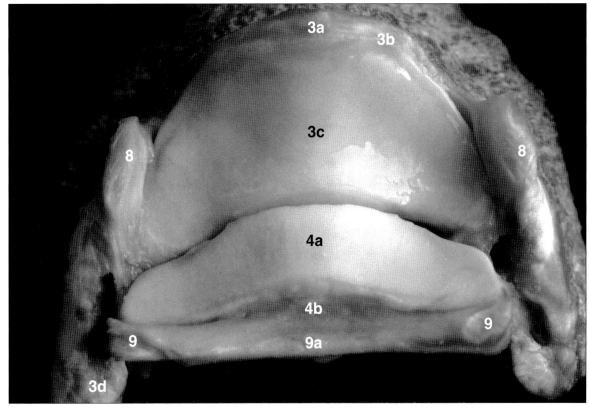

Proximal view
(the middle
phalanx has
been removed).

Dissection 16: Synovial Recesses of the Foot
(After Coloured Latex Injections)

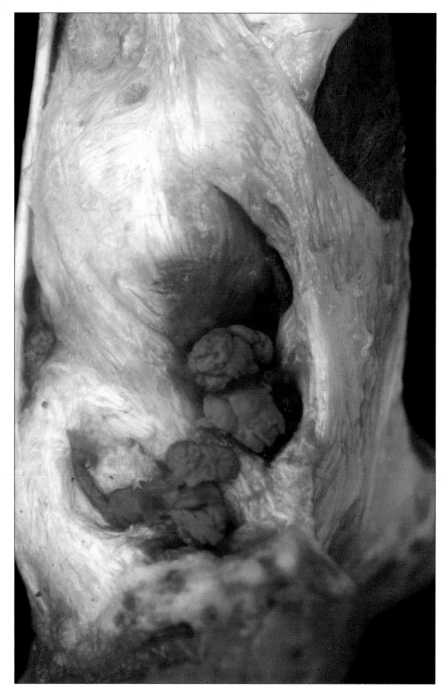

Lateral view.

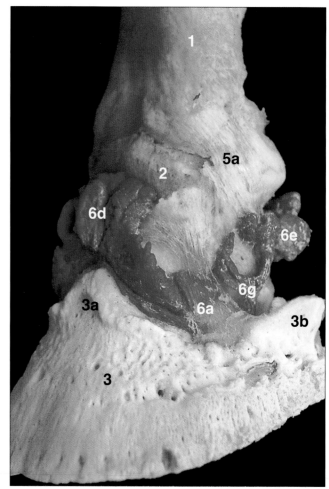

Casting preparation of the DIP joint cavity, dorsolateral view.

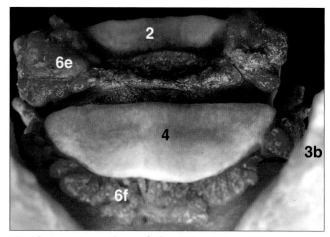

Casting preparation of the DIP joint cavity, palmarodistal view.

Dissection 16: Synovial Recesses of the Foot
(After Coloured Latex Injections)

1 Proximal phalanx
2 Middle phalanx
3 Distal phalanx
   3a Extensor process
   3b Palmar process
   3c Solar sulcus
   3d Flexor surface
4 Distal sesamoid bone
5 Proximal interphalangeal (PIP) joint
   5a Collateral ligament
   5b Distodorsocollateral recess
6 Distal interphalangeal (DIP) joint
   6a Collateral ligament
   6b Collateral sesamoidean ligament
   6c Impar distal sesamoidean ligament
   6d Dorsal recess
   6e Proximopalmar recess
   6f Distopalmar recess
   6g Collateral recess
7 Deep digital flexor tendon
8 Distal digital annular ligament
   8a Proximal attachment
   8b Distal attachment
9 Digital sheath synovial cavity
   9a Dorsal distal recess
   9b Palmar distal recess
10 Podotrochlear bursa

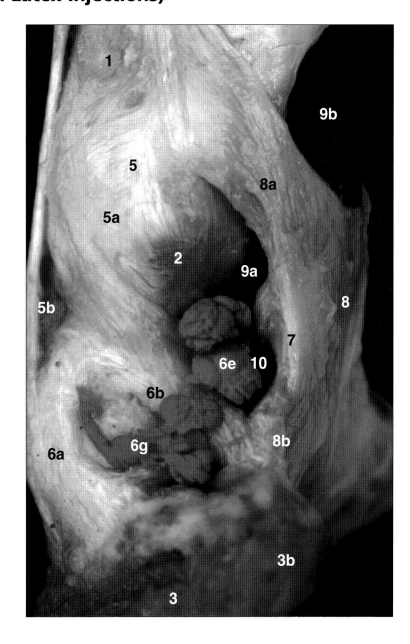

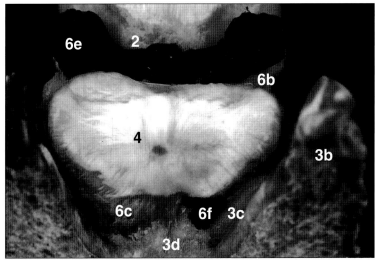

Palmar view.

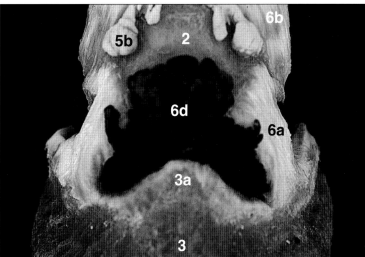

Dorsal view.

Sagittal and Parasagittal Sections of the Equine Foot

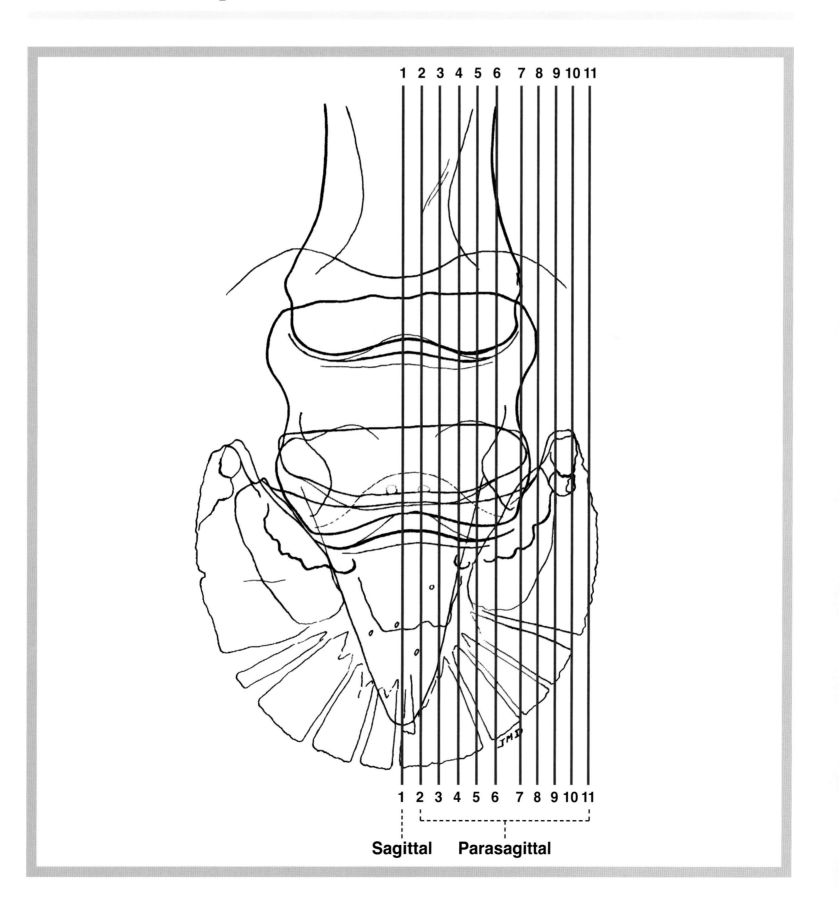

S1a: Sagittal Section of the Digit

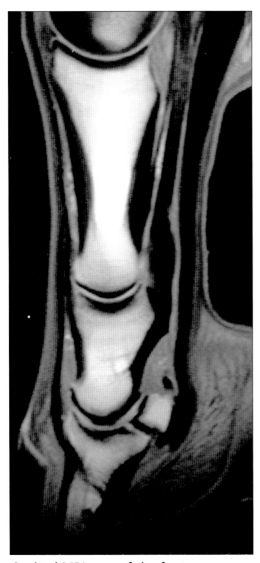

Sagittal MRI scan of the foot.

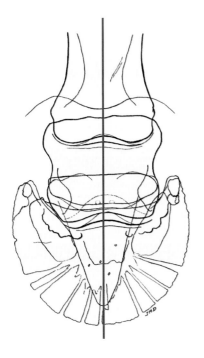

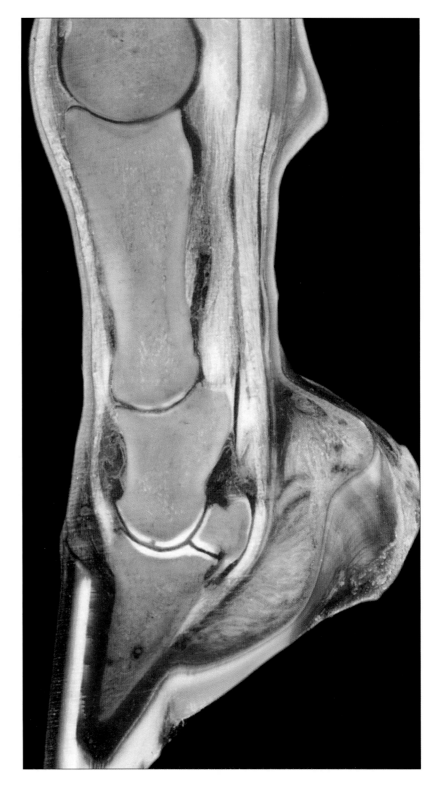

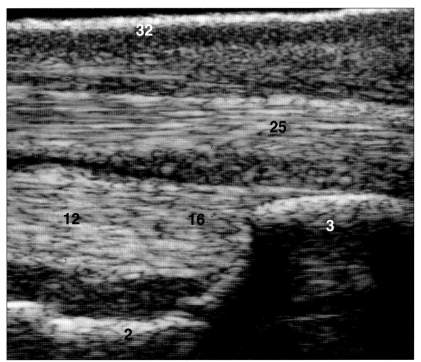

Sagittal ultrasound scan of the distal pastern, palmar approach (see dotted area in illustration at right).

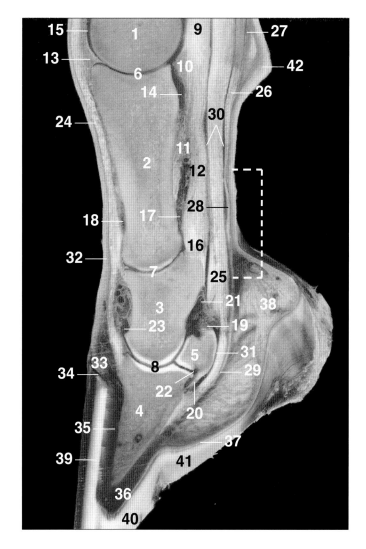

1	Third metacarpal bone	**22**	Distopalmar recess of the DIP joint
2	Proximal phalanx	**23**	Dorsal recess of the DIP joint
3	Middle phalanx	**24**	Dorsal digital extensor tendon
4	Distal phalanx	**25**	Deep digital flexor tendon
5	Distal sesamoid bone	**26**	Superficial digital flexor tendon
6	Metacarpophalangeal (MP) joint	**27**	Palmar annular ligament
7	Proximal interphalangeal (PIP) joint	**28**	Proximal digital annular ligament
8	Distal interphalangeal (DIP) joint	**29**	Distal digital annular ligament
9	Palmar (intersesamoidean) ligament	**30**	Digital sheath cavity
10	Cruciate sesamoidean ligament	**31**	Podotroclear bursa
11	Oblique sesamoidean ligament	**32**	Skin
12	Straight sesamoidean ligament	**33**	Pulvinus coronae
13	Dorsal articular capsule	**34**	Corium coronae
14	Distopalmar recess of the MP joint	**35**	Corium parietis
15	Dorsal recess of the MP joint	**36**	Corium soleae
16	Middle scutum	**37**	Corium cunei
17	Palmar recess of the PIP joint	**38**	Digital cushion
18	Dorsal recess of the PIP joint	**39**	Hoof wall
19	Collateral sesamoidean ligament	**40**	Sole
20	Impar distal sesamoidean ligament	**41**	Frog
21	Proximopalmar recess of the DIP joint	**42**	Ergot

S1b: Sagittal section of the Foot

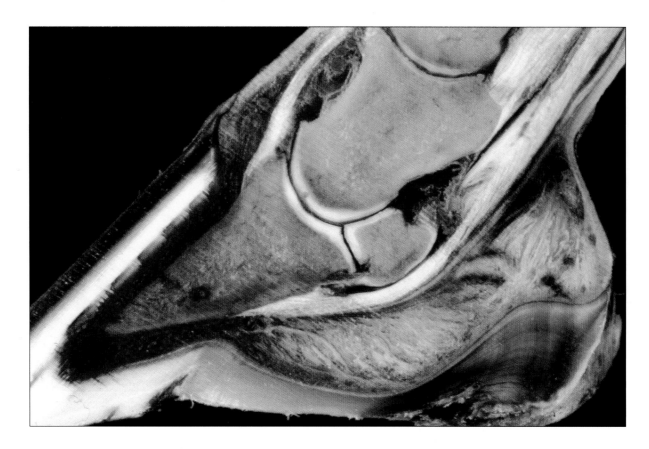

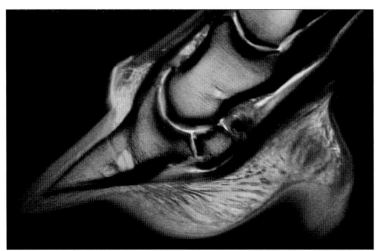

Sagittal MRI scan of the foot.

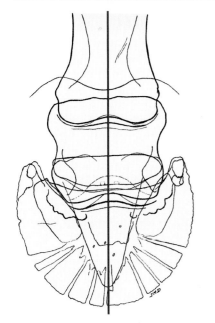

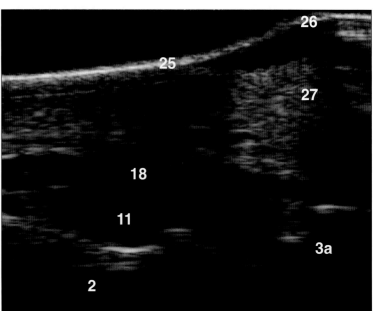

Sagittal ultrasound scan of the distal interphalangeal joint, dorsal approach (see dotted area in illustration at top of facing page).

S1b: Sagittal section of the Foot

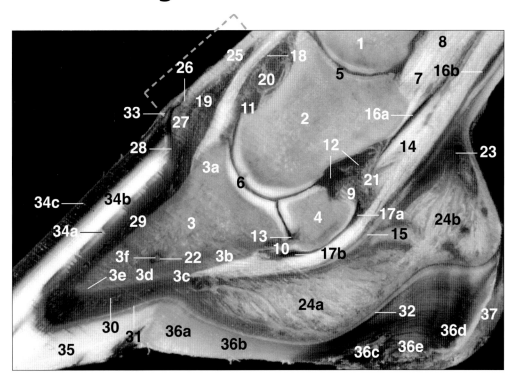

1 Proximal phalanx
2 Middle phalanx (P2)
3 Distal phalanx
   3a Extensor process
   3b Flexor surface
   3c Semilunar line
   3d Planum cutaneum
   3e Solar border
   3f Solar canal and terminal arch
4 Distal sesamoid bone
5 Proximal interphalangeal joint
6 Distal interphalangeal (DIP) joint
7 Middle scutum
8 Straight sesamoidean ligament
9 Collateral sesamoidean ligament
10 Impar distal sesamoidean ligament
11 Dorsal recess of the DIP joint
12 Proximopalmar recess of the DIP joint
13 Distopalmar recess of the DIP joint
14 Deep digital flexor tendon
15 Distal digital annular ligament
16 Digital sheath
   16a Dorsal distal recess
   16b Palmar distal recess
17 Podotrochlear bursa
   17a Proximal recess
   17b Distal recess
18 Dorsal digital extensor tendon
19 Coronal artery and vein

20 Dorsal rami of P2
21 Palmar ramus (artery) of P2
22 Terminal arch
23 Lateromedial palmar anastomosis
24 Digital cushion
   24a Cuneal part
   24b Toric part
25 Skin
26 Corium limbi
27 Pulvinus coronae
28 Corium coronae
29 Corium parietis
30 Solar subcutaneous layer
31 Corium soleae
32 Corium cunei
33 Periople
34 Hoof wall
   34a Stratum internum
   34b Stratum medium
   34c Stratum externum
35 Sole
36 Frog
   36a Apex
   36b Body
   36c Branch
   36d Base
   36e Central cuneal sulcus
37 Heel

S1c: Sagittal Section of the Interphalangeal Joints

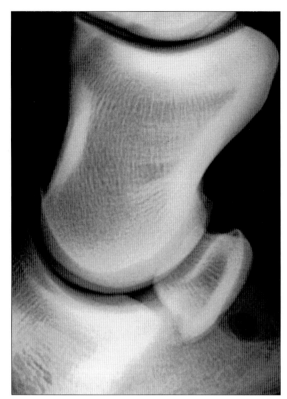

Lateromedial radiographic view of the interphalangeal joints.

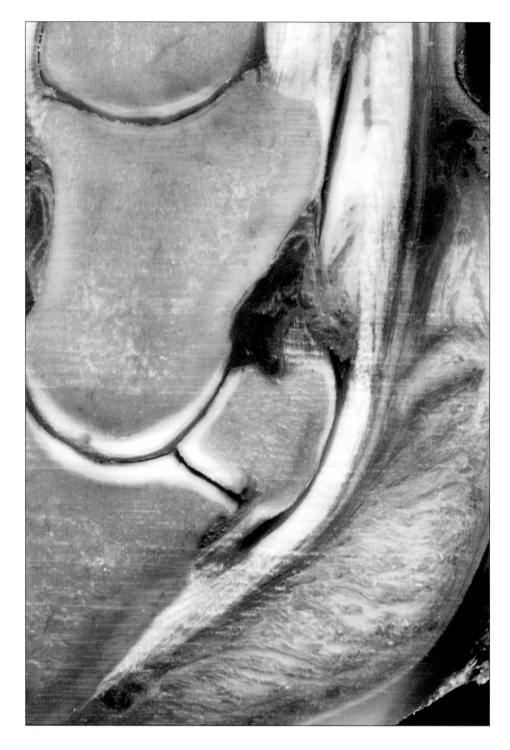

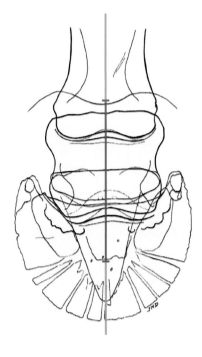

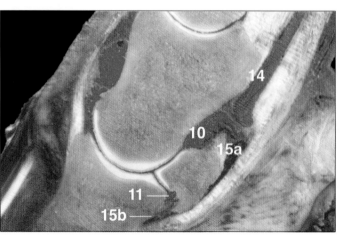

Sagittal section of the foot after injection of coloured latex in the synovial cavities.

1 Proximal phalanx
2 Middle phalanx (P2)
   2a Flexor tuberosity
   2b Distal condyle
3 Distal phalanx
   3a Articular surface
   3b Sesamoidean articular surface
   3c Flexor surface
   3d Distopalmar compact bone
4 Distal sesamoid bone
5 Proximal interphalangeal joint
6 Distal interphalangeal (DIP) joint
7 Middle scutum
8 Collateral sesamoidean ligament
9 Impar distal sesamoidean ligament
10 Proximopalmar recess of the DIP joint
11 Distopalmar recess of the DIP joint
12 Deep digital flexor tendon
   12a Fibrous parts
   12b Fibrocartilaginous parts
13 Distal digital annular ligament
14 Digital sheath (dorsal distal recess)
15 Podotrochlear bursa
   15a Proximal recess
   15b Distal recess
16 Palmar ramus (artery) of P2
17 Digital cushion
18 Skin
19 Corium cunei
20 Frog

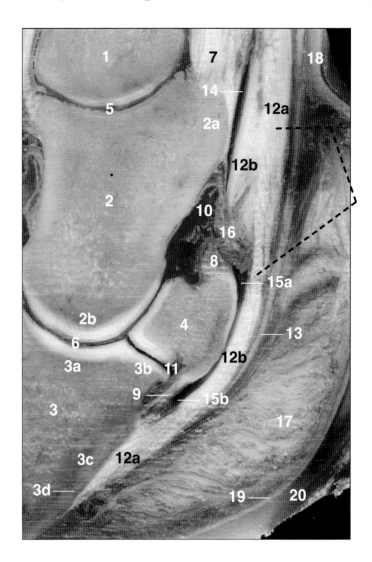

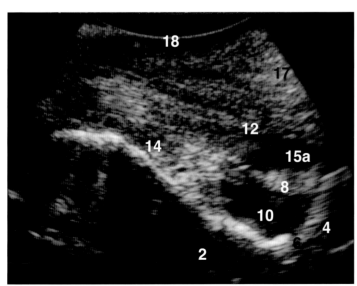

Sagittal ultrasound scan of the distal interphalangeal joint, palmar approach (see box above).

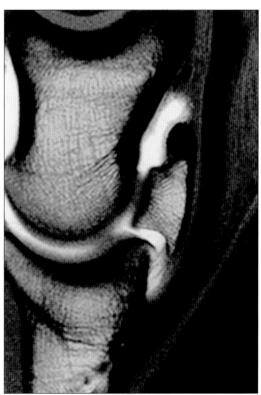

Sagittal MRI scan of the foot after injection of contrast material into the distal interphalangeal joint.

S1d: Sagittal Section of the Podotrochlear Apparatus

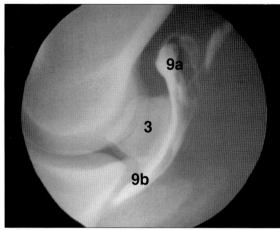

Double contrast radiographic study of the podotrochlear bursa (bursography), lateromedial view.

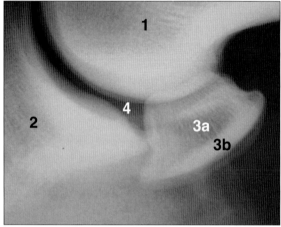

Lateromedial radiographic view of the distal sesamoid bone.

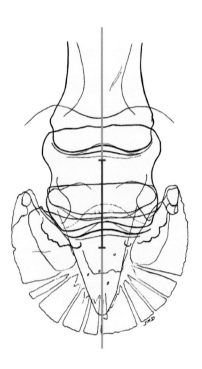

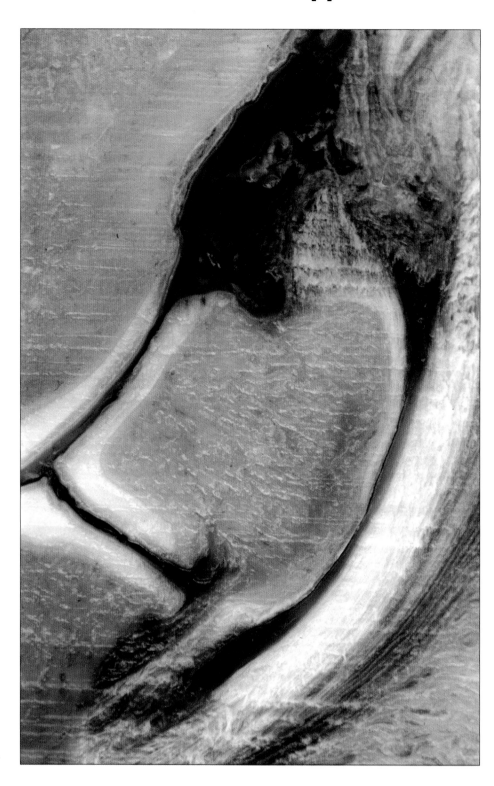

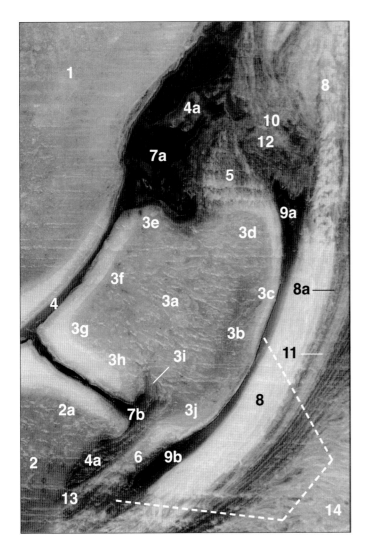

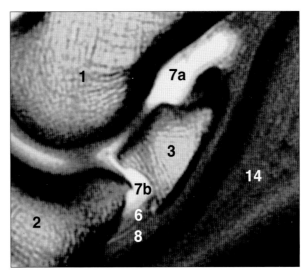

Sagittal MRI scan of the podotrochlear apparatus after injection of contrast material into the distal interphalangeal joint.

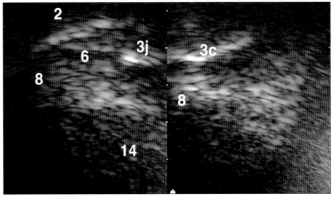

Sagittal ultrasound scan of the podotrochlear apparatus, palmarodistal (transcuneal) approach (see dotted area in illustration at left).

1 Middle phalanx (P2)
2 Distal phalanx (P3)
   2a Sesamoidean articular surface
3 Distal sesamoid bone
   3a Spongious bone
   3b Palmar compact bone
   3c Flexor surface
   3d Proximopalmar border
   3e Proximodorsal border
   3f Articular surface with P2
   3g Distodorsal border
   3h Articular surface with P3
   3i Synovial groove
   3j Distopalmar border
4 Distal interphalangeal (DIP) joint
   4a Synovial membrane and villi
5 Collateral sesamoidean ligament (sagittal reunion)

6 Impar distal sesamoidean ligament
7 Recesses of the DIP joint
   7a Proximopalmar recess
   7b Distopalmar recess
8 Deep digital flexor tendon
   8a Sagittal arterial supply
9 Podotrochlear bursa
   9a Proximal recess
   9b Distal recess
10 Synovial membranes of the podotrochlear bursa, DIP joint and digital sheath
11 Distal digital annular ligament
12 Proximal ramus (artery) of the distal sesamoid bone
13 Distal rami (artery and vein) of the distal sesamoid bone
14 Digital cushion (cuneal part)

S2: Parasagittal Section of the Foot

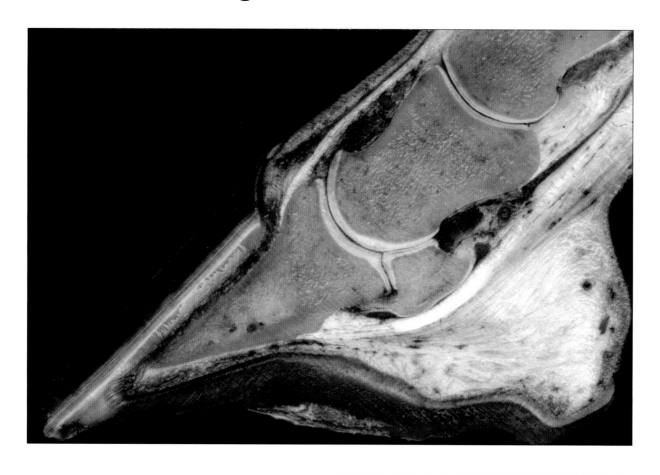

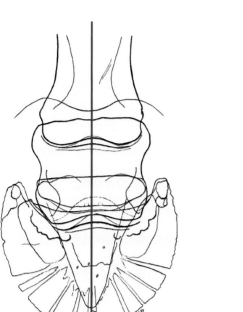

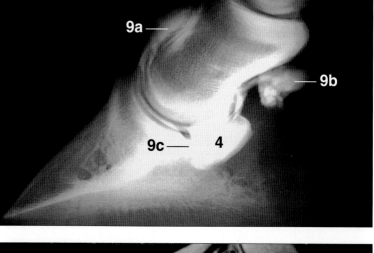

Contrast radiographic study of the distal interphalangeal joint (arthrography) lateromedial view.

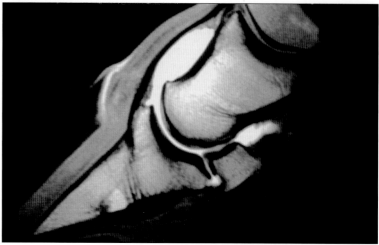

Parasagittal MRI scan of the foot after injection of contrast material into the distal interphalangeal joint.

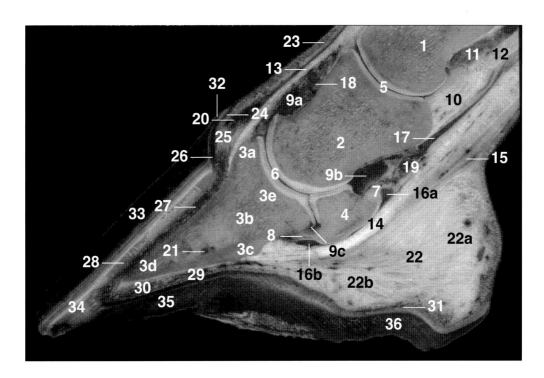

1 Proximal phalanx
2 Middle phalanx (P2)
3 Distal phalanx
  3a Extensor process
  3b Spongious bone
  3c Distopalmar compact bone
  3d Solar border
  3e Subchondral bone
4 Distal sesamoid bone
5 Proximal interphalangeal (PIP) joint
6 Distal interphalangeal (DIP) joint
7 Collateral sesamoidean ligament
8 Impar distal sesamoidean ligament
9 Articular recesses of the DIP joint cavity
  9a Dorsal recess
  9b Proximopalmar recess
  9c Distopalmar recess
10 Middle scutum
11 Palmar recess of the PIP joint
12 Straight sesamoidean ligament
13 Dorsal digital extensor tendon
14 Deep digital flexor tendon
15 Distal digital annular ligament
16 Podotrochlear bursa

16a Proximal recess
16b Distal recess
17 Digital sheath (dorsal distal recess)
18 Dorsal ramus (vein) of P2
19 Palmar rami (artery and vein) of P2
20 Coronal artery and vein
21 Terminal arch within the solar canal
22 Digital cushion
  22a Toric part
  22b Cuneal part
23 Skin
24 Corium limbi
25 Pulvinus coronae
26 Corium coronae
27 Corium parietis
28 Dermal and epidermal lamellae
29 Solar subcutaneous layer
30 Corium soleae
31 Corium cunei
32 Periople
33 Hoof wall
34 Zona alba (white zone)
35 Sole
36 Frog

S3: Parasagittal Section of the Foot

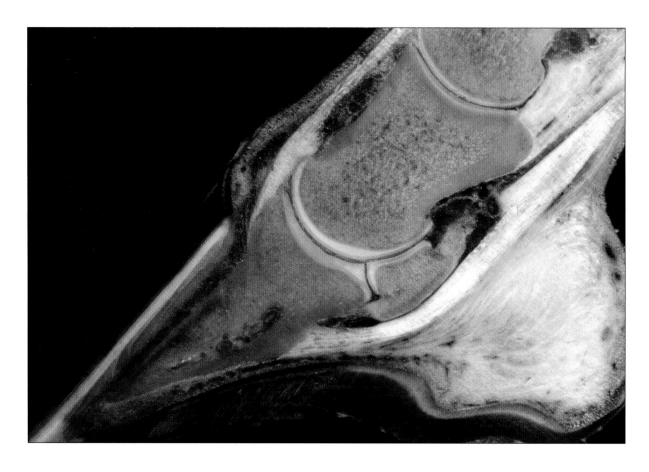

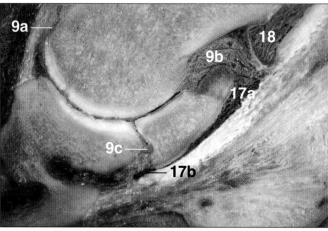

Parasagittal section of the foot after injection of coloured latex in the synovial cavities.

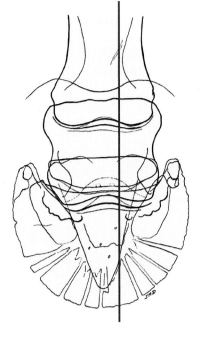

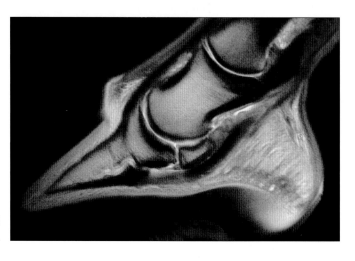

Parasagittal MRI scan of the foot.

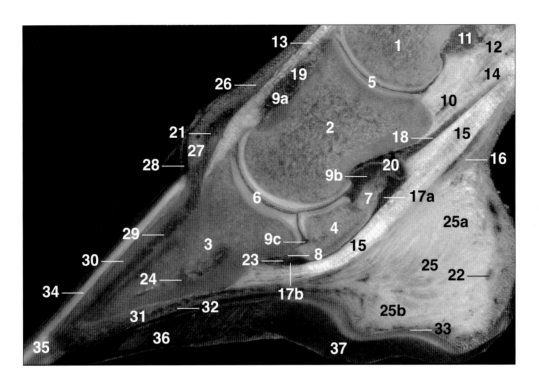

1 Proximal phalanx
2 Middle phalanx (P2)
3 Distal phalanx
4 Distal sesamoid bone
5 Proximal interphalangeal (PIP) joint
6 Distal interphalangeal (DIP) joint
7 Collateral sesamoidean ligament
8 Impar distal sesamoidean ligament
9 Articular recesses of the DIP joint cavity
   9a Dorsal recess
   9b Proximopalmar recess
   9c Distopalmar recess
10 Middle scutum
11 Palmar recess of the PIP joint
12 Straight sesamoidean ligament
13 Dorsal digital extensor tendon
14 Superficial digital flexor tendon
(distal branch)
15 Deep digital flexor tendon
16 Distal digital annular ligament
17 Podotrochlear bursa
   17a Proximal recess
   17b Distal recess

18 Digital sheath (dorsal distal recess)
19 Dorsal rami (artery and vein) of P2
20 Palmar rami (artery and vein) of P2
21 Coronal artery and vein
22 Ramus of the digital torus
23 Distal rami (artery and vein) of the distal sesamoid bone
24 Terminal arch
25 Digital cushion
   25a Toric part
   25b Cuneal part
26 Skin
27 Pulvinus coronae
28 Corium coronae
29 Corium parietis
30 Dermal and epidermal lamellae
31 Solar subcutaneous layer
32 Corium soleae
33 Corium cunei
34 Hoof wall
35 Zona alba (white zone)
36 Sole
37 Frog

S4: Parasagittal Section of the Foot

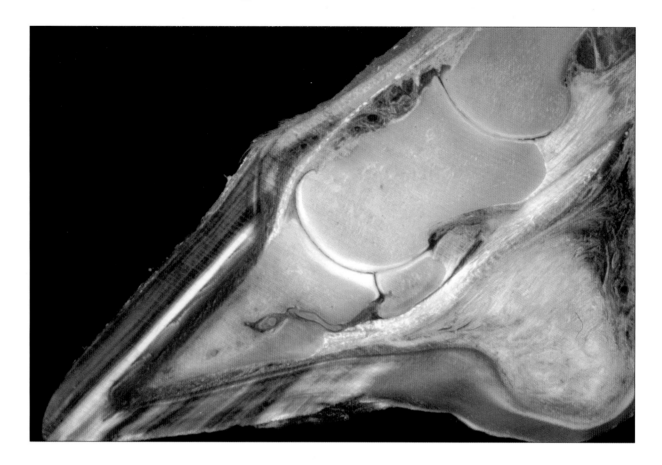

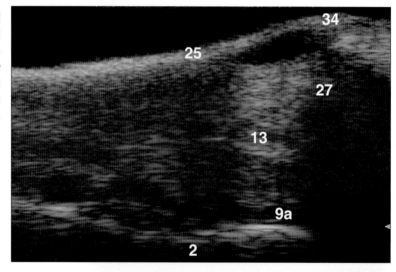

Parasagittal ultrasound scan of the distal interphalangeal joint, dorsal approach (see dotted area in illustration on facing page).

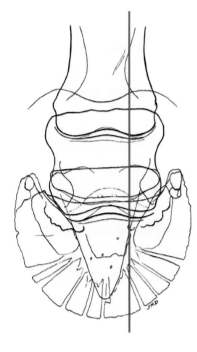

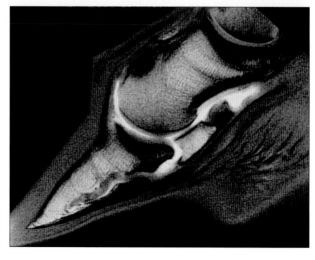

Parasagittal MRI scan of the foot after injection of contrast material in the distal interphalangeal joint.

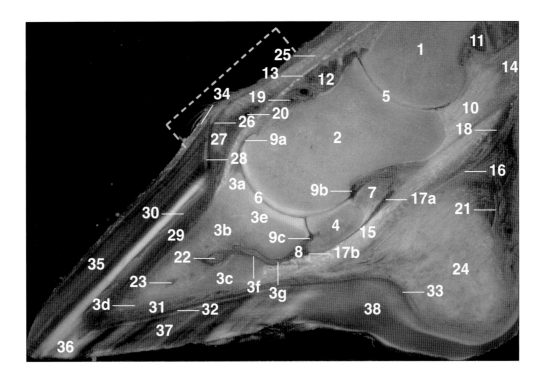

1 Proximal phalanx
2 Middle phalanx (P2)
3 Distal phalanx
   3a Coronal border
   3b Spongious bone
   3c Distopalmar compact bone
   3d Solar border
   3e Subchondral bone
   3f Solar canal
   3g Solar foramen
4 Distal sesamoid bone
5 Proximal interphalangeal (PIP) joint
6 Distal interphalangeal (DIP) joint
7 Collateral sesamoidean ligament
8 Impar distal sesamoidean ligament
9 Articular recesses of the DIP joint cavity
   9a Dorsal recess
   9b Proximopalmar recess
   9c Distopalmar recess
10 Middle scutum
11 Palmar recess of the PIP joint
12 Distodorsocollateral recess of the PIP joint
13 Dorsal digital extensor tendon
14 Superficial digital flexor tendon (distal branch)
15 Deep digital flexor tendon

16 Distal digital annular ligament
17 Podotrochlear bursa
   17a Proximal recess
   17b Distal recess
18 Digital sheath (palmar distal recess)
19 Dorsal rami (artery and vein) of P2
20 Coronal artery and vein
21 Ramus (artery) of the digital torus
22 Proper palmar digital artery and terminal arch within the solar canal
23 Perforating ramus
24 Digital cushion
25 Skin
26 Corium limbi
27 Pulvinus coronae
28 Corium coronae
29 Corium parietis
30 Dermal and epidermal lamellae
31 Solar subcutaneous layer
32 Corium soleae
33 Corium cunei
34 Periople
35 Hoof wall
36 Zona alba (white zone)
37 Sole
38 Frog

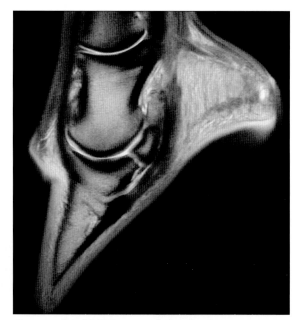

Parasagittal MRI scan of the foot.

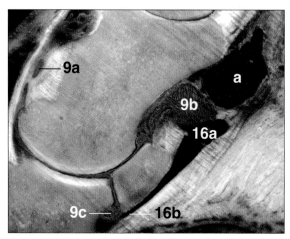

Parasagittal section of the foot after injection of coloured latex into the synovial cavities (**a** Dorsal distal recess of the digital sheath).

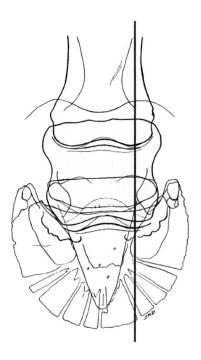

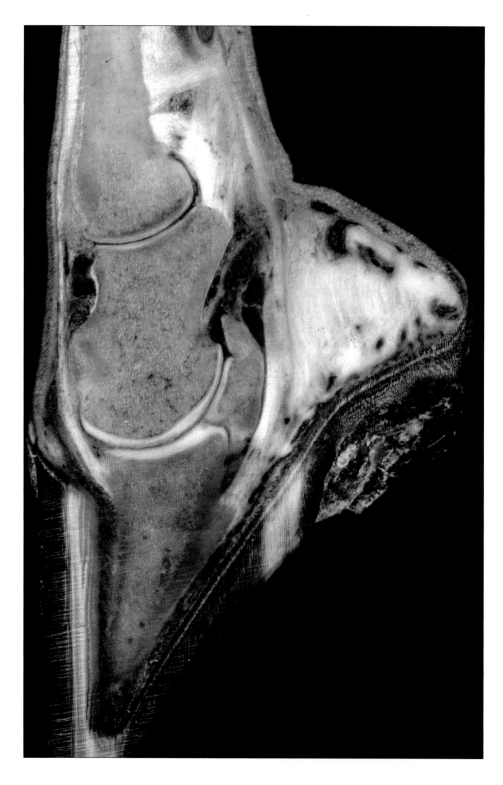

1 Proximal phalanx
2 Middle phalanx
3 Distal phalanx (P3)
4 Distal sesamoid bone
5 Proximal interphalangeal joint
   5a Distodorsocollateral recess
6 Distal interphalangeal (DIP) joint
   6a Collateral ligament
7 Collateral sesamoidean ligament
8 Impar distal sesamoidean ligament
9 Articular recesses of the DIP joint cavity
   9a Dorsal recess
   9b Proximopalmar recess
   9c Distopalmar recess
10 Middle scutum
11 Dorsal digital extensor tendon
12 Superficial digital flexor tendon
   (distal insertion)
13 Proximal digital annular ligament
   (distal insertion)
14 Deep digital flexor tendon
15 Distal digital annular ligament
16 Podotrochlear bursa
   16a Proximal recess
   16b Distal recess
17 Dorsal rami (artery and vein) of P2
18 Palmar rami (artery and vein) of P2
19 Ramus of the digital torus
20 Proper palmar digital artery
21 Perforating ramus
22 Deep ungular plexus
23 Digital cushion
24 Ungular cartilage
25 Skin
26 Corium limbi
27 Pulvinus coronae
28 Corium coronae
29 Corium parietis
30 Dermal and epidermal lamellae
31 Solar subcutaneous layer
32 Corium soleae
33 Corium cunei
34 Periople
35 Hoof wall
36 Sole (branch)
37 Frog (paracuneal sulcus)

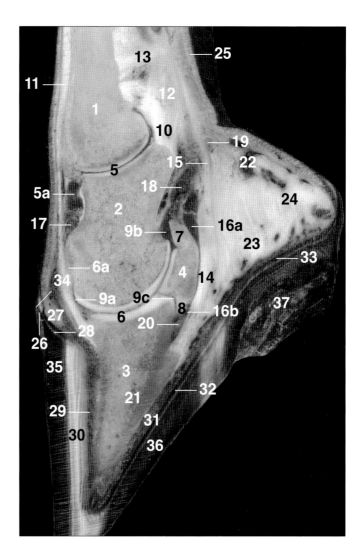

S6: Parasagittal Section of the Foot

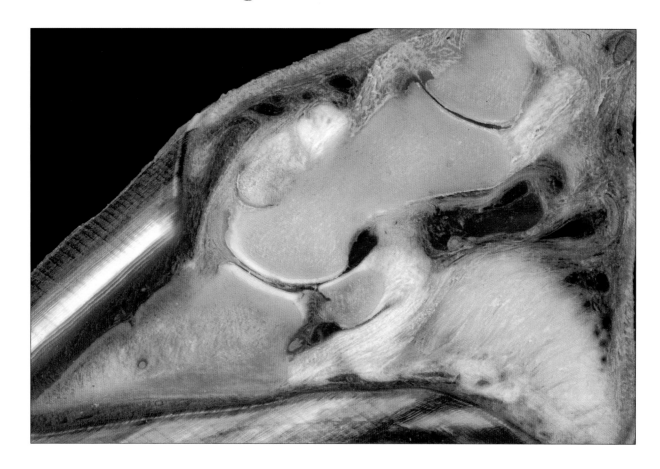

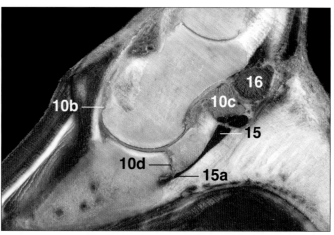

Parasagittal section of the foot after injection of coloured latex in the synovial cavities.

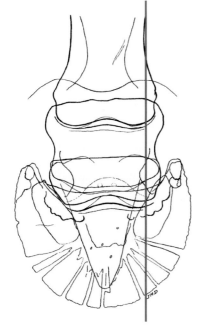

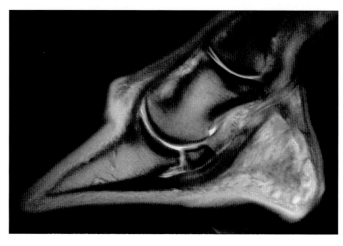

Parasagittal MRI scan of the foot.

S6: Parasagittal Section of the Foot

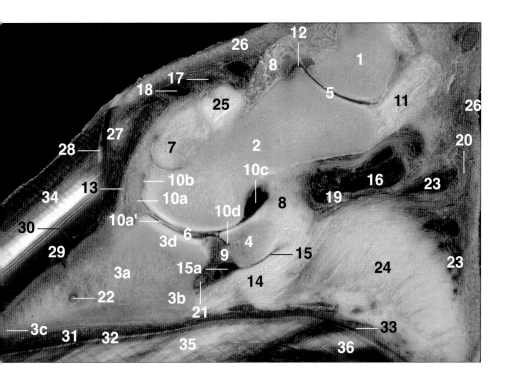

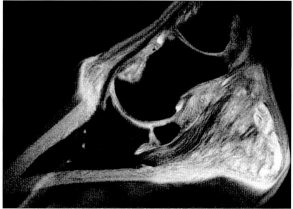

Parasagittal MRI scan of the foot.

1 Proximal phalanx	**15** Podotrochlear bursa
2 Middle phalanx (P2)	**15a** Distal recess
3 Distal phalanx	**16** Digital sheath (dorsal distal recess)
3a Spongious bone	**17** Dorsal rami (artery and vein) of P2
3b Distopalmar compact bone	**18** Coronal artery and vein
3c Solar border	**19** Palmar rami (artery and vein) of P2
3d Subchondral bone	**20** Ramus of the digital torus
4 Distal sesamoid bone	**21** Proper palmar digital artery
5 Proximal interphalangeal (PIP) joint	**22** Perforating ramus (from the terminal arch)
6 Distal interphalangeal (DIP) joint	**23** Deep ungular plexus
7 Collateral ligament of the DIP joint	**24** Digital cushion
8 Collateral sesamoidean ligament	**25** Ungular cartilage
9 Impar distal sesamoidean ligament	**26** Skin
10 Articular recesses of the DIP joint cavity	**27** Pulvinus coronae
10a Synovial membrane	**28** Corium coronae
10a' Synovial plica	**29** Corium parietis
10b Dorsal recess	**30** Dermal and epidermal lamellae
10c Proximopalmar recess	**31** Solar subcutaneous layer
10d Distopalmar recess	**32** Corium soleae
11 Middle scutum	**33** Corium cunei
12 PIP joint cavity	**34** Hoof wall
13 Dorsal digital extensor tendon	**35** Sole
14 Deep digital flexor tendon	**36** Frog

S7: Parasagittal Section of the Foot

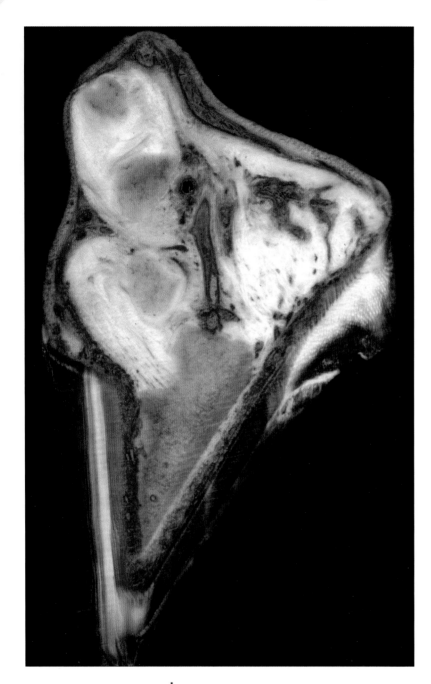

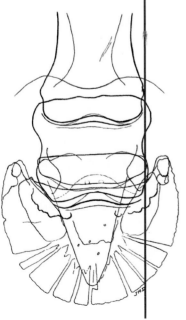

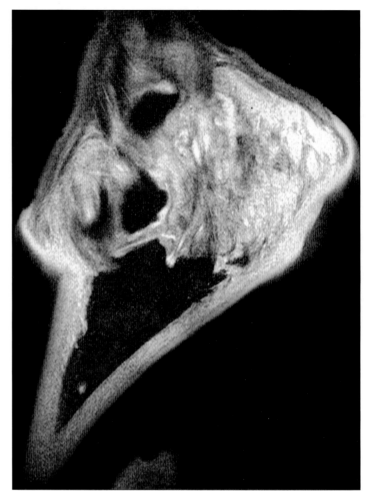

Parasagittal MRI scan of the foot.

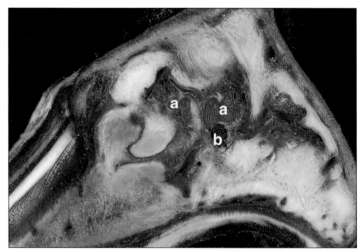

Parasagittal section of the foot after injection of coloured latex in the synovial cavities: **a** Distal interphalangeal joint cavity (collateral recess); **b** Podotrochlear bursa.

1 Proximal phalanx
2 Middle phalanx (P2)
    2a Flexor tuberosity
    2b Distal condyle
3 Distal phalanx (P3)
4 Collateral ligament of the distal interphalangeal joint
5 Collateral sesamoidean ligament
6 Ungular cartilage
7 Proper palmar digital artery
8 Perforating ramus
9 Dorsal rami (artery and vein) of P2
10 Palmar rami (artery and vein) of P2
11 Proper palmar digital vein
12 Deep ungular plexus
13 Skin
14 Corium limbi
15 Pulvinus coronae
16 Corium coronae
17 Corium parietis
18 Dermal and epidermal lamellae
19 Solar subcutaneous layer
20 Corium soleae
21 Periople
22 Hoof wall
    22a Collateral part (quarter)
    22b Inflex part (bar)
    22c Heel
23 Sole
24 Zona alba (white zone)

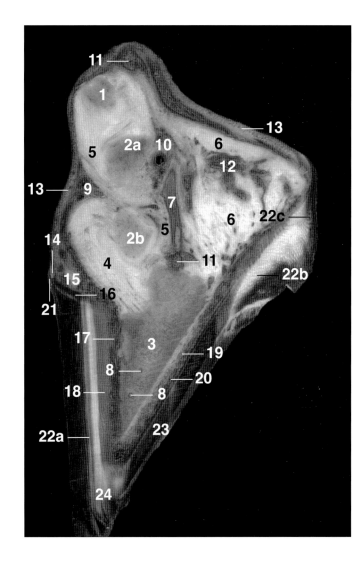

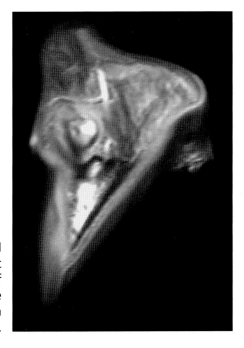

Parasagittal MRI scan of the foot after injection of fat material in the arteries and latex in the veins.

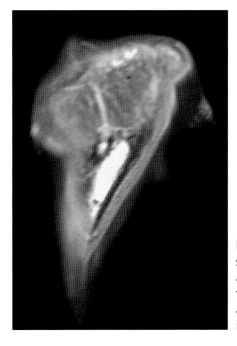

Parasagittal MRI scan of the foot after injection of fat material in the arteries and latex in the veins.

S8: Parasagittal Section of the Foot

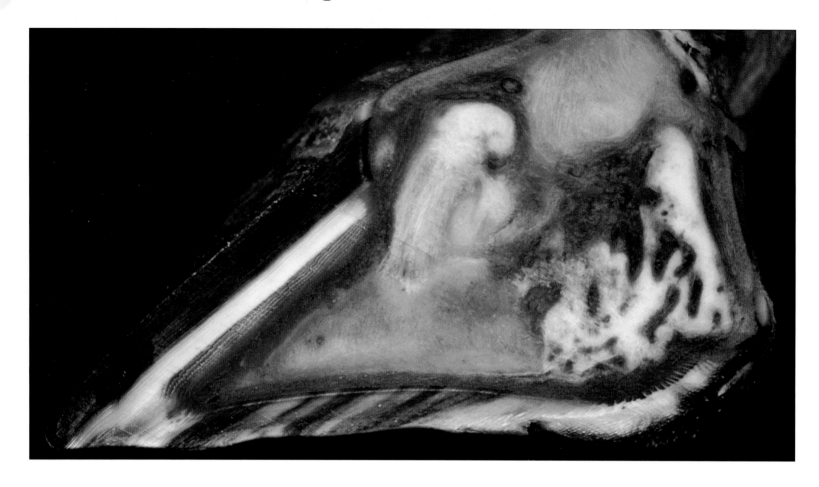

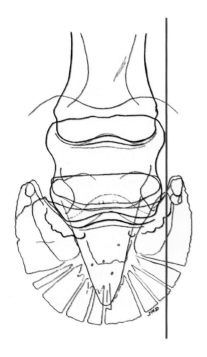

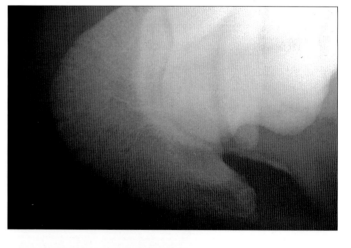

Proximolateral-distomedial oblique radiographic view of the palmar process of the distal phalanx.

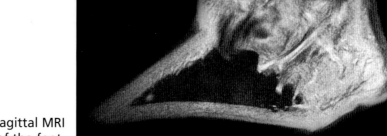

Parasagittal MRI scan of the foot.

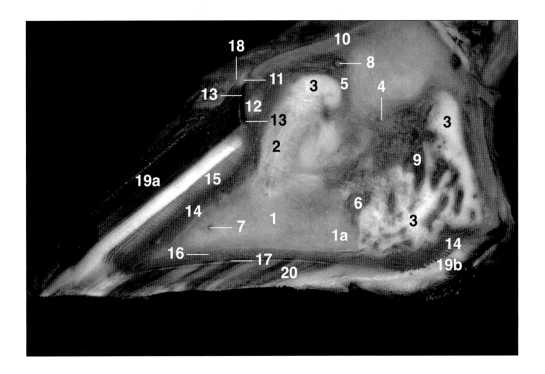

1 **Distal phalanx (P3)**
  1a Palmar process
2 **Collateral ligament of the distal interphalangeal joint**
3 **Ungular cartilage**
4 **Dorsal ramus (artery) of the middle phalanx**
5 **Coronal artery**
6 **Dorsal ramus (artery) of P3**
7 **Perforating ramus (from the terminal arch)**
8 **Coronal vein**
9 **Deep ungular plexus**
10 **Skin**

11 **Corium limbi**
12 **Pulvinus coronae**
13 **Corium coronae**
14 **Corium parietis**
15 **Dermal and epidermal lamellae**
16 **Solar subcutaneous layer**
17 **Corium soleae**
18 **Periople**
19 **Hoof wall**
  19a Collateral part (quarter)
  19b Inflex part (bar)
20 **Sole (angle)**

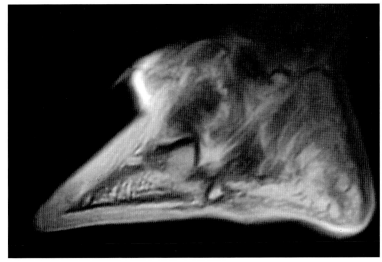

Parasagittal MRI scan of the foot.

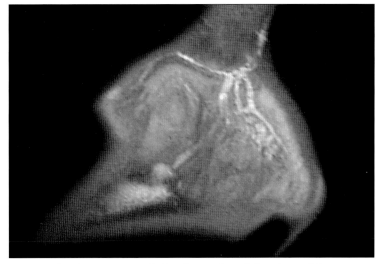

Parasagittal MRI scan of the foot after injection of latex into the arteries and fat material into the veins.

S9: Parasagittal Sections of the Foot

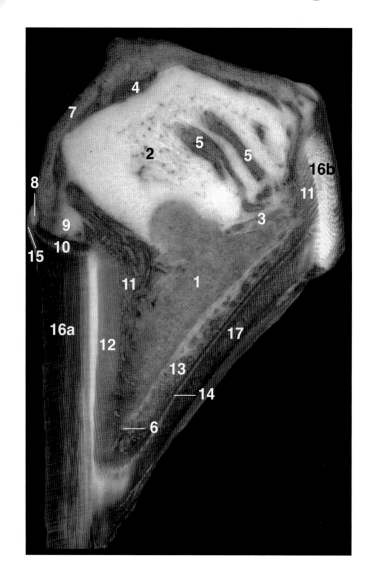

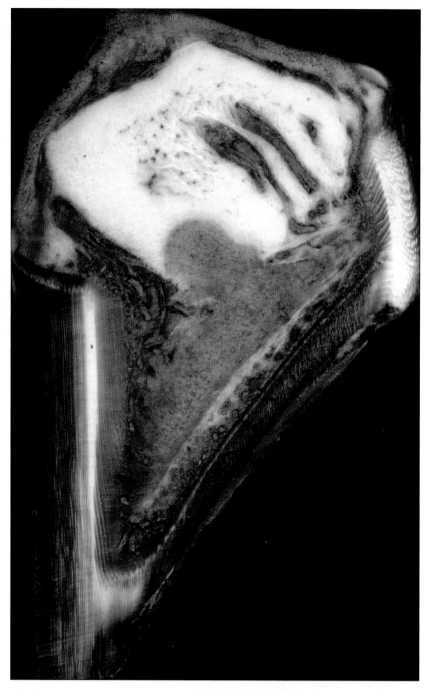

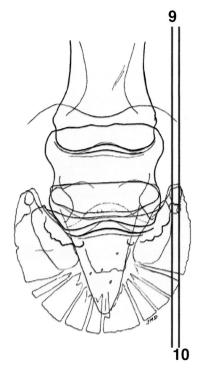

1 Distal phalanx
2 Ungular cartilage
3 Dorsal ramus of the distal phalanx
4 Coronal vein and artery
5 Ungular plexus
6 Circumflex artery and vein
7 Skin
8 Corium limbi
9 Pulvinus coronae
10 Corium coronae
11 Corium parietis with its venous plexus

12 Dermal and epidermal lamellae
13 Solar subcutaneous layer with its venous plexus
14 Corium soleae
15 Periople
16 Hoof wall
    16a Collateral part (quarter)
    16b Heel
    16c Inflex part (bar)
17 Sole (angle)

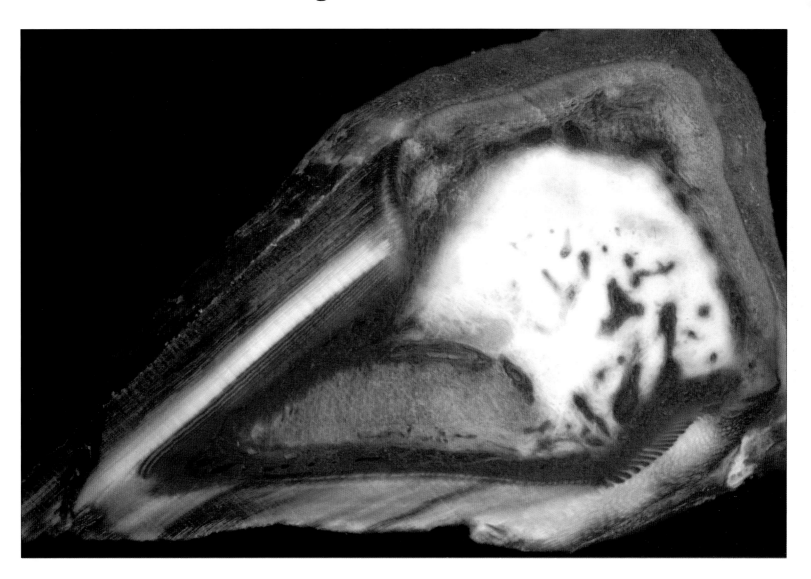

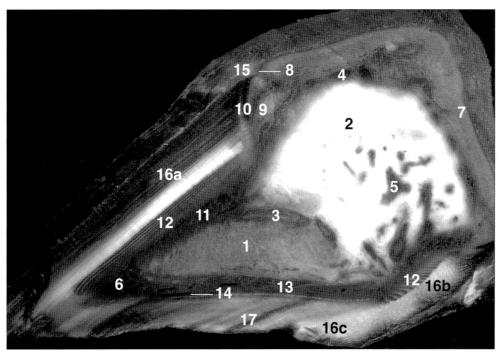

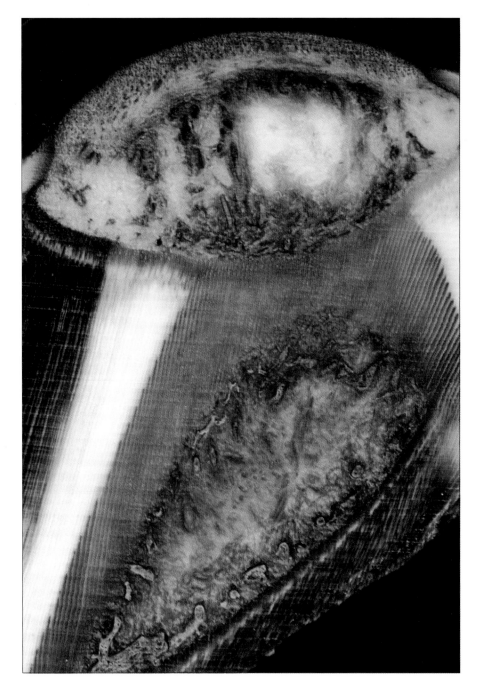

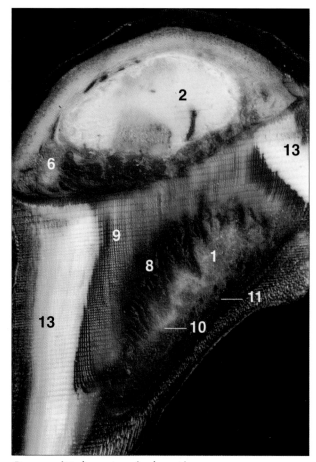

Parasagittal anatomical section.

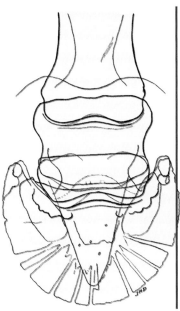

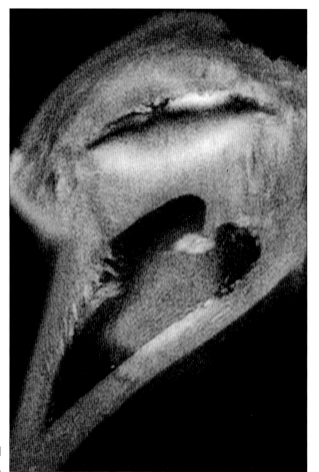

Parasagittal MRI
scan of the foot.

1 Distal phalanx
2 Ungular cartilage
3 Perforating ramus from the terminal arch
4 Skin
5 Corium limbi
6 Pulvinus coronae
7 Corium coronae with its venous plexus
8 Corium parietis with its venous plexus
9 Dermal and epidermal lamellae
10 Solar subcutaneous layer with its venous plexus
11 Corium soleae
12 Periople
13 Hoof wall (collateral part)
    13a Stratum internum
    13b Stratum medium
14 Sole (angle)

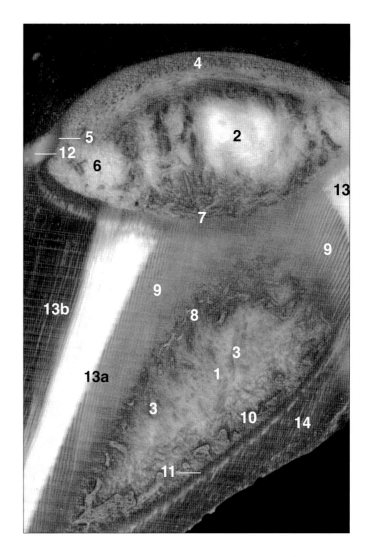

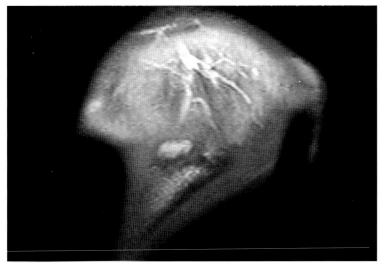

Parasagittal MRI scan of the foot after injection of latex into the arteries and fat material into the veins.

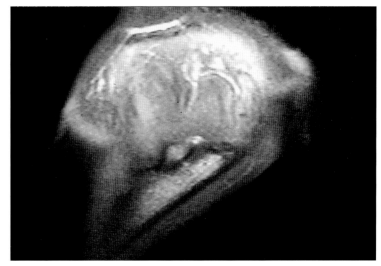

Parasagittal MRI scan of the foot after injection of latex into the arteries and fat material into the veins.

Transverse Sections of the Equine Foot

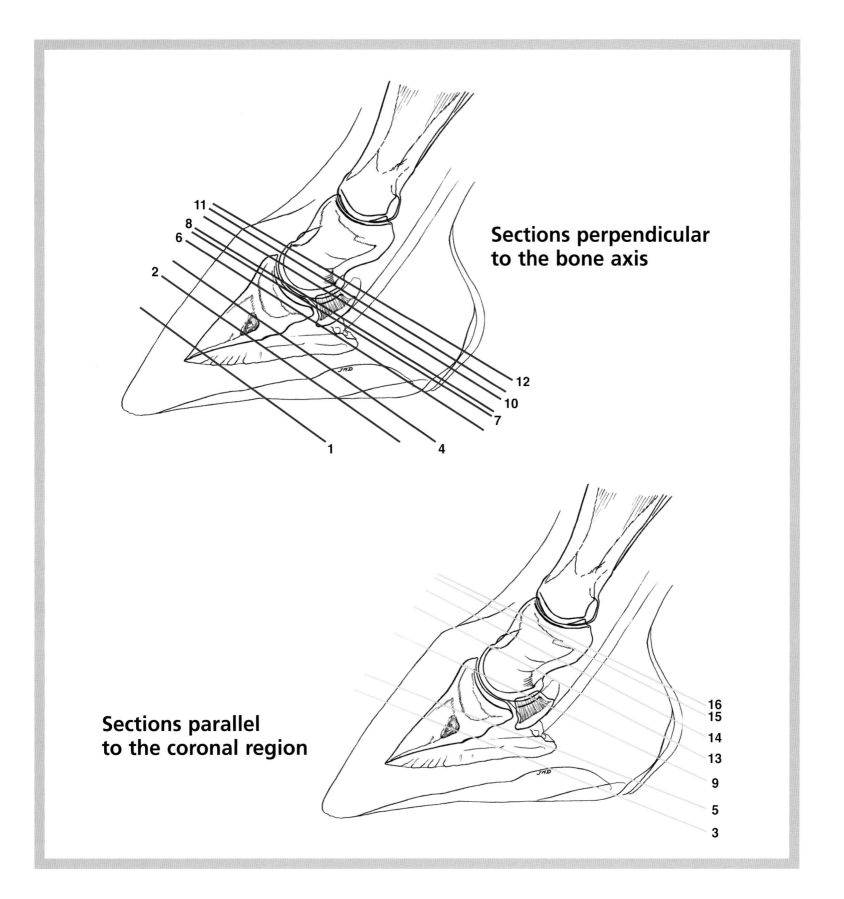

Sections perpendicular to the bone axis

Sections parallel to the coronal region

T1: Transverse Section of the Foot

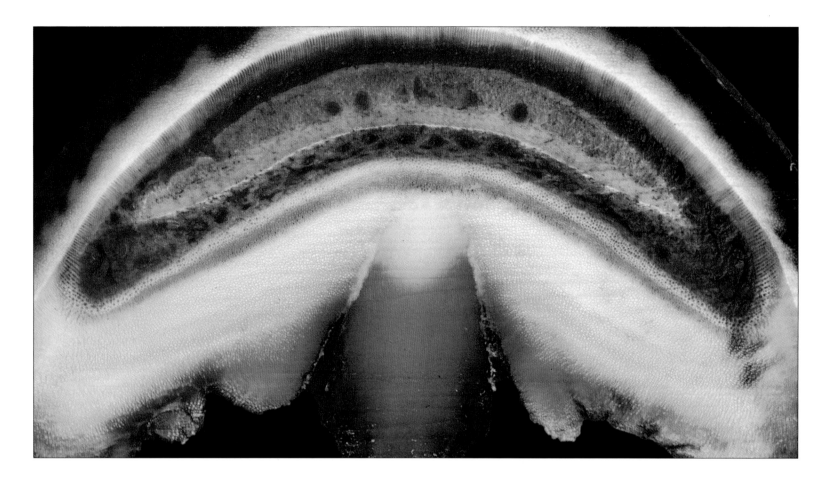

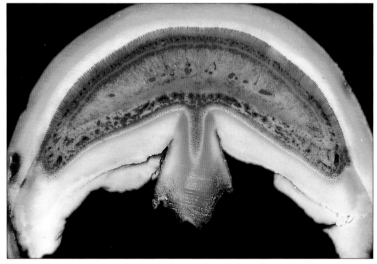

Transverse anatomical section after injection
of coloured latex into the vessels.

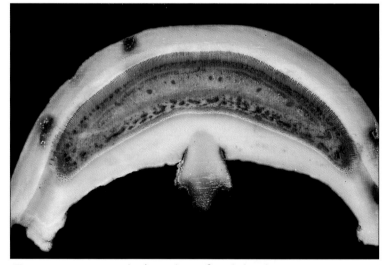

Transverse anatomical section after injection
of coloured latex into the vessels.

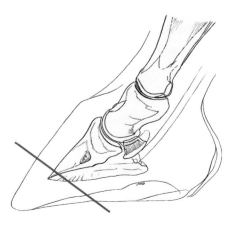

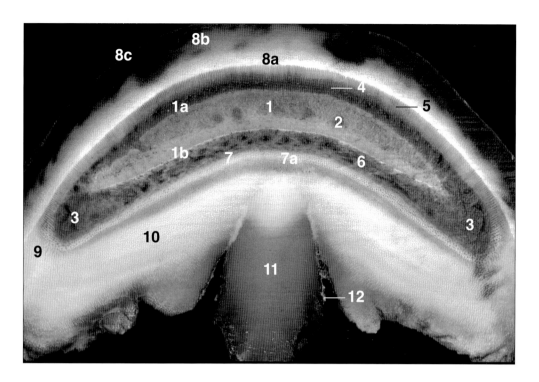

1 Distal phalanx (solar border)
  1a Parietal surface
  1b Planum cutaneum
2 Perforating ramus
3 Solar marginal artery (circumflex artery)
4 Corium parietis
5 Dermal and epidermal lamellae
6 Solar subcutaneous layer
7 Corium soleae
  7a Dermal papillae
8 Hoof wall
  8a Stratum internum
  8b Stratum medium
  8c Stratum externum
9 Zona alba (white zone)
10 Sole
11 Frog (apex)
12 Paracuneal sulcus

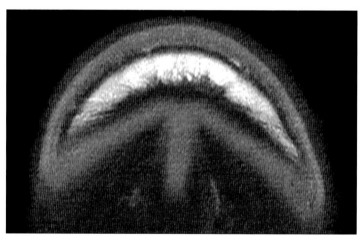

Parasagittal MRI scan of the foot after injection of latex into the arteries and veins.

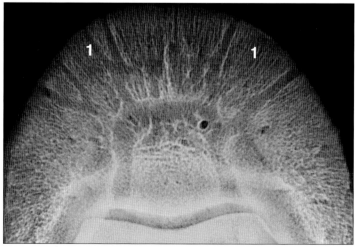

Dorsopalmar underexposed radiographic view of the solar border of the distal phalanx.

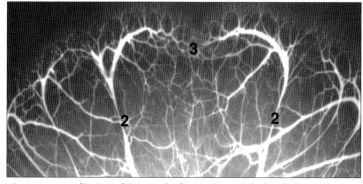

Contrast radiographic study (arteriography) of the solar marginal ('circumflex') artery, dorsopalmar view.

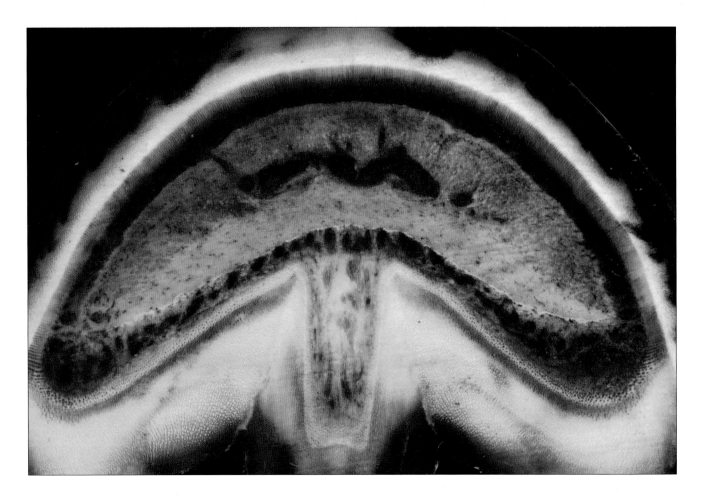

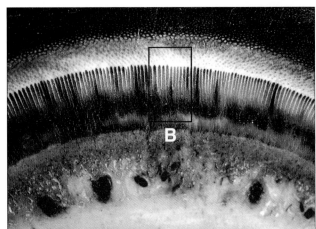

Close-up view of the lamellae (area A in illustration at top of facing page).

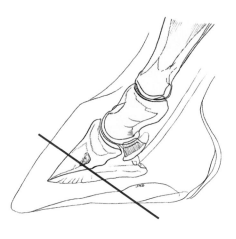

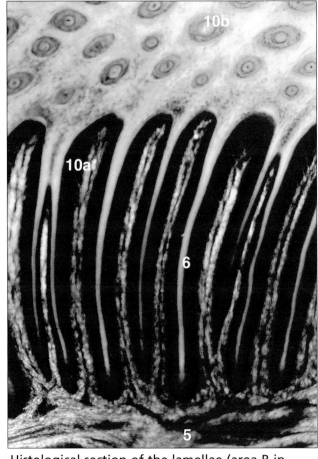

Histological section of the lamellae (area B in picture at left).

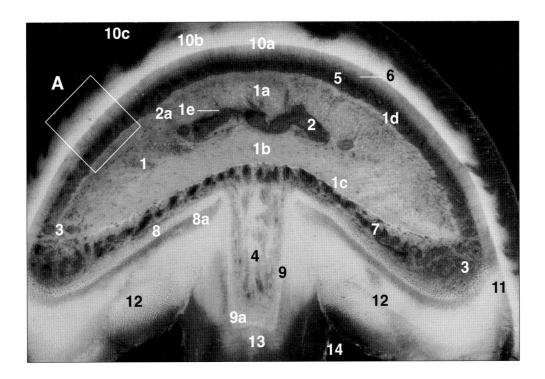

1 Distal phalanx
   1a Spongious bone
   1b Distopalmar compact bone
   1c Planum cutaneum
   1d Parietal surface
   1e Solar canal
2 Terminal arch
   2a Perforating ramus
3 Circumflex artery
4 Digital cushion (cuneal part)
5 Corium parietis
6 Dermal and epidermal lamellae
7 Solar subcutaneous layer

8 Corium soleae
   8a Dermal papillae
9 Corium cunei
   9a Dermal papillae
10 Hoof wall
   10a Stratum internum
   10b Stratum medium
   10c Stratum externum
11 Zone alba (white zone)
12 Sole
13 Frog (body)
14 Paracuneal sulcus

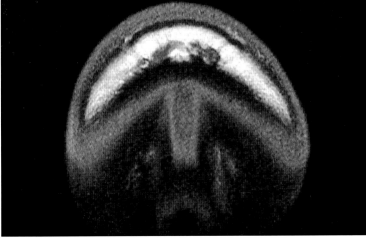

Transverse MRI scan of the foot after injection of latex into the arteries and veins.

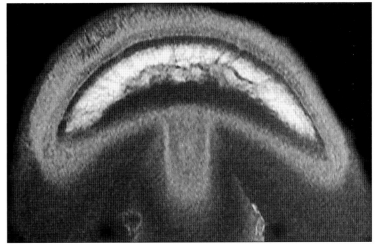

Transverse MRI scan of the foot after injection of fat material into the arteries and latex into the veins.

T3: Transverse Section of the Foot

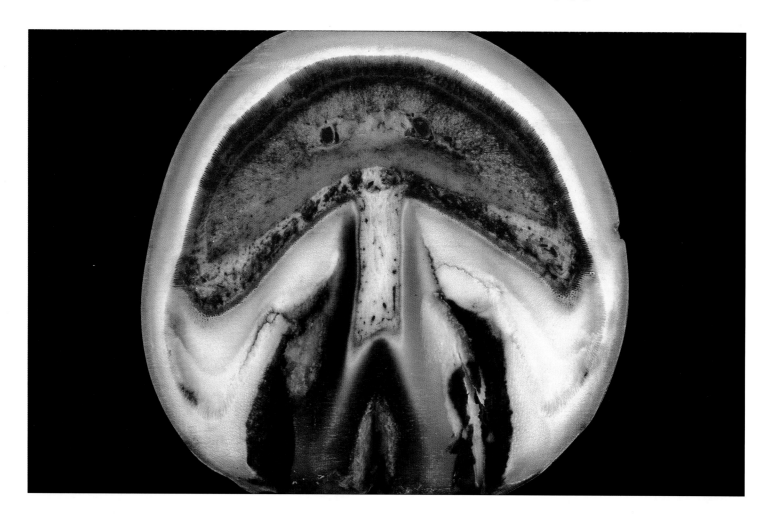

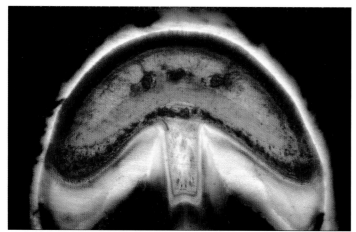

Transverse section of the foot.

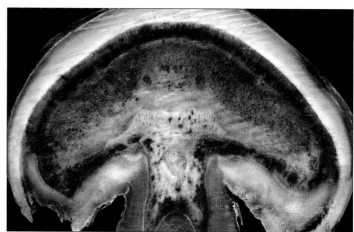

Transverse section of the foot.

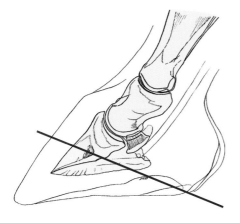

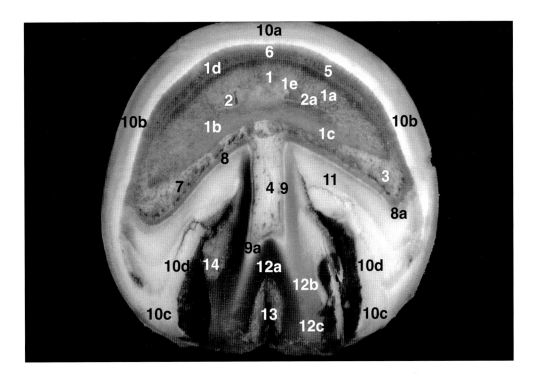

1 Distal phalanx
   1a Spongious bone
   1b Distopalmar compact bone
   1c Planum cutaneum
   1d Parietal surface
   1e Solar canal
2 Terminal arch
   2a Perforating rami
3 Circumflex artery
4 Digital cushion (cuneal part)
5 Corium parietis
6 Dermal and epidermal lamellae
7 Solar subcutaneous layer
8 Corium soleae
   8a Dermal papillae

9 Corium cunei
   9a Dermal papillae
10 Hoof wall
   10a Dorsal part (toe)
   10b Collateral part (quarter)
   10c Heel
   10d Inflex part (bar)
11 Sole
12 Frog
   12a Spine
   12b Branch
   12c Base
13 Central cuneal sulcus
14 Paracuneal sulcus

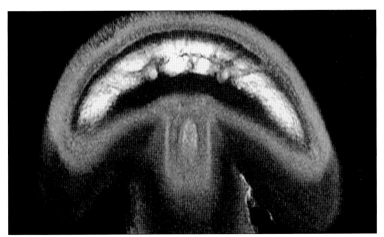

Transverse MRI scan of the foot after injection of fat material into the arteries and latex into the veins.

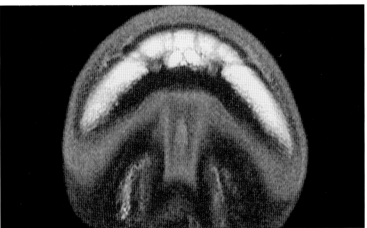

Transverse MRI scan of the foot after injection of latex into the arteries and veins.

T4: Transverse Section of the Foot

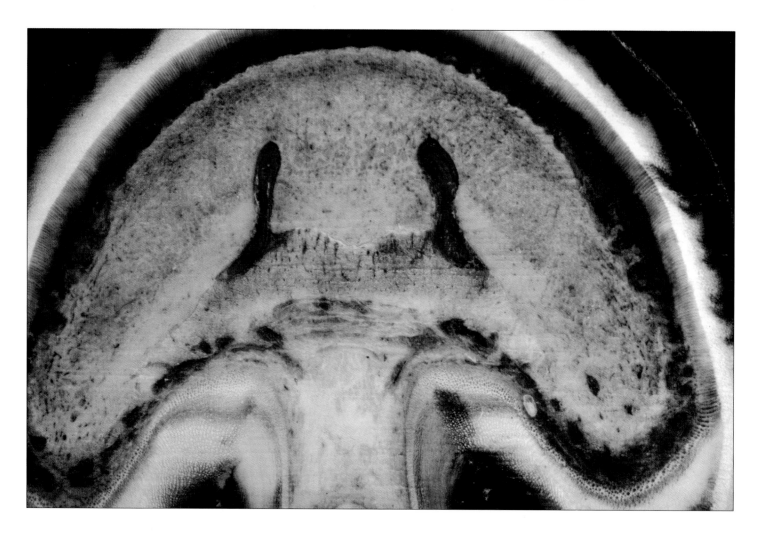

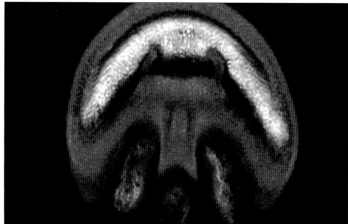

Transverse MRI scan of the foot after injection of latex into the arteries and veins.

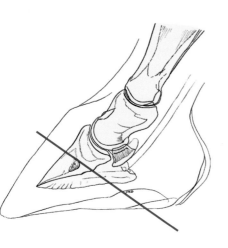

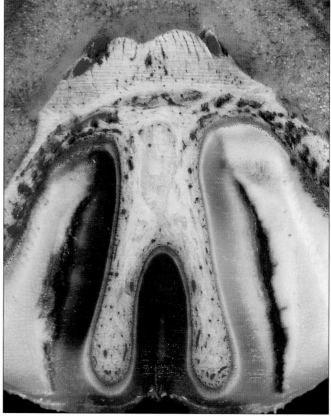

Transverse anatomical section of the foot after injection of coloured latex into the vessels.

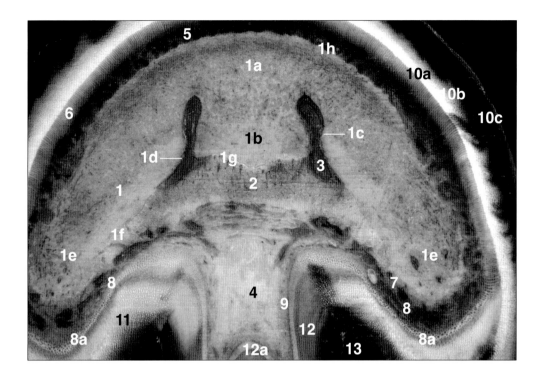

1 Distal phalanx
  1a Spongious bone
  1b Distopalmar compact bone
  1c Solar canal with terminal arch
  1d Solar foramen
  1e Palmar process
  1f Planum cutaneum
  1g Flexor surface
  1h Parietal surface
2 Deep digital flexor tendon
3 Proper palmar digital artery
4 Digital cushion (cuneal part)
5 Corium parietis

6 Dermal and epidermal lamellae
7 Solar subcutaneous layer
8 Corium soleae
  8a Dermal papillae
9 Corium cunei
10 Hoof wall
  10a Stratum internum
  10b Stratum medium
  10c Stratum externum
11 Sole
12 Frog (body)
  12a Spine
13 Paracuneal sulcus

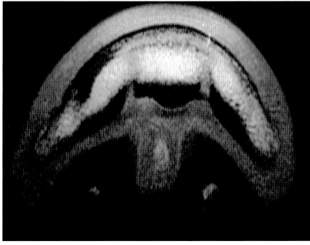

Transverse MRI scan of the foot.

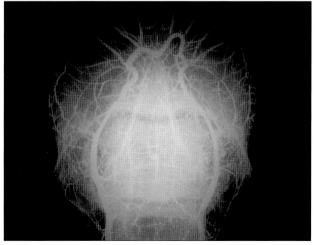

Contrast radiographic study of the arteries (arteriography) of the foot, dorsopalmar view.

T5: Transverse Section of the Foot

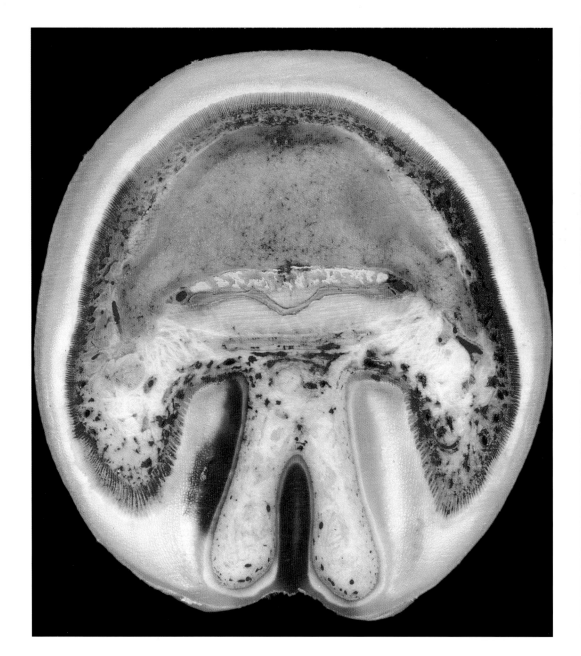

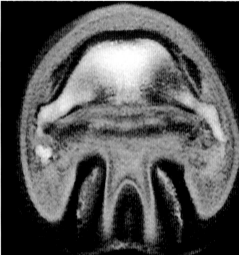

Transverse MRI scan of the foot after injection of latex into the arteries and veins.

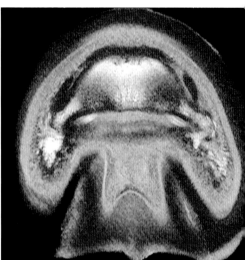

Transverse MRI scan of the foot after injection of fat material into the arteries and latex into the veins.

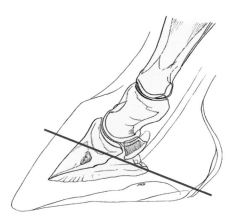

1 Distal phalanx (P3)
  1a Palmar process
  1b Parietal surface
  1c Insertion fossa for the collateral ligament
2 Collateral ligament of the distal interphalangeal joint
3 Impar distal sesamoidean ligament
4 Distopalmar recess of the distal interphalangeal joint
5 Deep digital flexor tendon
6 Podotrochlear bursa (distal recess)
7 Digital cushion (cuneal part)
8 Ungular cartilage
9 Proper palmar digital artery and vein
10 Dorsal ramus of P3
11 Corium parietis
12 Corium cunei
13 Hoof wall
  13a Dorsal part (toe)
  13b Collateral part (quarter)
  13c Heel
  13d Inflex part (bar)
14 Frog
  14a Spine
  14b Base
15 Bulb of the heel

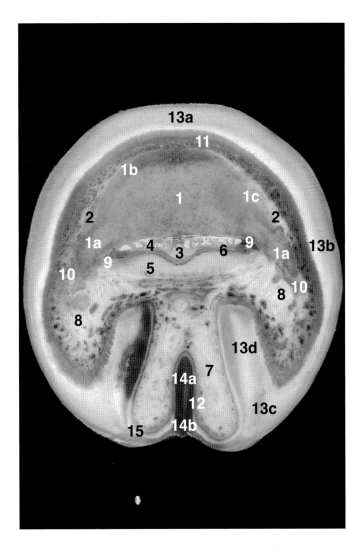

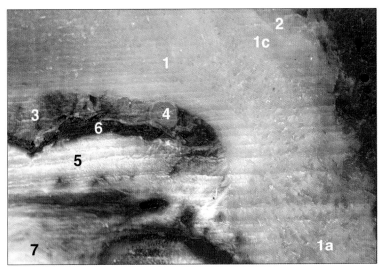

Transverse section of the foot after injection of coloured latex into the synovial cavities.

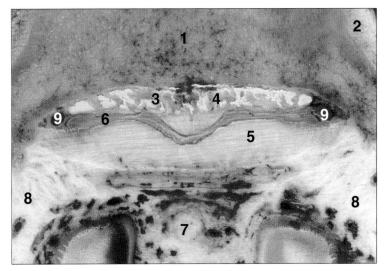

Transverse section of the foot after injection of coloured latex into the synovial cavities and vessels.

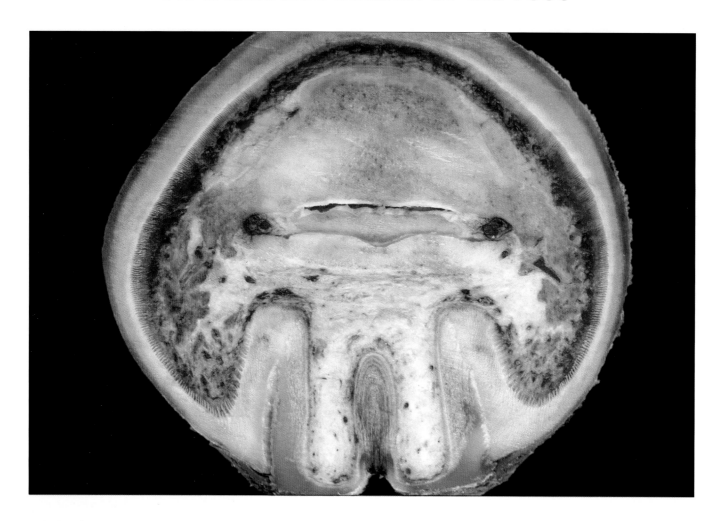

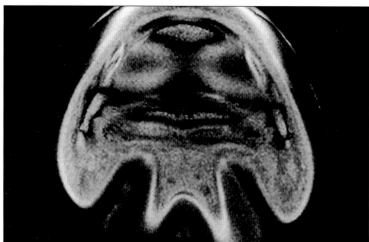

Transverse MRI scan of the foot.

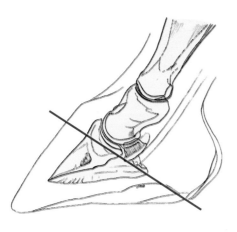

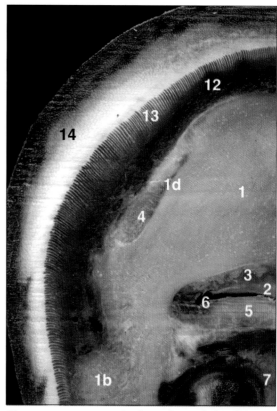

Transverse anatomical section of the foot after injection of coloured latex into the synovial cavities.

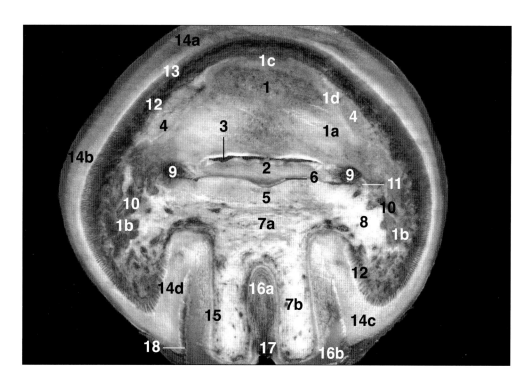

1 Distal phalanx (P3)
  1a Subchondral bone
  1b Palmar process
  1c Parietal surface
  1d Insertion fossa for the collateral ligament
2 Distal sesamoid bone (distal border)
3 Distal interphalangeal (DIP) joint (distopalmar recess)
4 Collateral ligament of the DIP joint
5 Deep digital flexor tendon
6 Podotrochlear bursa
7 Digital cushion
  7a Toric part
  7b Cuneal part
8 Ungular cartilage
9 Proper palmar digital artery and vein

10 Dorsal ramus of P3 (in the foramen of the palmar process)
11 Proper palmar digital nerve
12 Corium parietis
13 Dermal and epidermal lamellae
14 Hoof wall
  14a Dorsal part (toe)
  14b Collateral part (quarter)
  14c Heel
  14d Inflex part (bar)
15 Corium cunei
16 Frog
  16a Spine
  16b Base
17 Central cuneal sulcus
18 Paracuneal sulcus

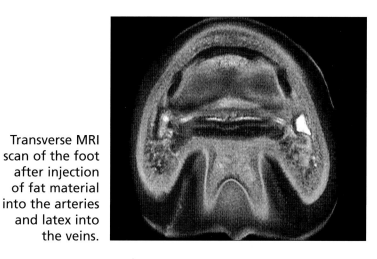

Transverse MRI scan of the foot after injection of fat material into the arteries and latex into the veins.

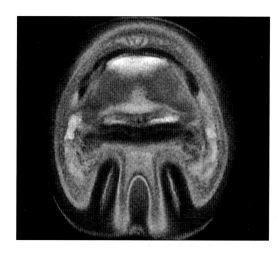

Transverse MRI scan of the foot after injection of latex into the arteries and veins.

T7: Transverse Section of the Foot

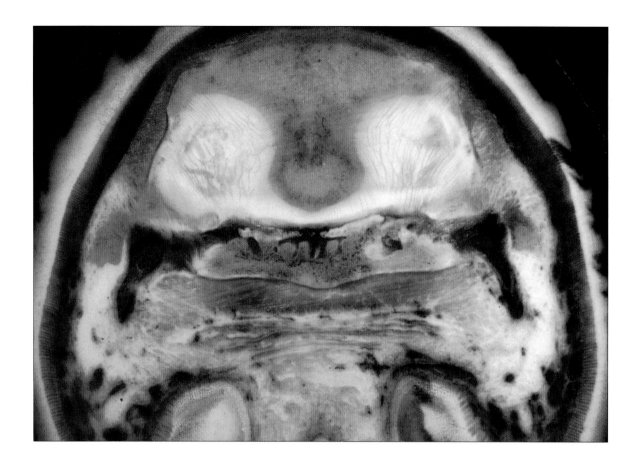

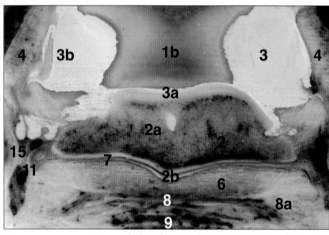

Transverse section of the foot after injection of coloured latex into the synovial cavities and vessels.

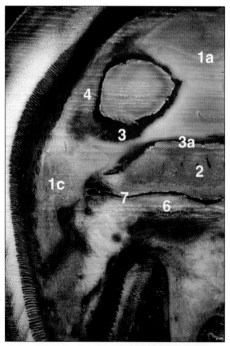

Transverse section of the foot after injection of coloured latex into the synovial cavities and vessels.

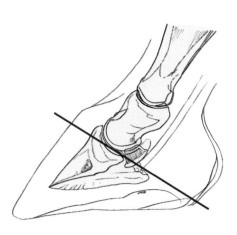

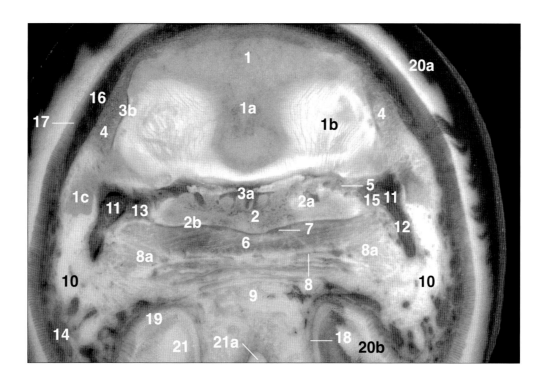

1 Distal phalanx (P3)
  1a Subchondral bone
  1b Articular cartilage of the DIP joint
  1c Palmar process
2 Distal sesamoid bone (distal border)
  2a Synovial fossa
  2b Flexor surface
3 Distal interphalangeal (DIP) joint
  3a Distopalmar recess
  3b Collateral recess
4 Collateral ligament of the DIP joint
5 Impar distal sesamoidean ligament
6 Deep digital flexor tendon
7 Podotrochlear bursa
8 Distal digital annular ligament
  8a Distal attachment

9 Digital cushion
10 Ungular cartilage
11 Proper palmar digital artery
12 Dorsal ramus of P3
13 Distal ramus (artery) of the distal sesamoid bone
14 Circumflex artery
15 Proper palmar digital nerve
16 Corium parietis
17 Dermal and epidermal lamellae
18 Corium cunei
19 Dermal papillae
20 Hoof wall
  20a Collateral part (quarter)
  20b Inflex part (bar)
21 Frog
  21a Spine

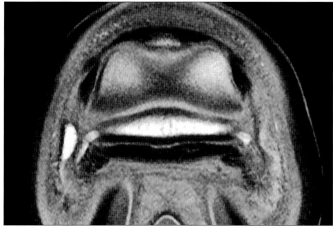

Transverse MRI scan of the foot after injection of fat material into the arteries and latex into the veins.

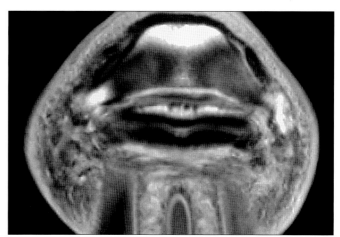

Transverse MRI scan of the foot.

T8: Transverse Section of the Foot

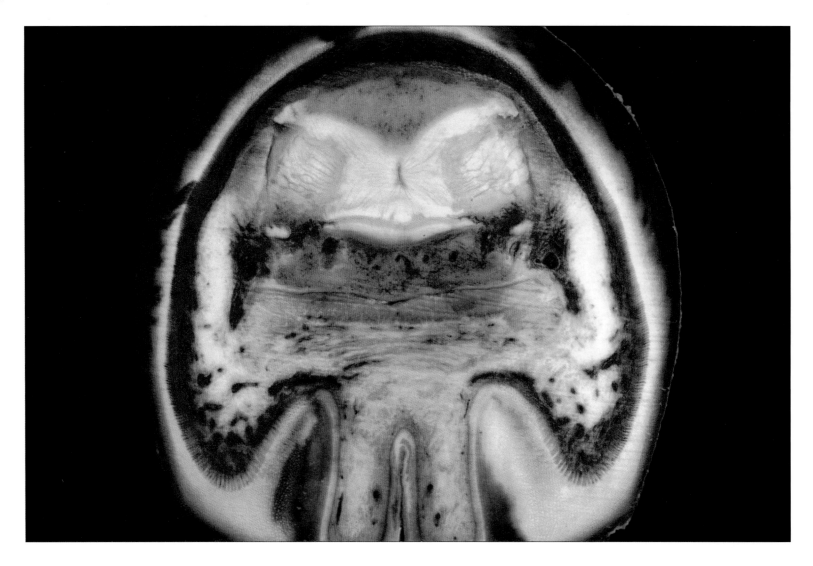

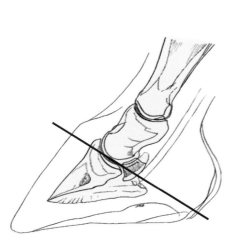

Transverse section of the foot after injection of coloured latex into the synovial cavities and vessels.

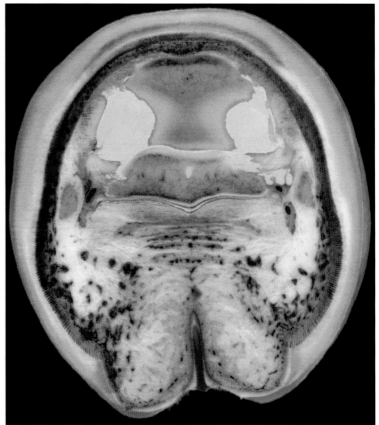

1 Distal phalanx
   1a Subchondral bone
   1b Articular cartilage
2 Distal condyle of the middle phalanx
3 Distal sesamoid bone
   3a Synovial fossa (enlarged)
   3b Flexor surface
4 Distal interphalangeal (DIP) joint
   4a Collateral recess
   4b Distopalmar recess
5 Collateral ligament of the DIP joint
6 Dorsal digital extensor tendon
7 Deep digital flexor tendon
8 Podotrochlear bursa
9 Distal digital annular ligament
   9a Distal attachment
10 Digital cushion
   10a Toric part
   10b Cuneal part
11 Ungular cartilage
12 Proper palmar digital artery and vein
13 Ramus of the digital torus
14 Proper palmar digital nerve
15 Corium coronae
16 Dermal papillae
17 Corium parietis
18 Corium cunei
19 Hoof wall
   19a Collateral part (quarter)
   19b Heel
   19c Inflex part (bar)
20 Frog
   20a Spine
   20b Base
21 Central cuneal sulcus
22 Paracuneal sulcus

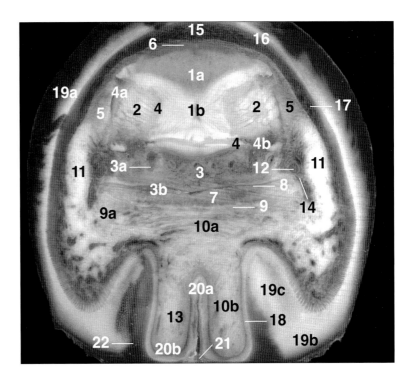

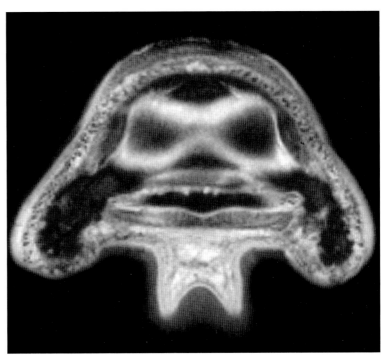

Transverse MRI scan of the foot.

T9: Transverse Section of the Foot

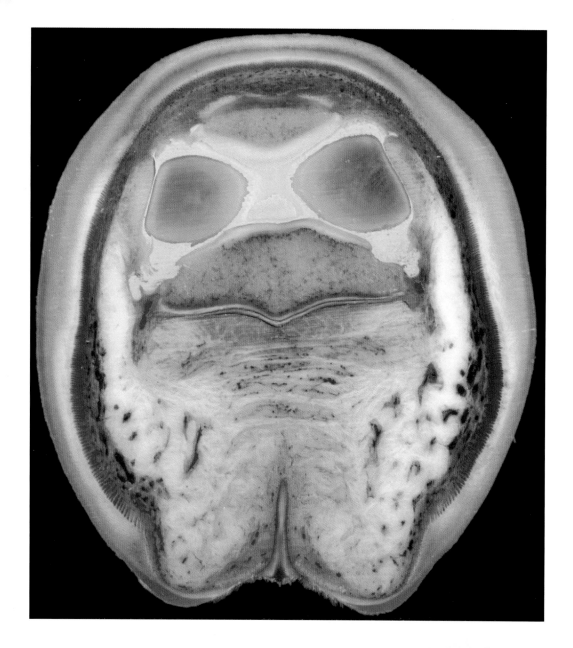

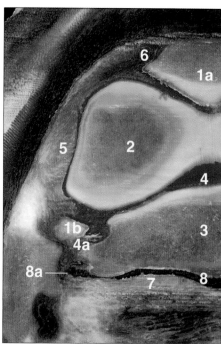

Transverse section of the foot after injection of coloured latex into the synovial cavities.

Transverse MRI scan of the foot after injection of contrast material into the DIP joint.

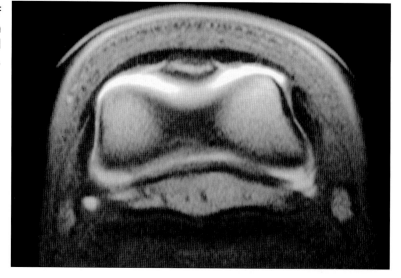

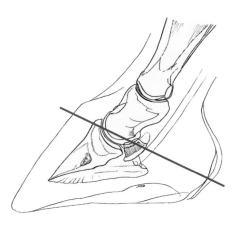

1 Distal phalanx
    1a Extensor process
    1b Articular cartilage
2 Middle phalanx (distal condyle)
    2a Articular cartilage
3 Distal sesamoid bone
    3a Articular surface
    3b Flexor surface
4 Distal interphalangeal (DIP) joint
    4a Collateral recess
5 Collateral ligament of the DIP joint
6 Dorsal digital extensor tendon
7 Deep digital flexor tendon
8 Podotrochlear bursa
    8a Collateral recess
9 Distal digital annular ligament
    9a Distal attachment
10 Digital cushion (toric part)
11 Ungular cartilage
12 Proper palmar digital artery, vein and nerve
13 Ramus of the digital torus
14 Superficial ungular plexus
15 Pulvinus coronae
16 Corium coronae
17 Dermal papillae
18 Corium parietis
19 Dermal and epidermal lamellae
20 Corium cunei
21 Hoof wall
22 Spine of the frog
23 Bulb of the heel

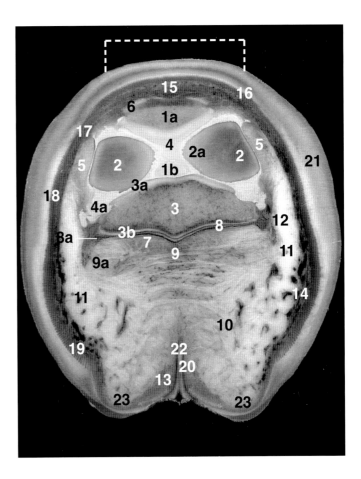

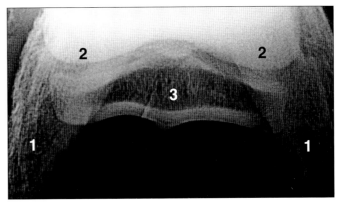

Proximopalmar-distodorsal radiographic projection (skyline view) of the palmar part of the foot.

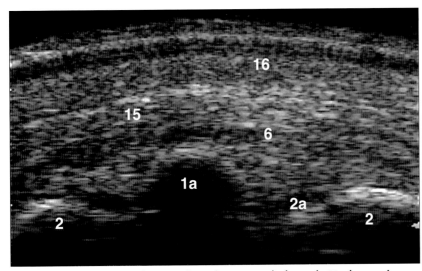

Transverse ultrasound scan, dorsal approach (see dotted area in illustration above, right).

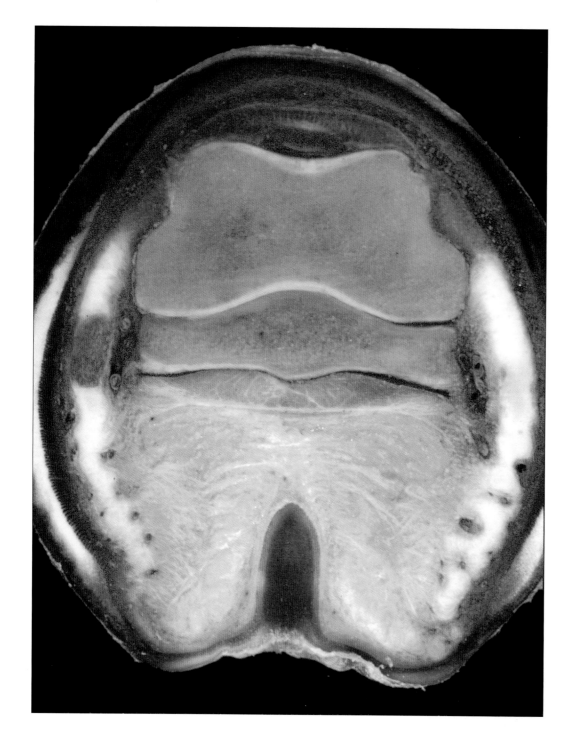

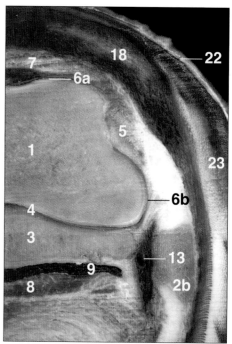

Transverse section of the foot after injection of coloured latex into the synovial cavities.

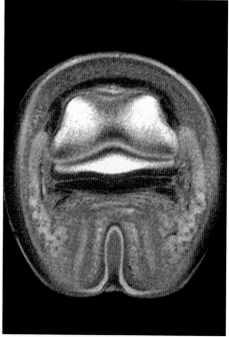

Transverse MRI scan of the foot after injection of latex into the arteries and veins.

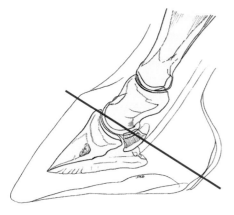

T10: Transverse Section of the Foot

1 Middle phalanx
2 Distal phalanx
   2a Extensor process
   2b Palmar process
3 Distal sesamoid bone
   3a Spongious bone
   3b Palmar compact bone
   3c Flexor surface
4 Distal interphalangeal (DIP) joint
5 Collateral ligament of the DIP joint
6 Recesses of the DIP joint
   6a Dorsal recess
   6b Collaterall recess
7 Dorsal digital extensor tendon
8 Deep digital flexor tendon
9 Podotrochlear bursa
10 Distal digital annular ligament
   10a Distal attachment
11 Digital cushion (toric part)
12 Ungular cartilage
13 Proper palmar digital artery and vein
14 Deep ungular plexus
15 Superficial ungular plexus
16 Proper palmar digital nerve
17 Corium limbi
18 Pulvinus coronae
19 Corium coronae
20 Corium parietis
21 Corium cunei
22 Periople
23 Hoof wall
24 Spine of the frog
25 Bulb of the heel

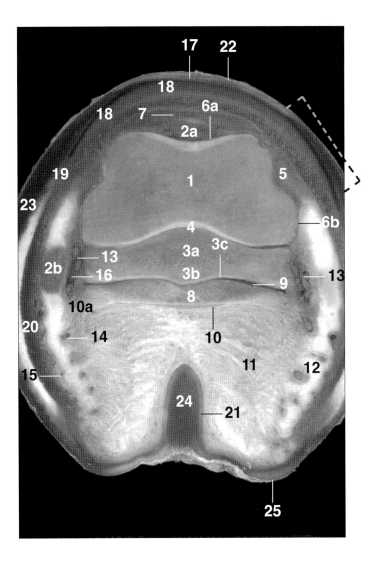

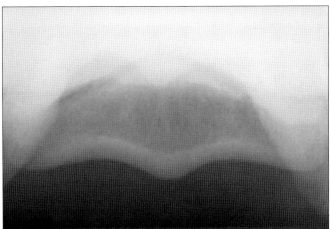

Palmaroproximal-dorsodistal oblique radiographic view (skyline view) of the distal sesamoid bone.

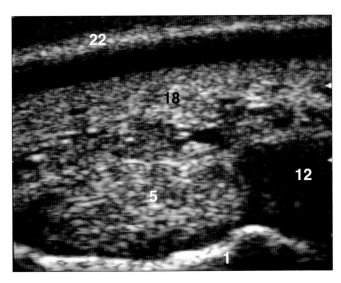

Transverse ultrasound scan of the collateral ligament of the DIP joint (see dotted area in illustration above, right).

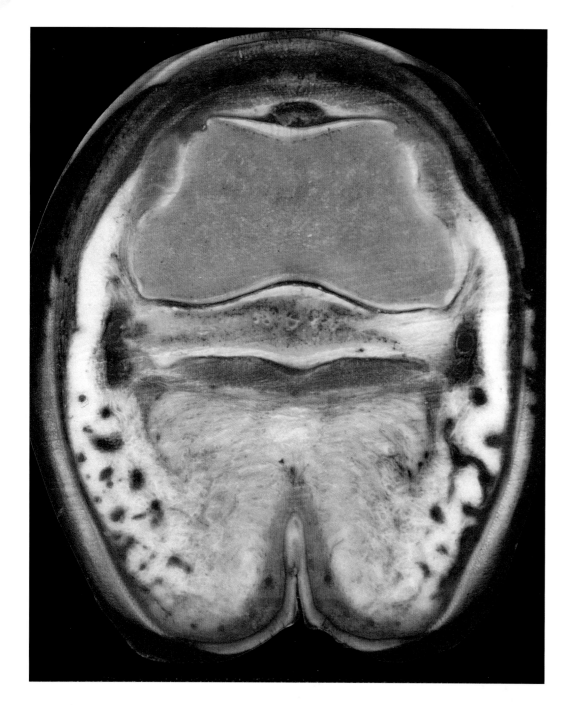

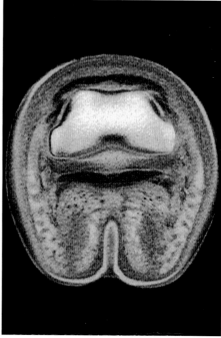

Transverse MRI scan of the foot after injection of latex into the arteries and veins.

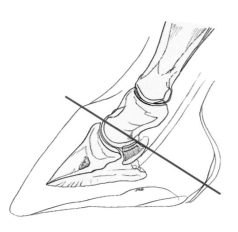

Transverse anatomical section of the foot after injection of coloured latex into the synovial cavities and vessels.

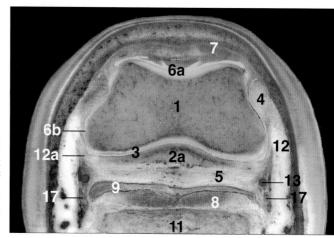

1 Middle phalanx
2 Distal sesamoid bone
   2a Proximal border
   2b Flexor surface
3 Distal interphalangeal (DIP) joint
4 Collateral ligament of the DIP joint
5 Collateral sesamoidean ligament
6 Recesses of the DIP joint
   6a Dorsal recess
   6b Collateral recess
7 Dorsal digital extensor tendon
8 Deep digital flexor tendon
9 Podotrochlear bursa
10 Distal digital annular ligament
11 Digital cushion (toric part)
12 Ungular cartilage
   12a Chondrosesamoidean ligament
13 Proper palmar digital artery (vein not injected
14 Ramus of the digital torus
15 Deep ungular plexus
16 Superficial ungular plexus
17 Proper palmar digital nerve
18 Corium limbi
19 Pulvinus coronae
20 Corium coronae
21 Periople
22 Hoof wall
23 Spine of the frog
24 Central cuneal sulcus
25 Bulb of the heel

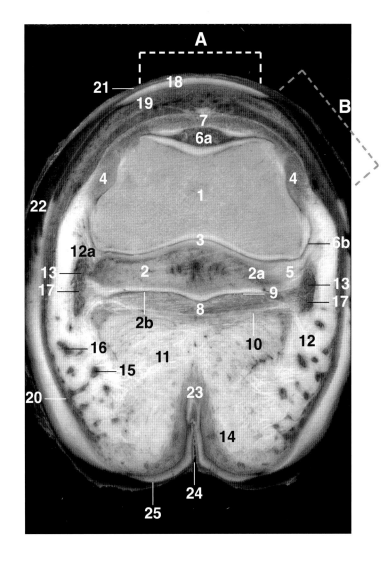

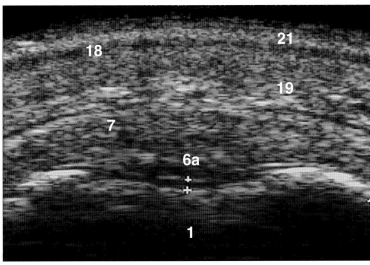

A Transverse ultrasound scan, dorsal approach (see dotted area in illustration above, right). Crosses show the articular cartilage.

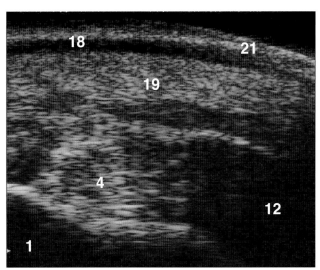

B Transverse ultrasound scan, dorsolateral approach (see dotted area in illustration above).

T11b: Transverse Section of the Foot

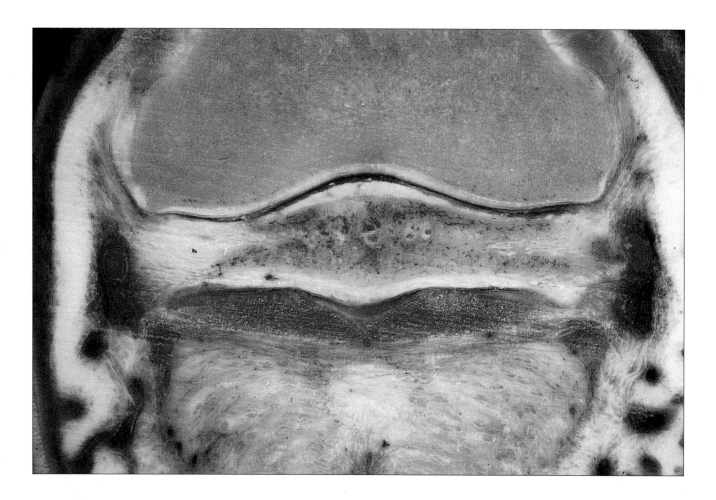

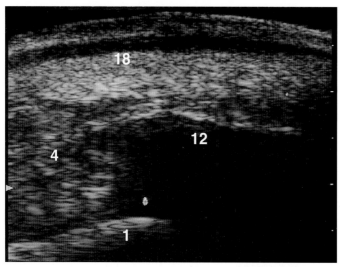

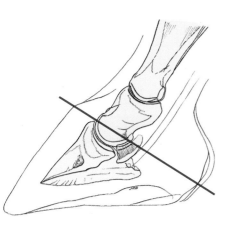

Transverse ultrasound scan of the coronet, dorsolateral approach (see dotted area in illustration on facing page).

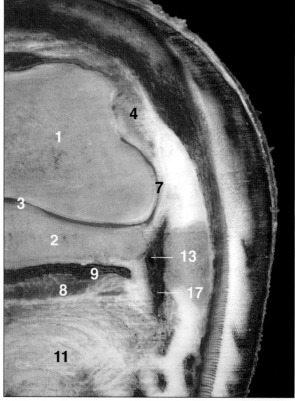

Transverse anatomical section of the foot after injection of coloured latex into the synovial cavities.

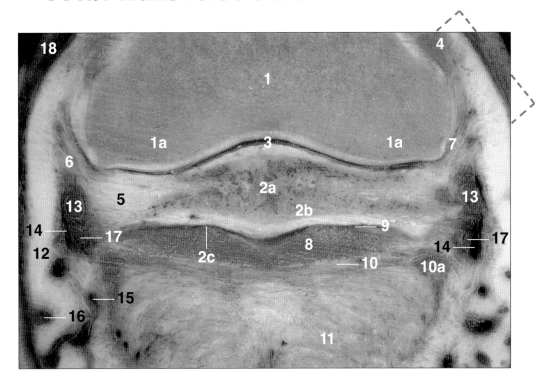

1 Middle phalanx
  1a Distal condyle
2 Distal sesamoid bone
  2a Spongious bone
  2b Palmar compact bone
  2c Flexor surface
3 Distal interphalangeal (DIP) joint
4 Collateral ligament of the DIP joint
5 Collateral sesamoidean ligament
6 Chondrosesamoidean ligament
7 Collateral recess of the DIP joint
8 Deep digital flexor tendon

9 Podotrochlear bursa
10 Distal digital annular ligament
  10a Distal attachment
11 Digital cushion (toric part)
12 Ungular cartilage
13 Proper palmar digital artery
14 Proper palmar digital vein (non-injected)
15 Deep ungular plexus
16 Superficial ungular plexus
17 Proper palmar digital nerve
18 Pulvinus coronae

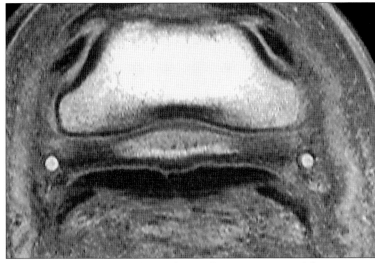

Transverse MRI scan of the foot after injection of fat material into the arteries and latex into the veins.

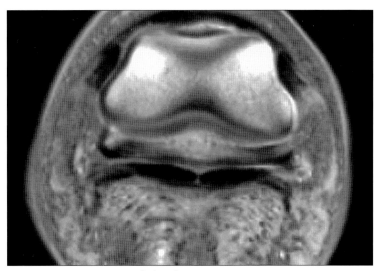

Transverse MRI scan of the foot.

T12: Transverse Section of the Foot

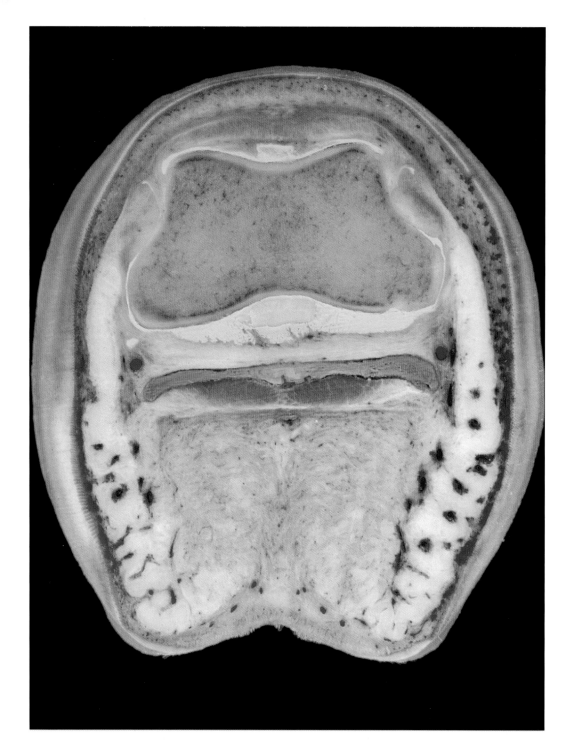

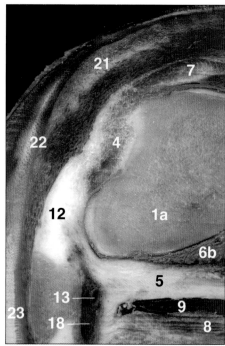

Transverse section of the foot after injection of coloured latex into the synovial cavities.

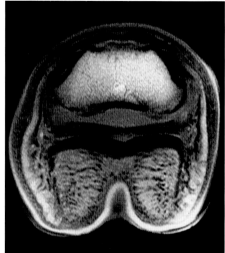

Transverse MRI scan of the foot.

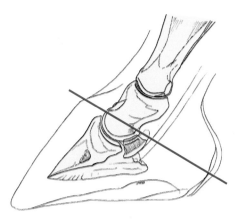

1 Middle phalanx
   1a Distal condyle
2 Distal sesamoid bone (proximal border)
3 Distal interphalangeal (DIP) joint
4 Collateral ligament of the DIP joint
5 Collateral sesamoidean ligament
6 Recesses of the DIP joint
   6a Dorsal recess
   6b Proximopalmar recess
   6c Collateral recess
7 Dorsal digital extensor tendon
8 Deep digital flexor tendon
9 Podotrochlear bursa
   9a Collateral recess
10 Distal digital annular ligament
11 Digital cushion (toric part)
12 Ungular cartilage
13 Proper palmar digital artery
14 Ramus of the digital torus
15 Proper palmar digital vein
16 Deep ungular plexus
17 Superficial ungular plexus
18 Proper palmar digital nerve
19 Skin
20 Corium limbi
21 Pulvinus coronae
22 Corium coronae
23 Corium parietis
24 Periople
25 Hoof wall
26 Bulb of the heel

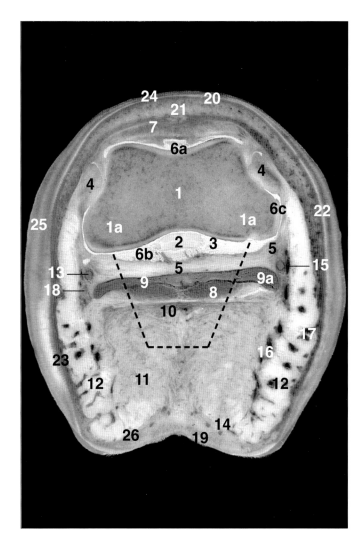

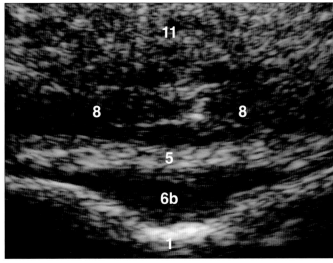

Transverse ultrasound scan oblique dorsodistally of the palmar part of the foot (see dotted area in illustration above right).

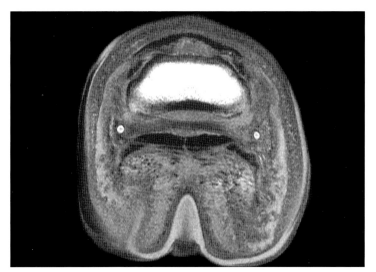

Transverse MRI scan of the foot after injection of fat material into the arteries and latex into the veins.

T13: Transverse Section of the Foot

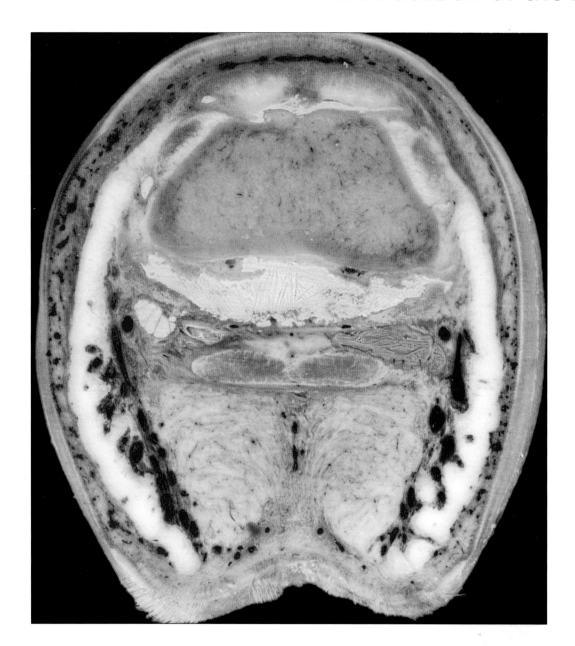

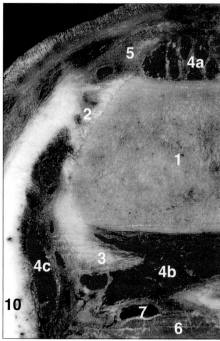

Transverse section of the foot after injection of coloured latex into the synovial cavities.

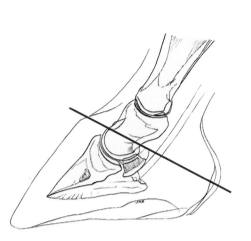

Transverse MRI scan of the foot after injection of latex into the arteries and fat material into the veins.

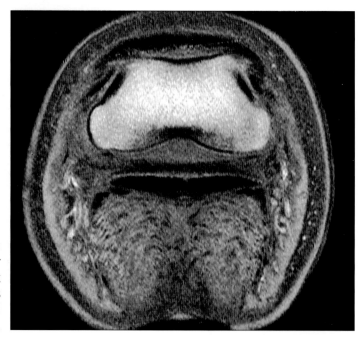

1 Middle phalanx (P2)
2 Collateral ligament of the distal interphalangeal (DIP) joint
3 Collateral sesamoidean ligament
4 Recesses of the DIP joint
    4a Dorsal recess
    4b Proximopalmar recess
    4c Collateral recess
5 Dorsal digital extensor tendon
6 Deep digital flexor tendon
    6a Fibrous part
    6b Fibrocartilaginous part
7 Podotrochlear bursa (proximal recess)
8 Distal digital annular ligament
9 Digital cushion (toric part)
10 Ungular cartilage
11 Proper palmar digital artery
12 Ramus of the digital torus
13 Palmar ramus of P2
14 Coronal artery
15 Deep ungular plexus
16 Proper palmar digital nerve
17 Skin
18 Corium limbi
19 Pulvinus coronae
20 Corium coronae
21 Periople
22 Hoof wall
23 Bulb of the heel

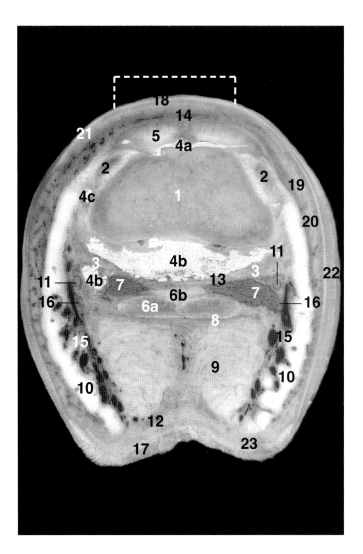

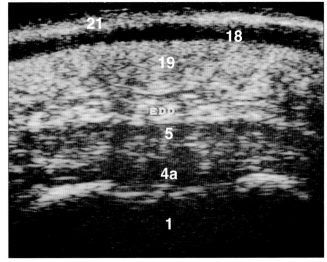

Transverse ultrasound scan of the dorsal part of the coronet, dorsal approach (see dotted area in illustration above, right).

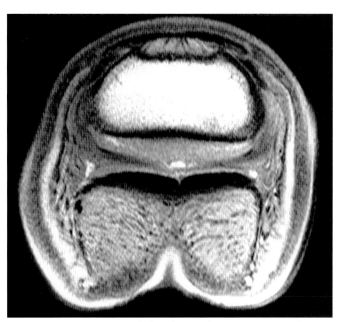

Transverse MRI scan of the foot after injection of latex into the arteries and fat material into the veins.

T14: Transverse Section of the Foot

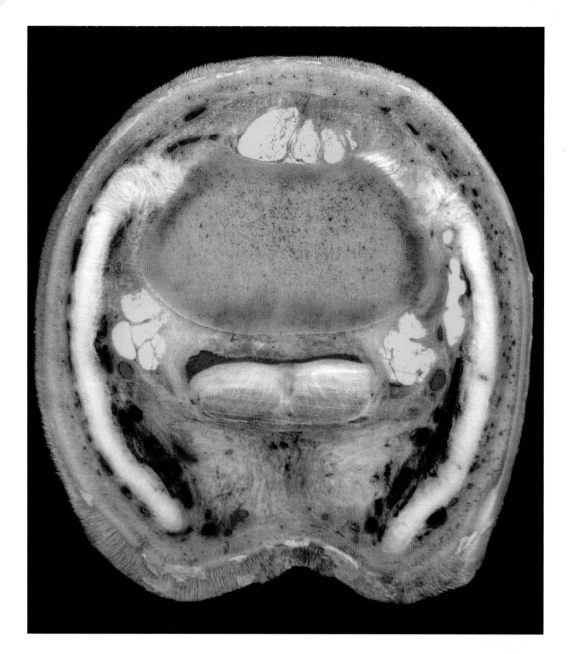

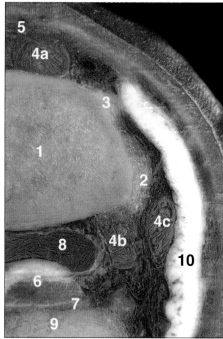

Transverse section of the foot after injection of coloured latex into the synovial cavities.

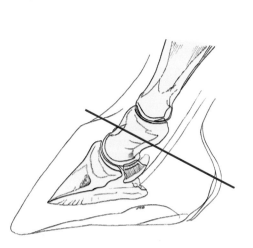

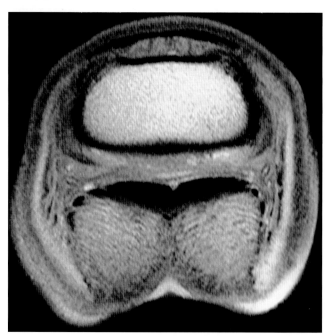

Transverse MRI scan of the foot.

1 Middle phalanx (P2)
2 Collateral sesamoidean ligament
3 Chondrocoronal ligament
4 Recesses of the distal interphalangeal joint
    4a Dorsal recess
    4b Proximopalmar recess
    4c Collateral recess
5 Dorsal digital extensor tendon
6 Deep digital flexor tendon
    6a Fibrous part
    6b Fibrocartilaginous part
7 Distal digital annular ligament
8 Dorsal distal recess of the digital sheath
9 Digital cushion (toric part)
10 Ungular cartilage
11 Proper palmar digital artery
12 Ramus of the digital torus
13 Dorsal ramus of P2
14 Deep ungular plexus
15 Superficial ungular plexus
16 Proper palmar digital nerve
17 Skin
18 Periople
19 Bulb of the heel

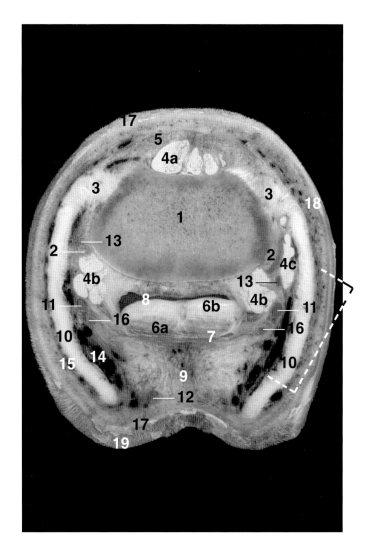

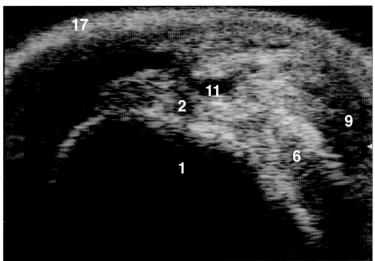

Transverse ultrasound scan of the coronet, palmarolateral approach (see dotted area in illustration above, right).

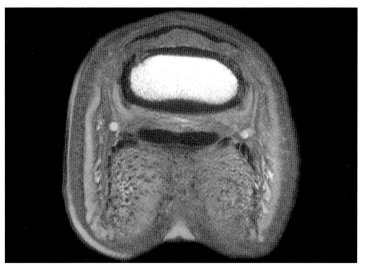

Transverse MRI scan of the foot after injection of fat material into the arteries and latex into the veins.

T15: Transverse Section of the Foot

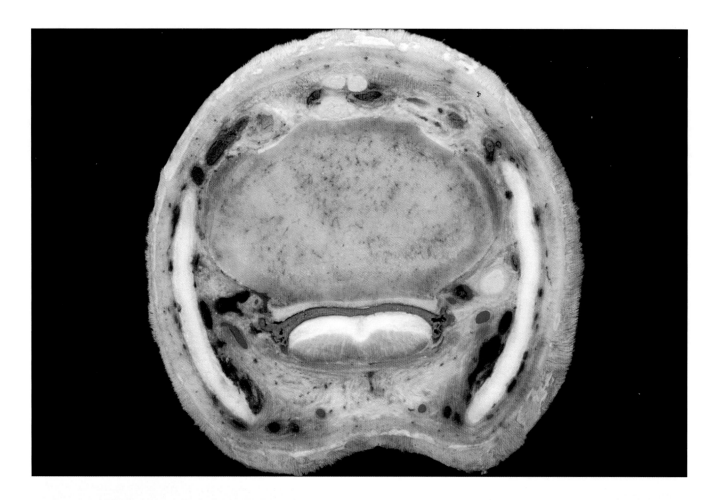

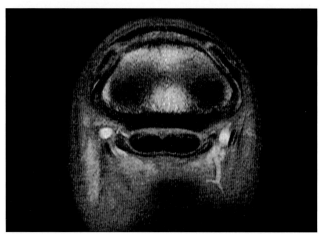

Transverse MRI scan of the foot after injection of fat material into the arteries and latex into the veins.

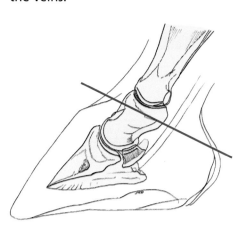

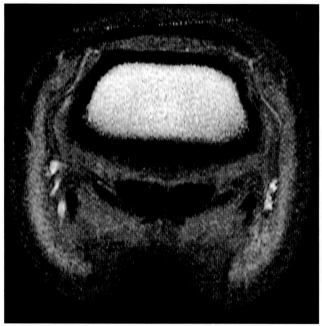

Transverse MRI scan of the foot after injection of latex into the arteries and fat material into the veins.

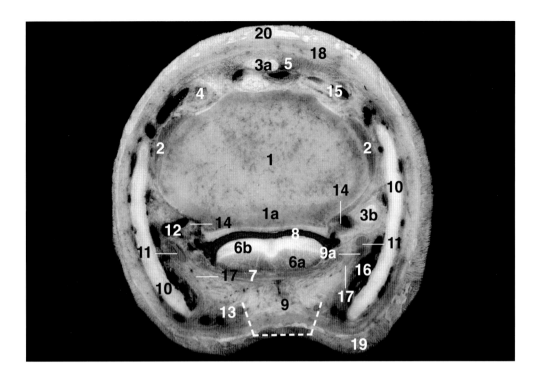

1 Middle phalanx (P2)
   1a Flexor tuberosity
2 Collateral sesamoidean ligament
3 Recesses of the distal interphalangeal joint
   3a Dorsal recess
   3b Proximopalmar recess
4 Distodorsocollateral recess of the proximal interphalangeal joint
5 Dorsal digital extensor tendon
6 Deep digital flexor tendon
   6a Fibrous part
   6b Fibrocartilaginous part
7 Distal digital annular ligament

8 Dorsal distal recess of the digital sheath
9 Digital cushion (toric part)
   9a Proximal attachment
10 Ungular cartilage
11 Proper palmar digital artery
12 Proper palmar digital vein
13 Rami (artery and vein) of the digital torus
14 Palmar rami (artery and vein) of P2
15 Dorsal rami (artery and vein) of P2
16 Deep ungular plexus
17 Proper palmar digital nerve
18 Skin
19 Bulb of the heel
20 Coronal region

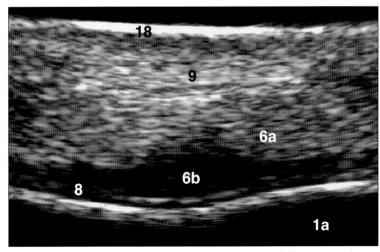

Transverse ultrasound scan of the deep digital flexor tendon, palmar approach (see dotted area in illustration above).

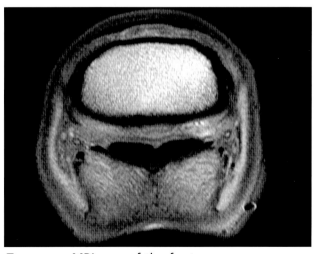

Transverse MRI scan of the foot.

T16: Transverse Section of the Foot

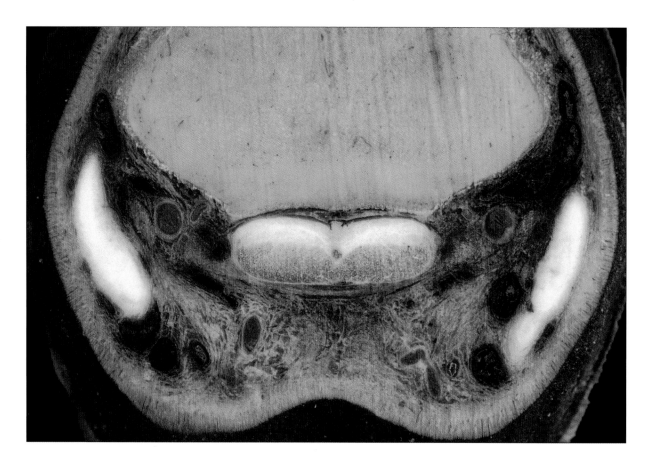

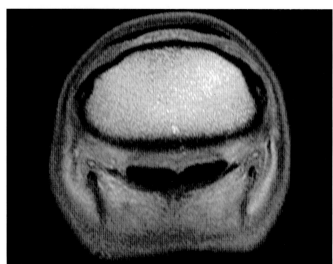

Transverse MRI scan of the foot.

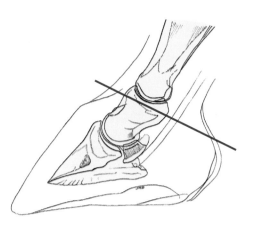

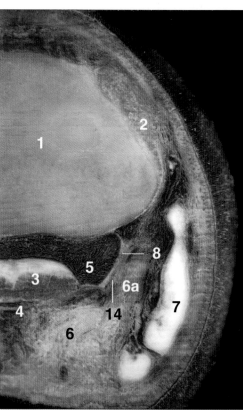

Transverse section of the foot after injection of coloured latex into the synovial cavities.

T16: Transverse Section of the Foot

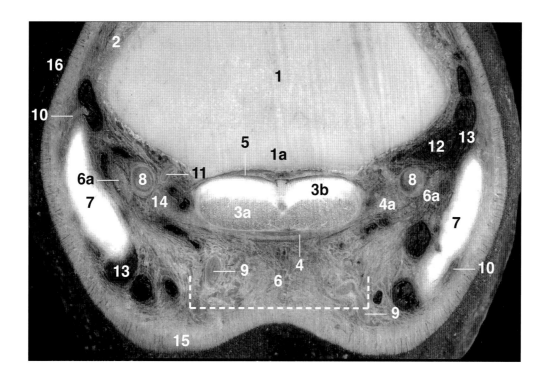

1 Middle phalanx (P2)
  1a Flexor tuberosity
2 Collateral ligament of the proximal interphalangeal joint
3 Deep digital flexor tendon
  3a Fibrous part
  3b Fibrocartilaginous part
4 Distal digital annular ligament
  4a Proximal attachment
5 Dorsal distal recess of the digital sheath
6 Digital cushion (toric part)

6a Proximal attachment
7 Ungular cartilage
8 Proper palmar digital artery
9 Ramus of the digital torus
10 Coronal artery
11 Palmar ramus of P2
12 Proper palmar digital vein
13 Ungular plexus
14 Proper palmar digital nerve
15 Skin
16 Coronal region

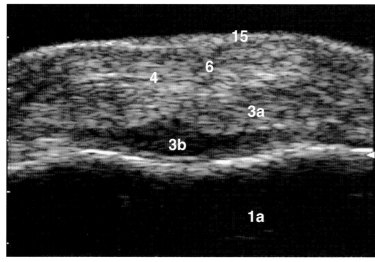

Transverse ultrasound scan of the pastern, palmar approach (see dotted area in illustration at top of page).

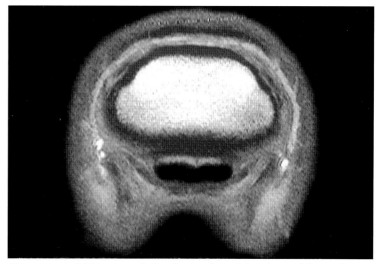

Transverse MRI scan of the foot after injection of latex into the arteries and fat material into the veins.

Frontal Sections of the Equine Foot

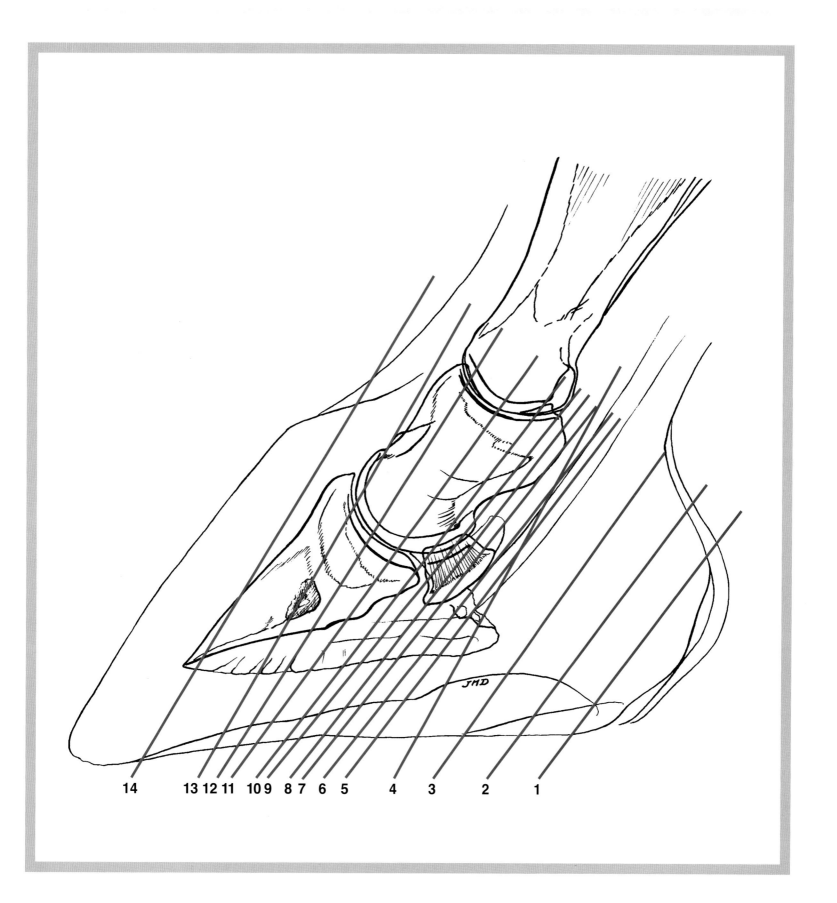

F1: Frontal Section of the Foot

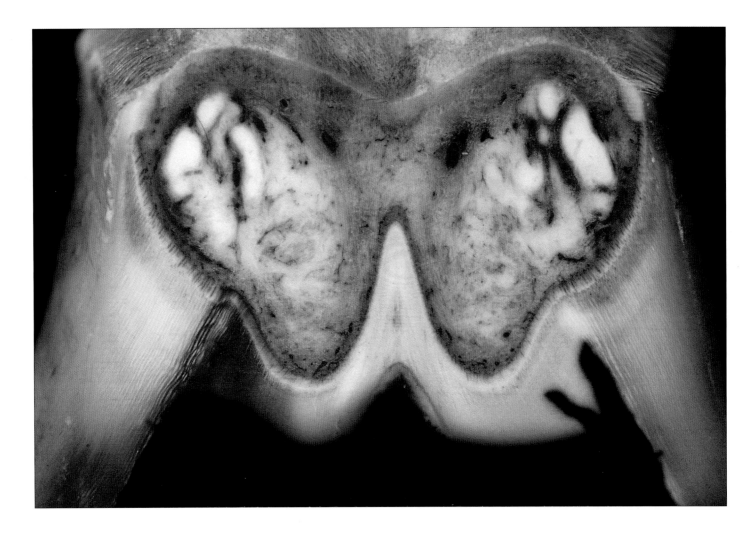

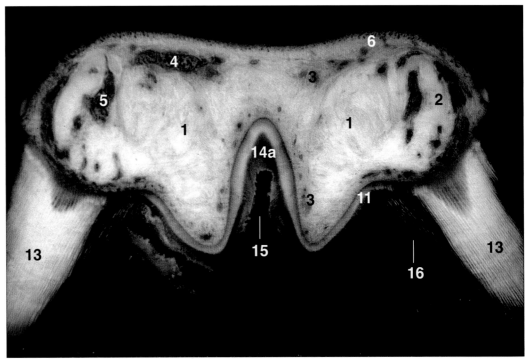

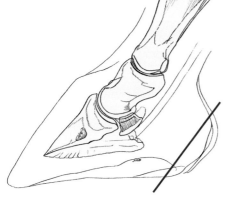

Frontal anatomical section of the equine foot, dorsal view.

F1: Frontal Section of the Foot

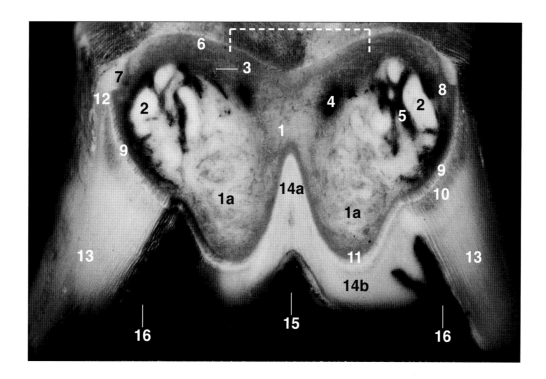

1 Digital cushion
  1a Cuneal part
2 Ungular cartilage
3 Ramus of the digital torus
4 Lateromedial palmar anastomosis
5 Deep ungular plexus
6 Skin
7 Corium limbi
8 Pulvinus coronae
9 Corium coronae

10 Dermal papillae
11 Corium cunei
12 Periople
13 Hoof wall (heel)
14 Frog
  14a Spine
  14b Base
15 Central cuneal sulcus
16 Paracuneal sulcus

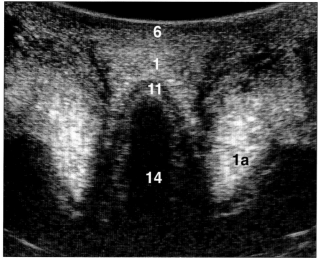

Frontal ultrasound scan of the palmar part of the foot, proximopalmar approach (see dotted area in illustration at top of page).

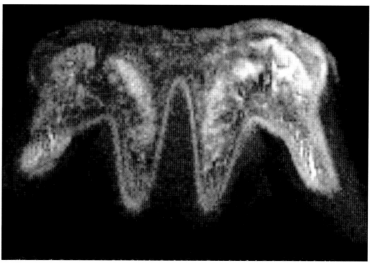

Frontal MRI scan of the foot after injection of latex into the arteries and fat material into the veins.

F2: Frontal Section of the Foot

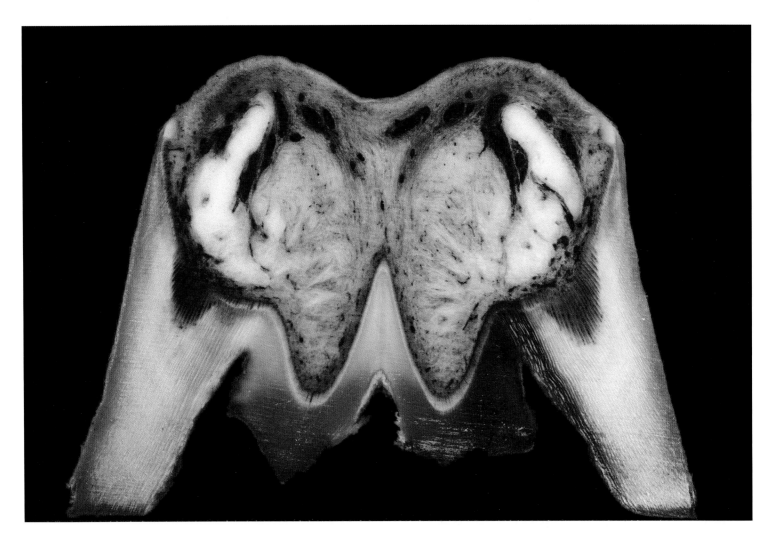

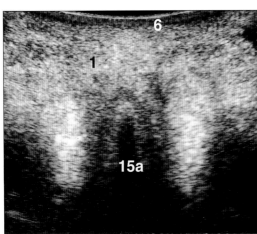

Frontal ultrasound scan of the palmar part of the foot, proximopalmar approach (see dotted area in illustration at top of facing page).

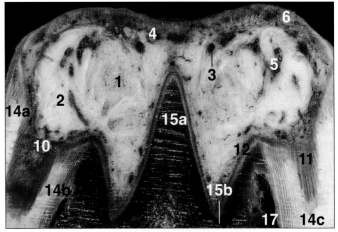

Frontal anatomical section of the equine foot after injection of coloured latex into the vessels, dorsal view.

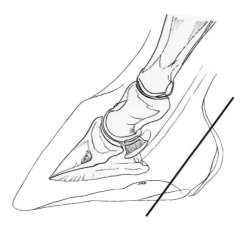

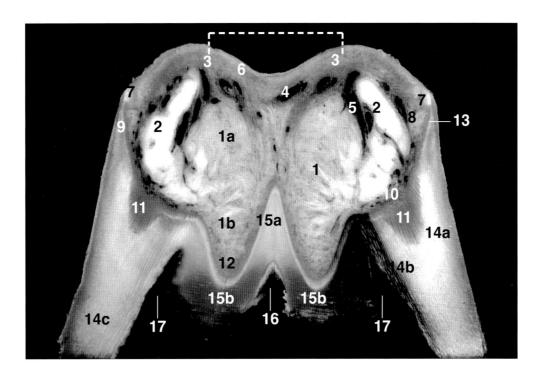

1 Digital cushion	11 Dermal and epidermal lamellae
1a Toric part	12 Corium cunei
1b Cuneal part	13 Periople
2 Ungular cartilage	14 Hoof wall
3 Ramus of the digital torus	**14a** Collateral part (quarter)
4 Lateromedial palmar anastomosis	**14b** Inflex part (bar)
5 Deep ungular plexus	**14c** Heel
6 Skin	15 Frog
7 Corium limbi	**15a** Spine
8 Pulvinus coronae	**15b** Branch
9 Corium coronae	16 Central cuneal sulcus
10 Corium parietis	17 Paracuneal sulcus

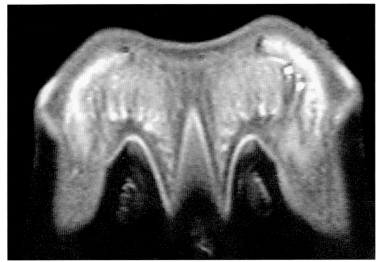

Frontal MRI scan of the foot after injection of latex into the arteries and fat material into the veins.

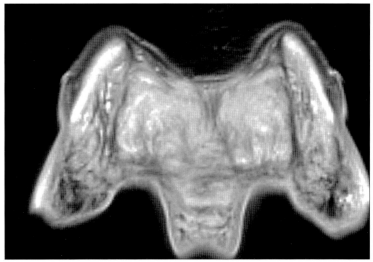

Frontal MRI scan of the foot.

F3: Frontal Section of the Foot

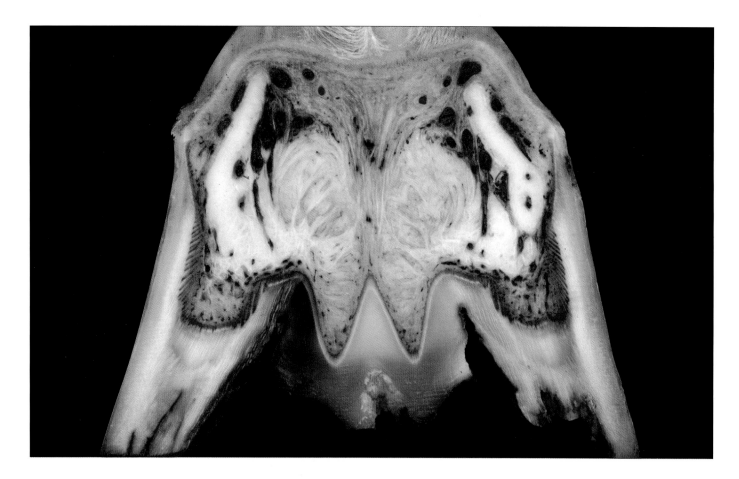

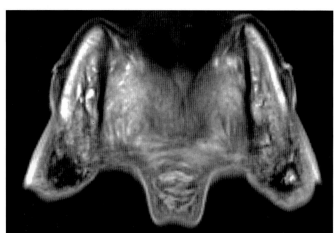

Frontal MRI scan of the foot.

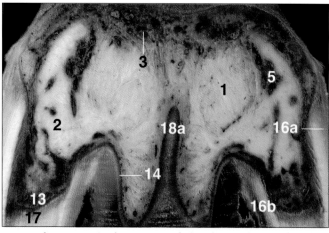

Frontal anatomical section of the foot after injection of coloured latex into the vessels, palmar view.

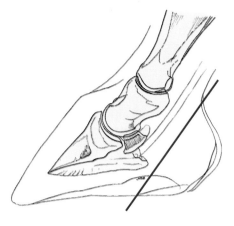

F3: Frontal Section of the Foot

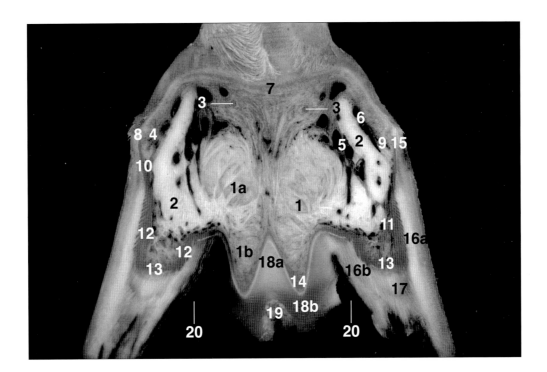

1 **Digital cushion**
   1a Toric part
   1b Cuneal part
2 **Ungular cartilage**
3 **Ramus of the digital torus**
4 **Coronal artery**
5 **Deep ungular plexus**
6 **Superficial ungular plexus**
7 **Skin**
8 **Corium limbi**
9 **Pulvinus coronae**
10 **Corium coronae**
11 **Corium parietis**

12 **Dermal and epidermal lamellae**
13 **Corium soleae**
14 **Corium cunei**
15 **Periople**
16 **Hoof wall**
   16a Collateral part (quarter)
   16b Inflex part (bar)
17 **Sole (angle)**
18 **Frog**
   18a Spine
   18b Branch
19 **Central cuneal sulcus**
20 **Paracuneal sulcus**

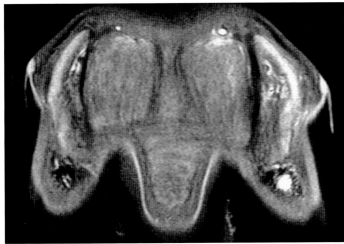

Frontal MRI scan of the foot after injection of fat material into the arteries and latex into the veins.

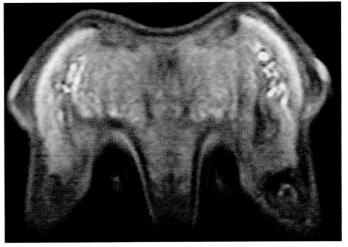

Frontal MRI scan of the foot after injection of latex into the arteries and fat material into the veins.

F4: Frontal Section of the Foot

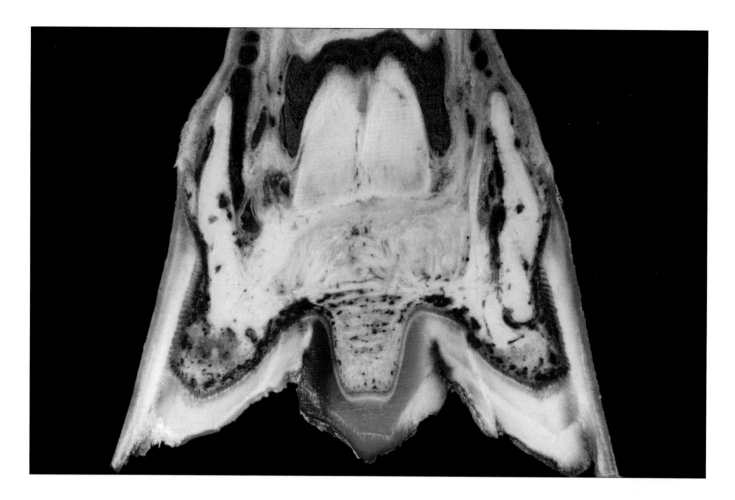

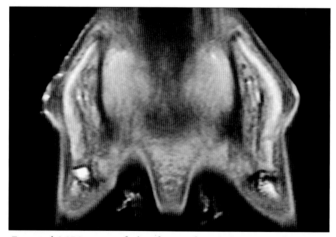

Frontal MRI scan of the foot after injection of latex into the arteries and veins.

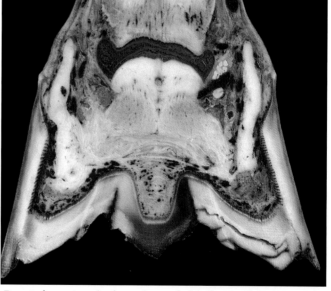

Frontal anatomical section of the foot after injection of coloured latex into the vessels and synovial cavities.

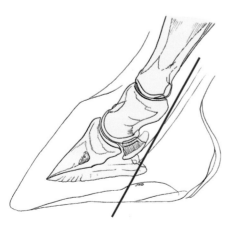

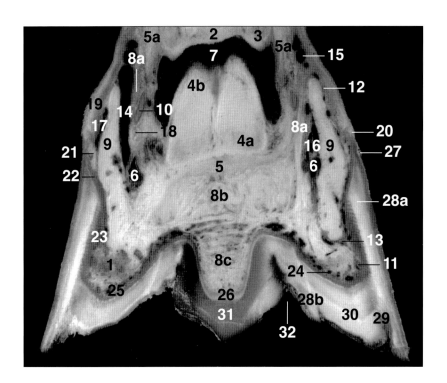

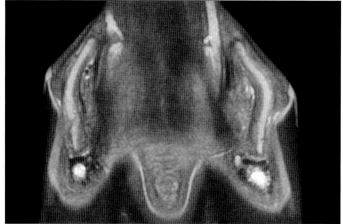

Frontal MRI scan of the foot after injection of fat material into the arteries and latex into the veins.

1 Palmar process of the distal phalanx (P3)
2 Middle scutum
3 Superficial digital flexor tendon
   (distal branch)
4 Deep digital flexor tendon
      4a Fibrous part
      4b Fibrocartilaginous part
5 Distal digital annular ligament
      5a Proximal attachment
6 Podotrochlear bursa (proximal recess)
7 Dorsal distal recess of the digital sheath
8 Digital cushion
      8a Proximal attachment
      8b Toric part
      8c Cuneal part
9 Ungular cartilage
10 Proper palmar digital artery
11 Circumflex artery
12 Coronal artery
13 Dorsal ramus of P3
14 Proper palmar digital vein

15 Coronal vein
16 Deep ungular plexus
17 Superficial ungular plexus
18 Proper palmar digital nerve
19 Skin
20 Corium limbi
21 Pulvinus coronae
22 Corium coronae
23 Corium parietis
24 Solar subcutaneous layer
25 Corium solae
26 Corium cunei
27 Periople
28 Hoof wall
      28a Collateral part (quarter)
      28b Inflex part (bar)
29 Zona alba
30 Sole (branch)
31 Frog (body)
32 Paracuneal sulcus

F5: Frontal Section of the Foot

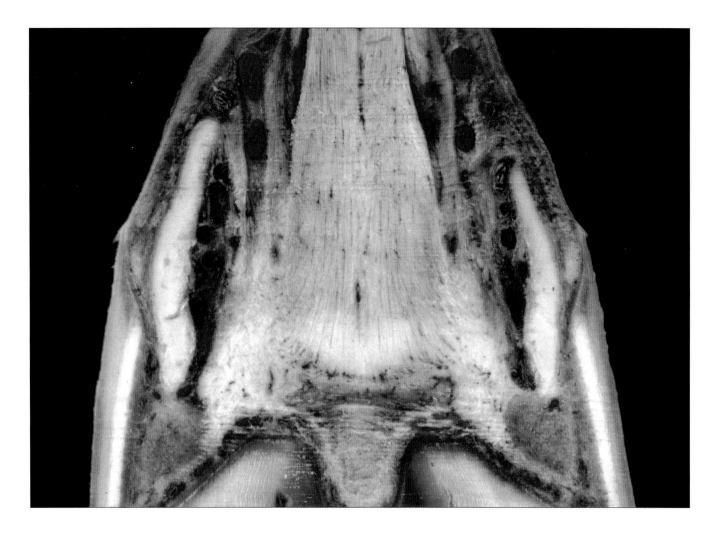

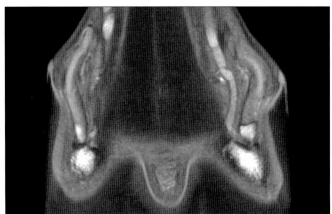

Frontal MRI scan of the foot after injection of fat material into the arteries and latex into the veins.

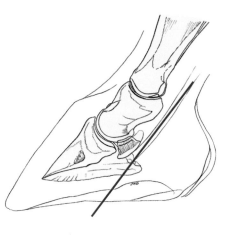

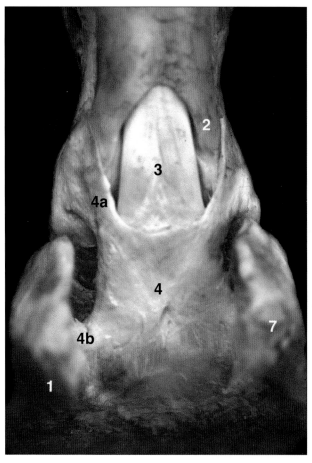

Dissected specimen, palmar aspect.

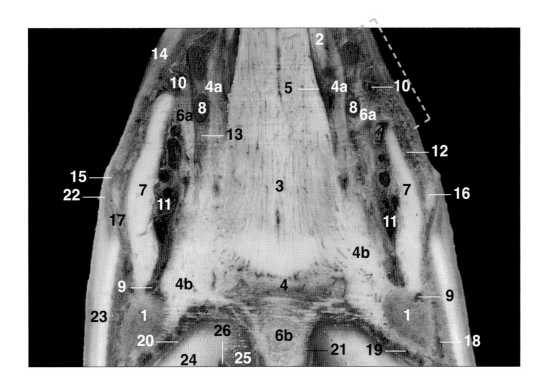

1 Palmar process of the distal phalanx
2 Superficial digital flexor tendon (distal branch)
3 Deep digital flexor tendon (fibrous part)
4 Distal digital annular ligament
   4a Proximal attachment
   4b Distal attachment
5 Dorsal distal recess of the digital sheath
6 Digital cushion
   6a Proximal insertion
   6b Cuneal part
7 Ungular cartilage
8 Proper palmar digital artery
9 Dorsal ramus of the distal phalanx
10 Proper palmar digital vein
11 Deep ungular plexus

12 Superficial ungular plexus
13 Proper palmar digital nerve
14 Skin
15 Corium limbi
16 Pulvinus coronae
17 Corium coronae
18 Corium parietis
19 Solar subcutaneous layer
20 Corium soleae
21 Corium cunei
22 Periople
23 Hoof wall (quarter)
24 Sole (branch)
25 Frog (body)
26 Paracuneal sulcus

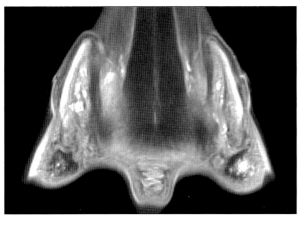

Frontal MRI scan of the foot.

Frontal ultrasound scan of the deep digital flexor tendon, lateral approach (see dotted area in illustration at top of page).

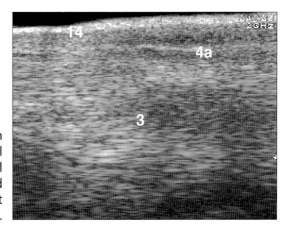

F6: Frontal Section of the Foot

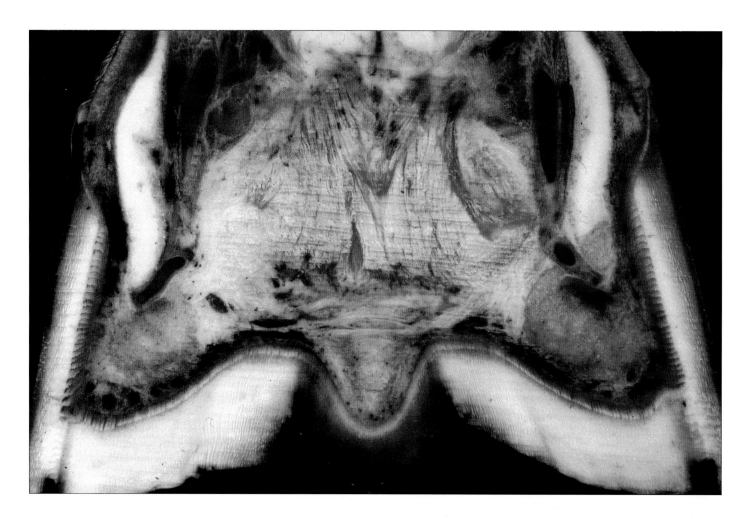

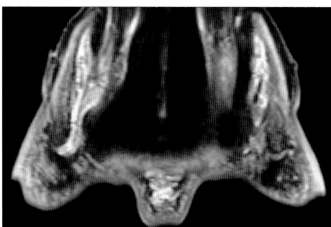

Frontal MRI scan of the foot.

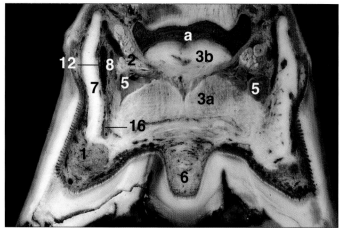

Frontal anatomical section of the foot after injection of coloured latex into the vessels and synovial cavities. **a** Digital sheath (dorsal distal recess).

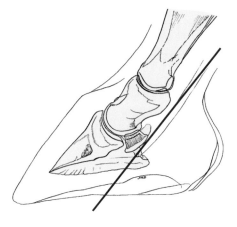

F6: Frontal Section of the Foot

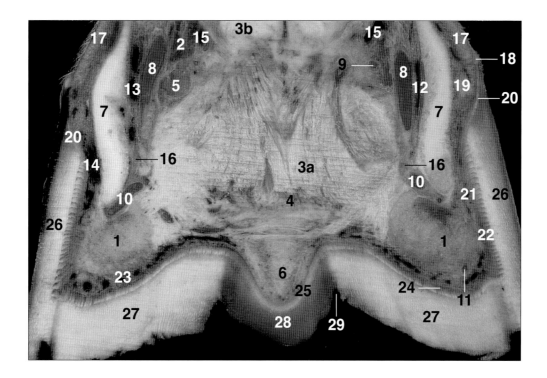

1 Palmar process of the distal phalanx (P3)
2 Proximopalmar recess of the distal interphalangeal joint
3 Deep digital flexor tendon
   3a Fibrous part
   3b Fibrocartilaginous part
4 Distal digital annular ligament
5 Podotrochlear bursa
6 Digital cushion (cuneal part)
7 Ungular cartilage
8 Proper palmar digital artery
9 Palmar ramus (artery) of middle phalanx
10 Dorsal ramus of P3
11 Circumflex artery
12 Proper palmar digital vein
13 Deep ungular plexus

14 Superficial ungular plexus
15 Palmar ramus (vein) of middle phalanx
16 Proper palmar digital nerve
17 Skin
18 Corium limbi
19 Pulvinus coronae
20 Corium coronae
21 Corium parietis
22 Dermal and epidermal lamellae
23 Solar subcutaneous layer
24 Corium soleae
25 Corium cunei
26 Hoof wall (collateral part – quarter)
27 Sole (branch)
28 Frog (body)
29 Paracuneal sulcus

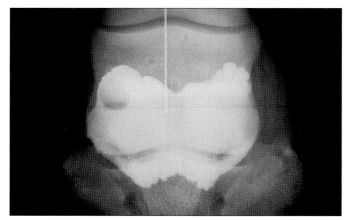

Contrast radiographic study of the podotrochlear bursa (bursography), dorsopalmar view.

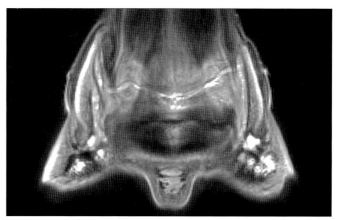

Frontal MRI scan of the foot.

F7: Frontal Section of the Foot

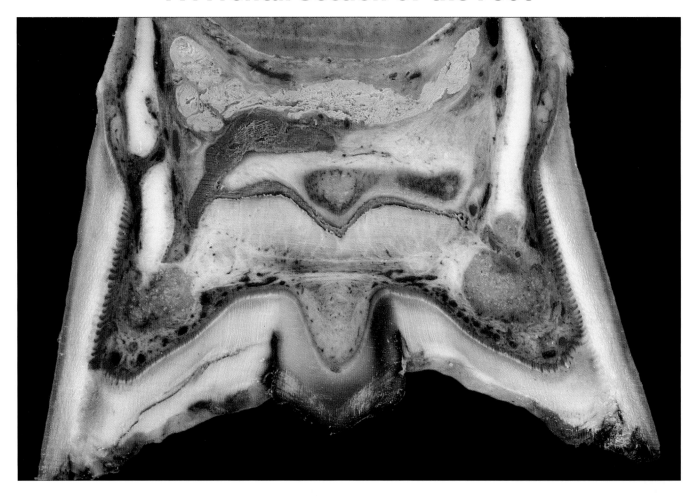

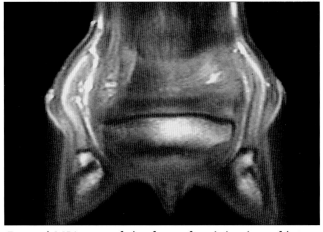

Frontal MRI scan of the foot after injection of latex into the arteries and fat material into the veins.

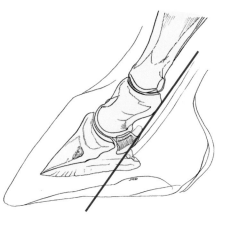

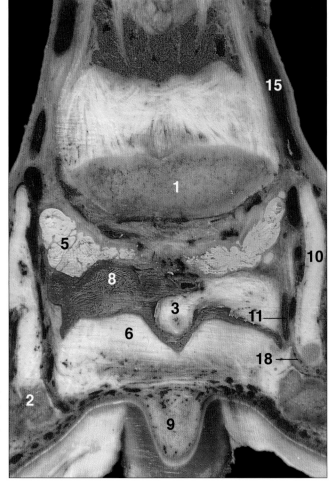

Frontal anatomical section of the foot after injection of coloured latex into the vessels and synovial cavities.

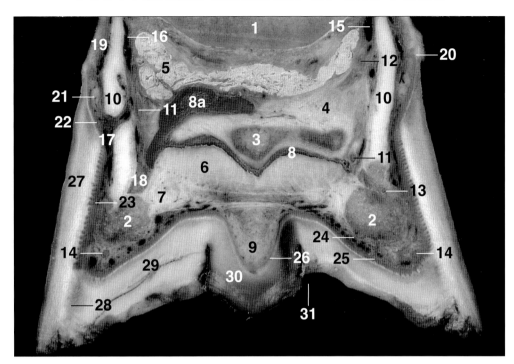

1 Middle phalanx (flexor tuberosity)	**15** Proper palmar digital vein
2 Palmar process of the distal phalanx	**16** Deep ungular plexus
3 Distal sesamoid bone	**17** Superficial ungular plexus
4 Collateral sesamoidean ligament	**18** Proper palmar digital nerve
5 Proximopalmar recess of the distal interphalangeal joint	**19** Skin
	20 Corium limbi
6 Deep digital flexor tendon	**21** Pulvinus coronae
7 Distal digital annular ligament (distal attachment)	**22** Corium coronae
	23 Corium parietis
8 Podotrochlear bursa	**24** Solar subcutaneous layer
8a Proximal recess	**25** Corium soleae
9 Digital cushion (cuneal part)	**26** Corium cunei
10 Ungular cartilage	**27** Hoof wall (quarter)
11 Proper palmar digital artery	**28** Zona alba
12 Dorsal ramus of the middle phalanx	**29** Sole (branch)
13 Dorsal ramus of the distal phalanx	**30** Frog (body)
14 Circumflex artery	**31** Paracuneal sulcus

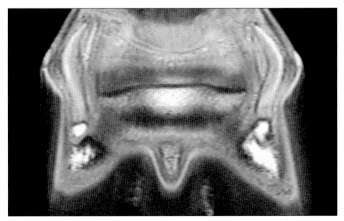

Frontal MRI scan of the foot after injection of latex into the arteries and veins.

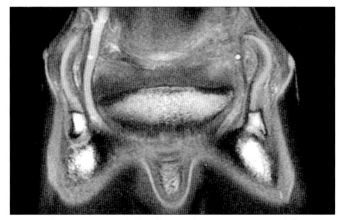

Frontal MRI scan of the foot after injection of fat material into the arteries and latex into the veins.

F8: Frontal Section of the Foot

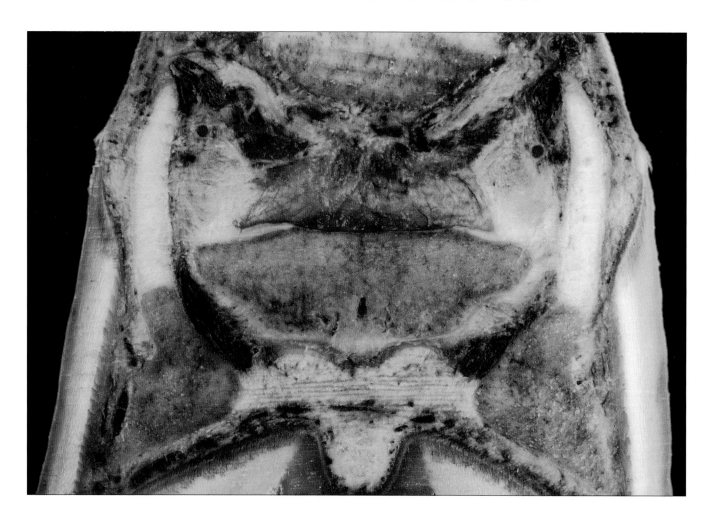

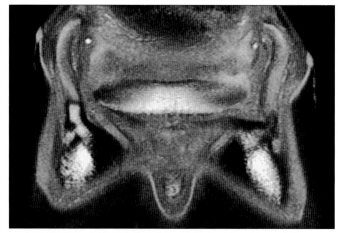

Frontal MRI scan of the foot after injection of fat
material into the arteries and latex into the veins.

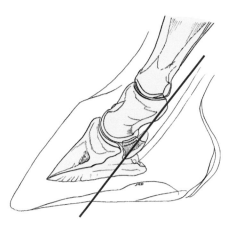

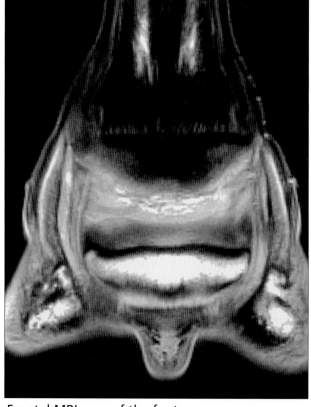

Frontal MRI scan of the foot.

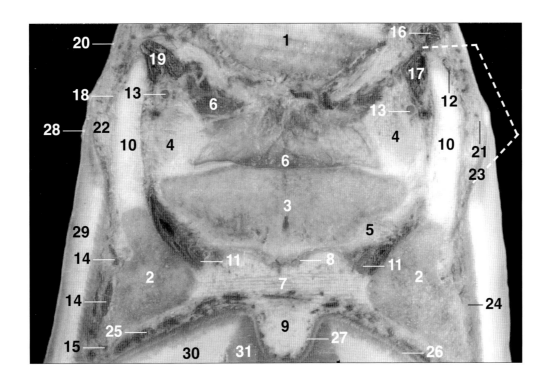

1 Middle phalanx, P2 (flexor tuberosity)
2 Palmar process of the distal phalanx (P3)
3 Distal sesamoid bone
4 Collateral sesamoidean ligament
5 Impar distal sesamoidean ligament
6 Proximopalmar recess of the distal interphalangeal joint
7 Deep digital flexor tendon
8 Podotrochlear bursa (distal recess)
9 Digital cushion (cuneal part)
10 Ungular cartilage
11 Proper palmar digital artery
12 Coronal artery
13 Dorsal ramus of P2
14 Dorsal ramus of P3
15 Circumflex artery

16 Proper palmar digital vein
17 Deep ungular plexus
18 Superficial ungular plexus
19 Palmar ramus (vein) of P2
20 Skin
21 Corium limbi
22 Pulvinus coronae
23 Corium coronae
24 Corium parietis
25 Solar subcutaneous layer
26 Corium soleae
27 Corium cunei
28 Periople
29 Hoof wall (quarter)
30 Sole (branch)
31 Frog (body)

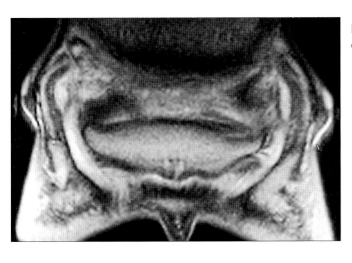

Frontal MRI scan of the foot.

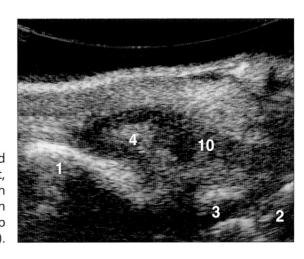

Frontal ultrasound scan of the foot, collateral approach (see dotted area in illustration at top of page).

F9: Frontal Section of the Foot

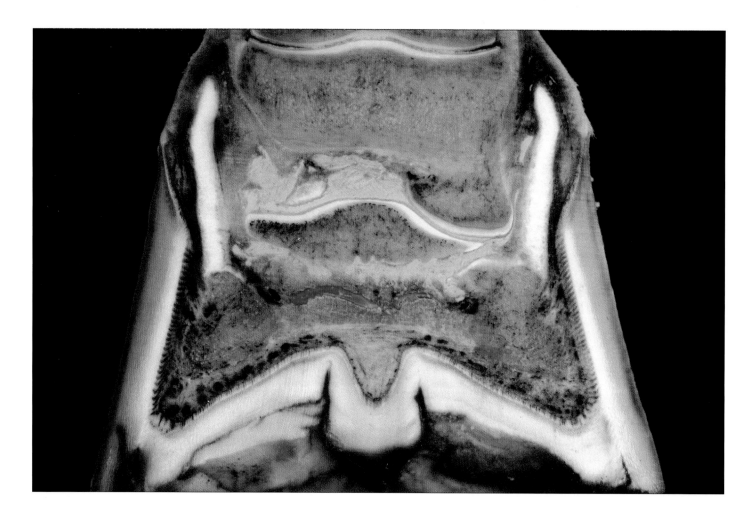

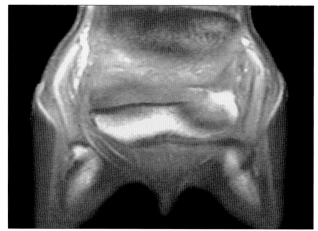

Frontal MRI scan of the foot after injection of latex into the arteries and fat material into the veins.

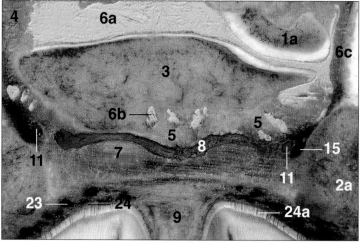

Frontal anatomical section of the foot after injection of coloured latex in the vessels and synovial cavities.

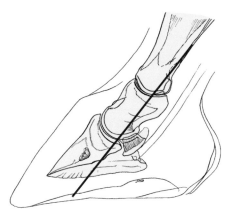

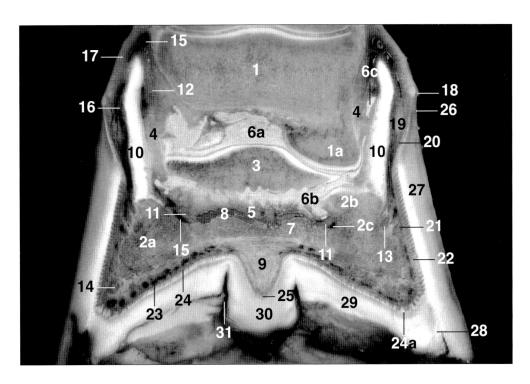

1 Middle phalanx (P2)
  1a Distal condyle
2 Distal phalanx (P3)
  2a Palmar process
  2b Articular surface
  2c Solar sulcus
3 Distal sesamoid bone
4 Collateral sesamoidean
  ligament
5 Impar distal sesamoidean
  ligament
6 Recesses of the distal
  interphalangeal joint
  6a Proximopalmar recess
  6b Distopalmar recess
  6c Collateral recess
7 Deep digital flexor tendon
8 Podotrochlear bursa (distal
  recess)
9 Digital cushion (cuneal part)
10 Ungular cartilage
11 Proper palmar digital artery

12 Dorsal ramus of P2
13 Dorsal ramus of P3
14 Circumflex artery
15 Proper palmar digital vein
16 Superficial ungular plexus
17 Skin
18 Corium limbi
19 Pulvinus coronae
20 Corium coronae
21 Corium parietis
22 Dermal and epidermal
  lamellae
23 Solar subcutaneous layer
24 Corium soleae
    24a Dermal papillae
25 Corium cunei
26 Periople
27 Hoof wall (quarter)
28 Zona alba
29 Sole (branch)
30 Frog (apex)
31 Paracuneal sulcus

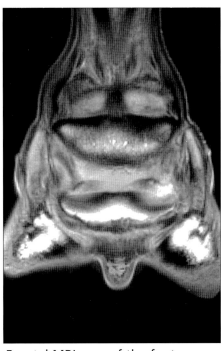

Frontal MRI scan of the foot.

F10: Frontal Section of the Foot

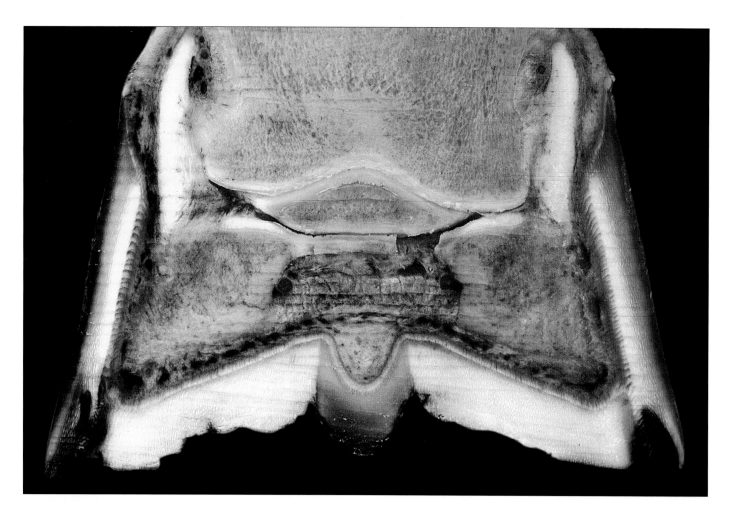

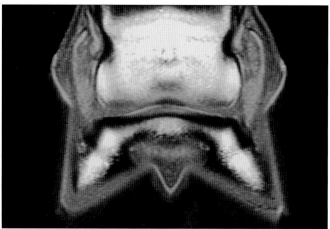

Frontal MRI scan of the foot after injection of latex into the arteries and veins.

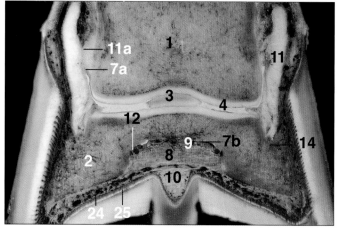

Frontal anatomical section of the foot after injection of coloured latex into the vessels and synovial cavities.

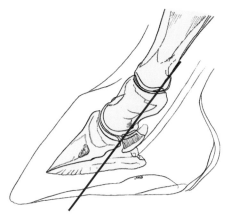

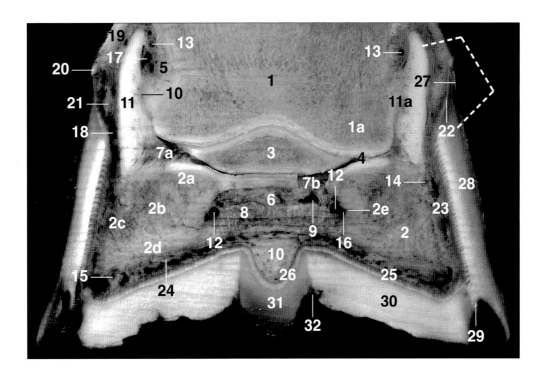

1 Middle phalanx (P2)
  1a Distal condyle
2 Distal phalanx (P3)
  2a Subchondral bone
  2b Palmar process
  2c Parietal surface
  2d Planum cutaneum
  2e Solar sulcus
3 Distal sesamoid bone
4 Distal interphalangeal (DIP) joint
5 Collateral sesamoidean ligament
6 Impar distal sesamoidean ligament
7 Recesses of the DIP joint
  7a Collateral recess
  7b Distopalmar recess
8 Deep digital flexor tendon
9 Podotrochlear bursa (distal recess)
10 Digital cushion (cuneal part)
11 Ungular cartilage
  11a Chondrocoronal ligament
12 Proper palmar digital artery
13 Dorsal ramus (artery) of P2
14 Dorsal ramus (artery) of P3
15 Circumflex artery
16 Proper palmar digital vein
17 Dorsal ramus (vein) of P2
18 Superficial ungular plexus
19 Skin

20 Corium limbi
21 Pulvinus coronae
22 Corium coronae
23 Corium parietis
24 Solar subcutaneous layer
25 Corium soleae
26 Corium cunei
27 Periople
28 Hoof wall (quarter)
29 Zona alba
30 Sole
31 Frog (apex)
32 Paracuneal sulcus

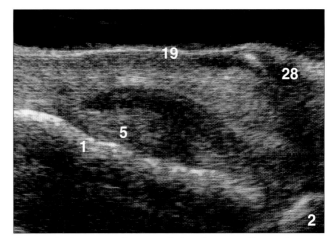

Frontal ultrasound scan of the foot, collateral approach (see dotted area in illustration at top of page).

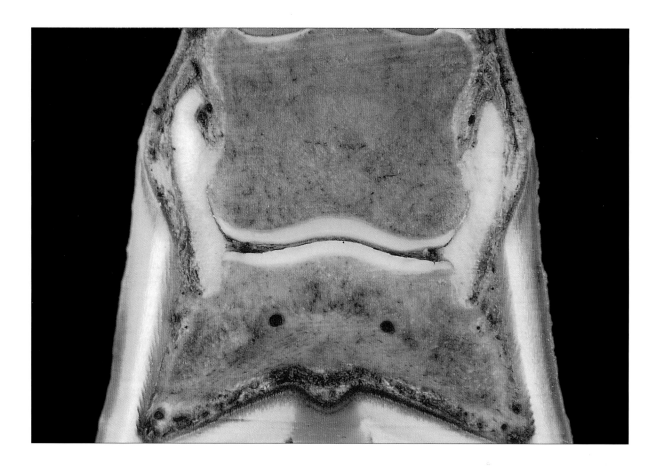

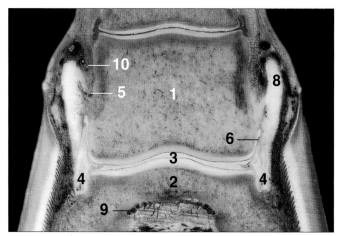

Frontal anatomical section of the foot after injection of coloured latex into the vessels and synovial cavities.

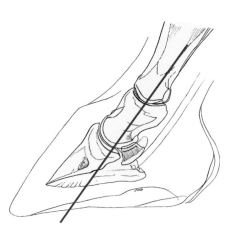

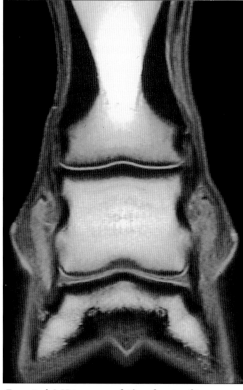

Frontal MRI scan of the foot after injection of latex into the arteries and veins.

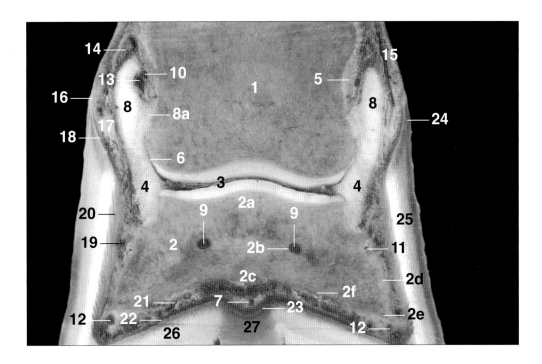

1 Middle phalanx (P2)
2 Distal phalanx (P3)
  2a Subchondral bone
  2b Solar canal
  2c Distopalmar compact bone
  2d Parietal surface
  2e Solar border
  2f Planum cutaneum
3 Distal interphalangeal (DIP) joint
4 Collateral ligament of the DIP joint
5 Collateral sesamoidean ligament
6 Collateral recess of the DIP joint
7 Digital cushion (cuneal part)
8 Ungular cartilage
  8a Chondrocoronal ligament
9 Proper palmar digital artery (terminal arch)
10 Dorsal ramus (artery) of P2

11 Dorsal ramus (artery) of P3
12 Circumflex artery
13 Dorsal ramus (vein) of P2
14 Coronal vein
15 Skin
16 Corium limbi
17 Pulvinus coronae
18 Corium coronae
19 Corium parietis
20 Dermal and epidermal lamellae
21 Solar subcutaneous layer
22 Corium soleae
23 Corium cunei
24 Periople
25 Hoof wall (quarter)
26 Sole
27 Frog (apex)

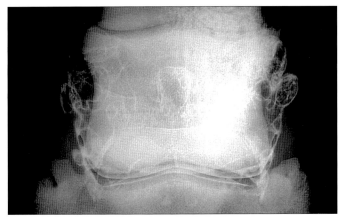

Double contrast radiographic study of the DIP joint (arthrography), dorsopalmar projection.

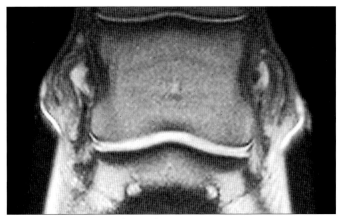

Frontal MRI scan of the foot.

F12: Frontal Section of the Foot

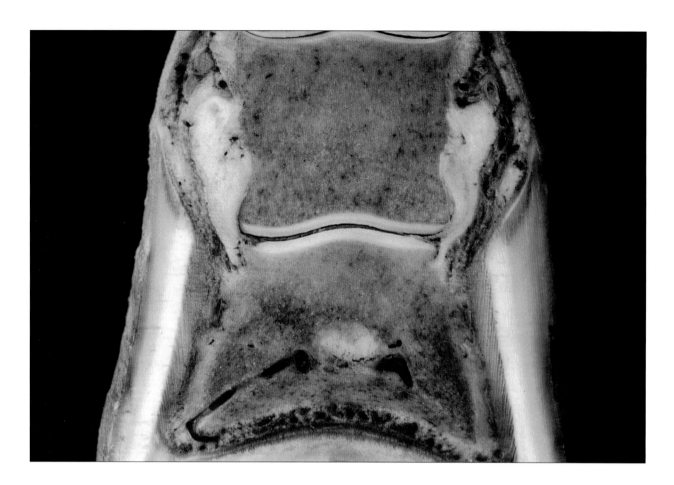

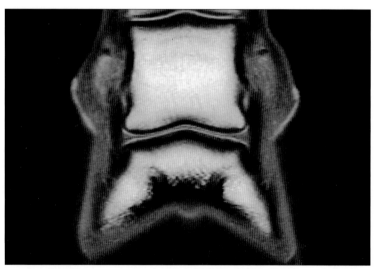

Frontal MRI scan of the foot after injection of latex into the arteries and veins.

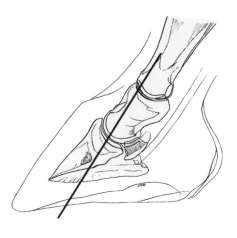

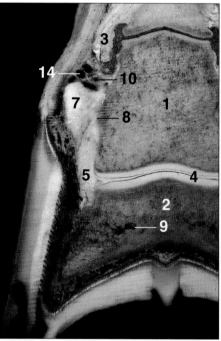

Frontal anatomical section of the foot after injection of coloured latex into the vessels and synovial cavities.

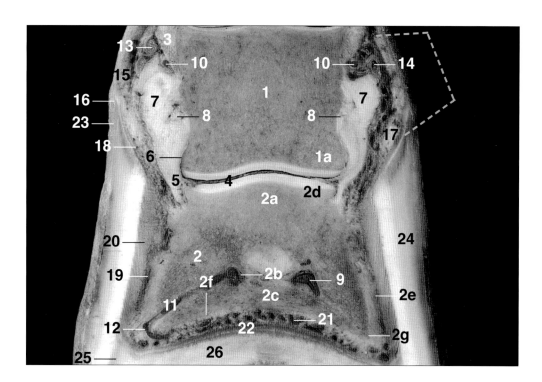

1 **Middle phalanx (P2)**
  1a Distal condyle
2 **Distal phalanx (P3)**
  2a Subchondral bone
  2b Solar canal
  2c Distopalmar compact bone
  2d Articular surface
  2e Parietal surface
  2f Planum cutaneum
  2g Solar border
3 Collateral ligament of the proximal interphalangeal joint joint and collateral sesamoidean ligament
4 Distal interphalangeal (DIP) joint
5 Collateral ligament of the DIP joint
6 Collateral recess of the DIP joint
7 Ungular cartilage
8 Chondrocoronal ligament
9 Proper palmar digital artery (terminal arch)
10 Dorsal ramus of P2
11 Perforating ramus
12 Circumflex artery
13 Dorsal ramus (vein) of P2
14 Coronal vein
15 Skin
16 Corium limbi

17 Pulvinus coronae
18 Corium coronae
19 Corium parietis
20 Dermal and epidermal lamellae
21 Solar subcutaneous layer
22 Corium soleae
23 Periople
24 Hoof wall (quarter)
25 Zona alba
26 Sole (body)

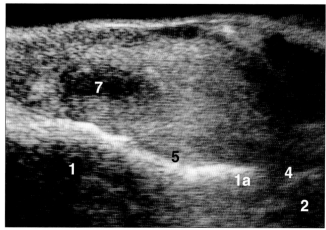

Frontal ultrasound scan of the coronet, collateral approach (see dotted area in illustration at top of page).

F13: Frontal Section of the Foot

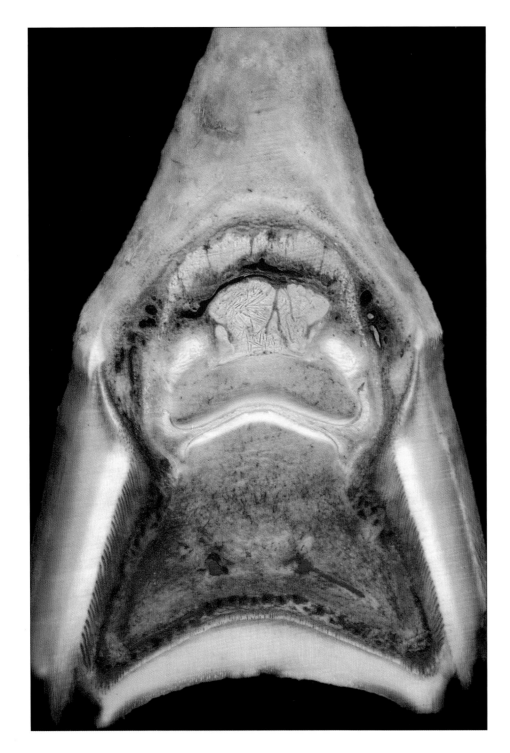

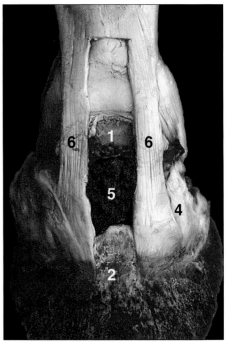

Anatomical specimen after injection of coloured latex into the synovial cavities, dorsal view.

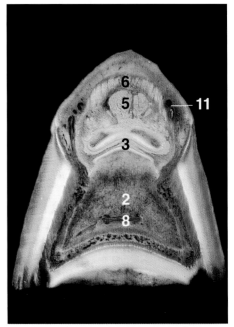

Frontal anatomical section of the foot after injection of coloured latex into the vessels and synovial cavities.

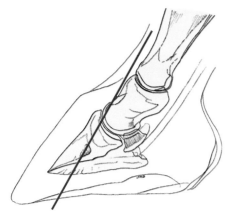

1 Middle phalanx, P2 (distal condyle)
2 Distal phalanx
    2a Articular surface
    2b Parietal surface
    2c Planum cutaneum
    2d Solar border
    2e Solar canal
3 Distal interphalangeal (DIP) joint
4 Collateral ligament of the DIP joint
5 Dorsal recess of the DIP joint
6 Dorsal digital extensor tendon
7 Chondrocoronal ligament
8 Proper palmar digital artery (terminal arch)
9 Perforating ramus
10 Circumflex artery
11 Coronal artery and vein
12 Dorsal ramus (artery and vein) of P2
13 Skin
14 Pulvinus limbi
15 Corium limbi
16 Pulvinus coronae
17 Corium coronae
18 Dermal papillae
19 Corium parietis
20 Dermal and epidermal lamellae
21 Solar subcutaneus layer
22 Corium soleae
23 Dermal papillae
24 Periople
25 Hoof wall
26 Zona alba
27 Sole (body)

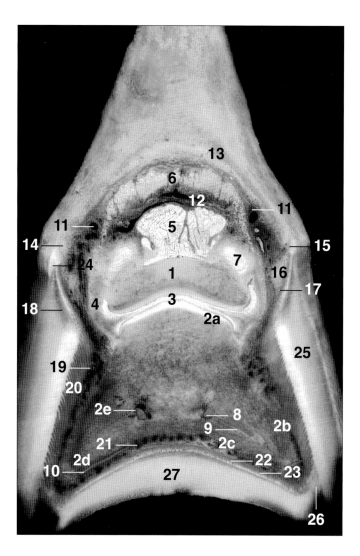

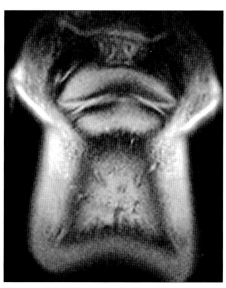

Frontal MRI scan of the foot.

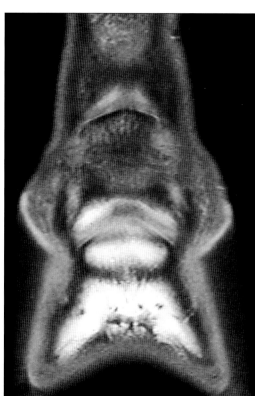

Frontal MRI scan of the foot after injection of latex into the arteries and veins.

F14: Frontal Section of the Foot

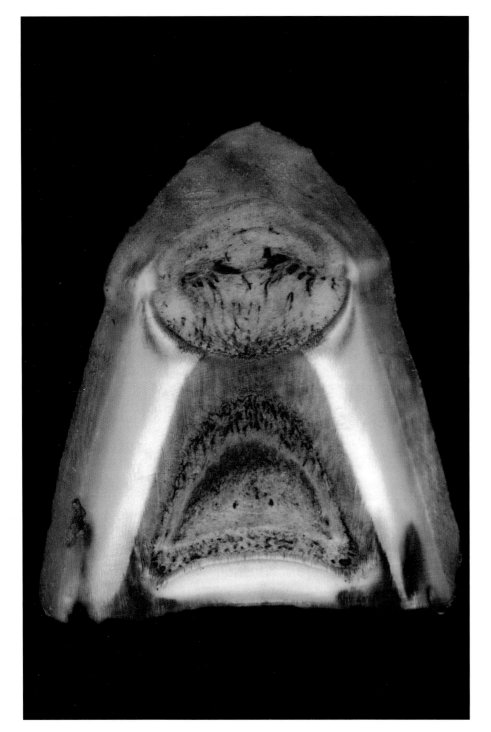

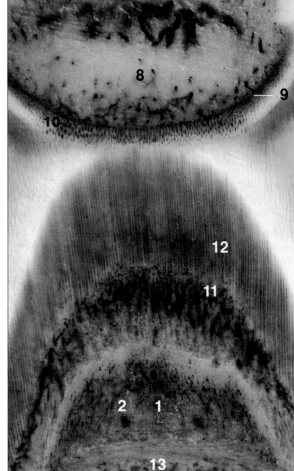

Frontal anatomical section of the foot after injection of coloured latex into the vessels.

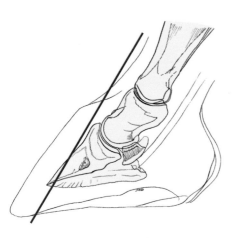

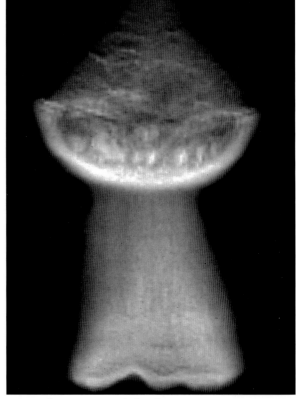

Frontal MRI scan of the foot.

1 Distal phalanx
   1a Parietal surface
   1b Planum cutaneum
2 Perforating ramus
3 Circumflex artery
4 Coronal vein
5 Skin
6 Pulvinus limbi
7 Corium limbi
8 Pulvinus coronae
9 Corium coronae
10 Dermal papillae
11 Corium parietis
12 Dermal and epidermal lamellae
13 Solar subcutaneous layer
14 Corium solae
15 Dermal papillae
16 Periople
17 Hoof wall
   17a Stratum externum
   17b Stratum medium
   17c Stratum internum
18 Sole (body)

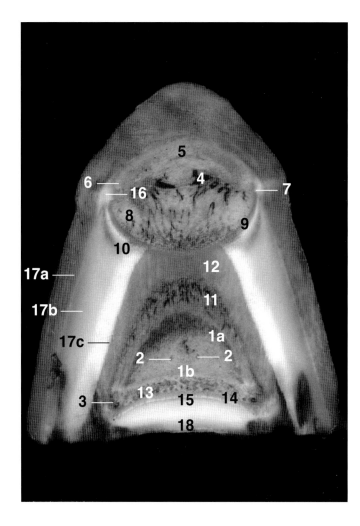

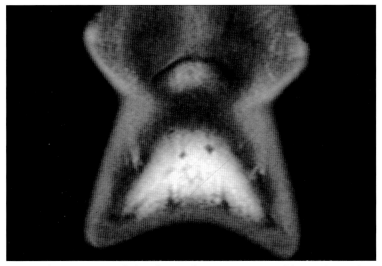

Frontal MRI scan of the foot after injection of latex into the arteries and veins.

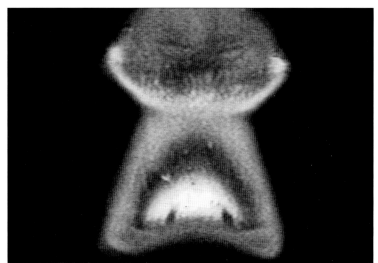

Frontal MRI scan of the foot after injection of latex into the arteries and veins.

The Equine Pastern

Dissections of the Equine Pastern

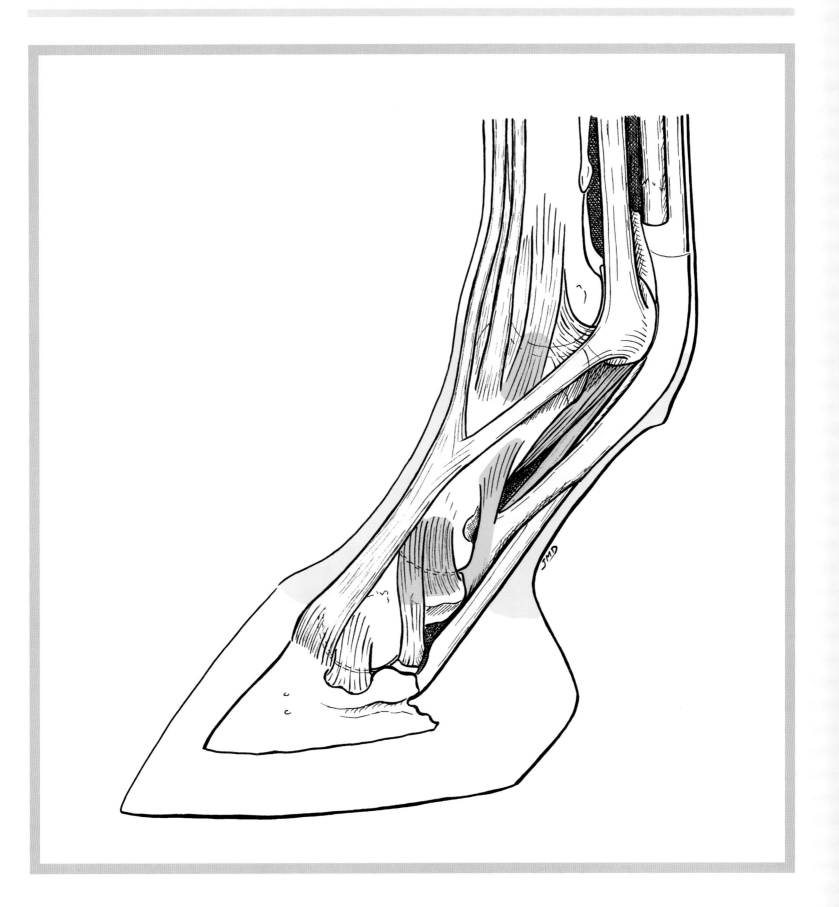

Dissection 1: Vessels and Nerves of the Digit – Dorsomedial View

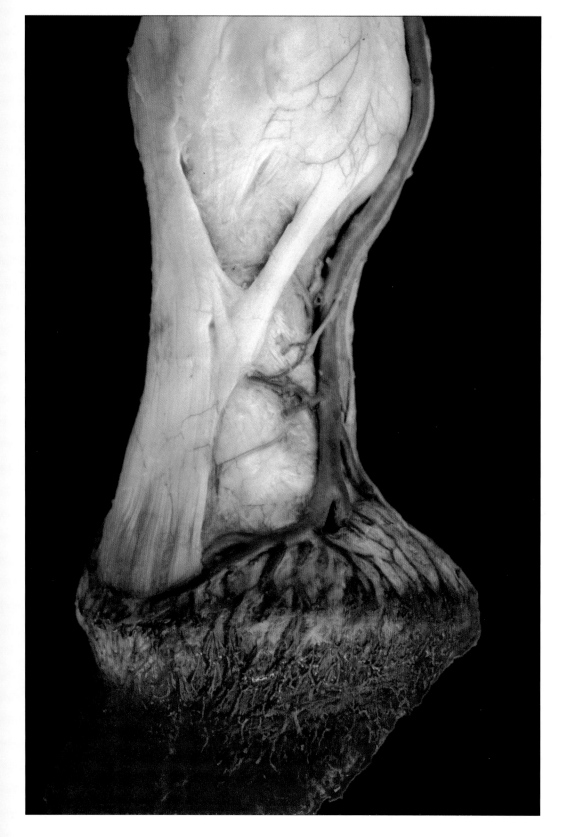

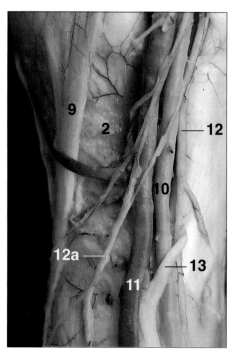

Vessels and nerves of the pastern, lateral view.

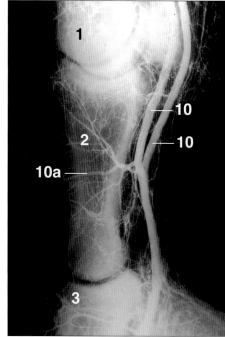

Contrast radiographic study of the arteries (arteriography) of the digit, lateromedial view.

Dissection 1: Vessels and Nerves of the Digit – Dorsomedial View

1 Third metacarpal bone
2 Proximal phalanx (P1)
3 Middle phalanx (P2)
4 Distal phalanx (P3)
   4a Parietal surface
   4b Solar border
5 Metacarpophalangeal (MP) joint
6 Proximal interphalangeal (PIP) joint
7 Dorsal capsule of the MP joint
8 Dorsal digital extensor tendon
9 Extensor branch of the third interosseus muscle
10 Proper palmar digital artery
   10a Dorsal ramus of P1
11 Proper palmar digital vein
   11a Parietal plexus
   11b Superficial ungular plexus
   11c Coronal vein
   11d Dorsal ramus of P2
   11e Dorsal ramus of P1
12 Proper palmar digital nerve
   12a Dorsal ramus
13 Ergot ligament
14 Ungular cartilage
15 Heel

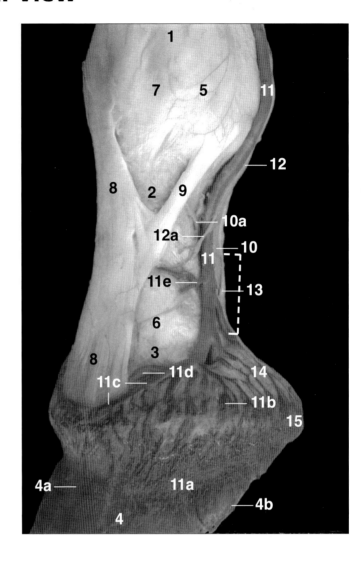

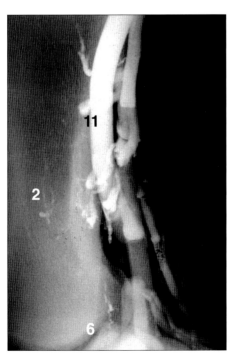

Contrast radiographic study of the digital veins demonstrating numerous valves, lateromedial view.

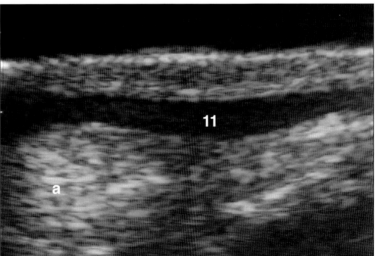

Frontal ultrasound scan of the proper palmar digital vein (see dotted area in illustration above, right). a Superficial digital flexor tendon (distal branch).

Dissection 2: Vessels of the Digit – Palmar View

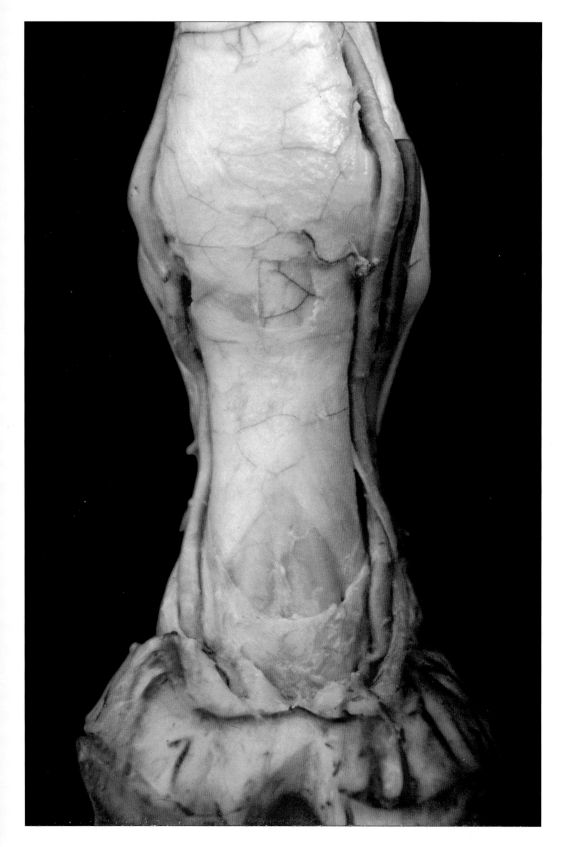

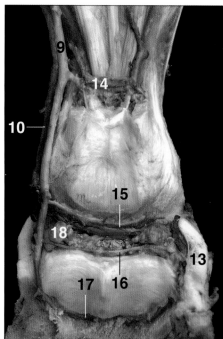

Dissected specimen after removal of the flexor tendons, palmar view.

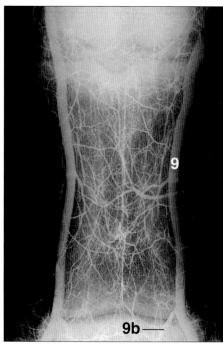

Contrast radiographic study of the arteries (arteriography) of the digit, dorsopalmar view.

Dissection 2: Vessels of the Digit – Palmar View

1 Proximal phalanx (P1), palmar eminence
2 Third interosseus muscle extensor branch
3 Superficial digital flexor tendon
   3a Distal branch
4 Deep digital flexor tendon
5 Palmar annular ligament
6 Proximal digital annular ligament
   6a With window cut into it
7 Distal digital annular ligament
8 Digital sheath
   8a Wall
   8b Cavity
   8c Mesotendon
9 Proper palmar digital artery
   9a Ergot ramus
   9b Ramus of the digital torus
10 Proper palmar digital vein
   10a Superficial ungular plexus
   10b Lateromedial palmar anastomosis
11 Ergot ligament
12 Digital cushion
13 Ungular cartilage
14 Palmar rami (artery and vein) of P1
15 Palmar rami (artery and vein) of the middle phalanx
16 Proximal ramus of the distal sesamoid bone
17 Distal ramus of the distal sesamoid bone
18 Proximopalmar recess of the distal interphalangeal joint

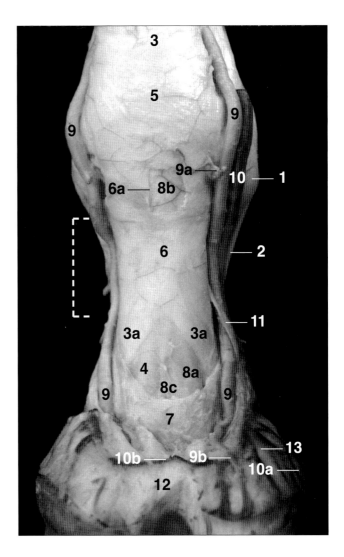

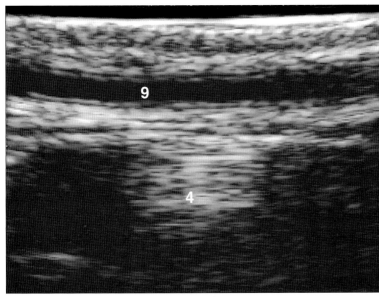

Frontal ultrasound scan of the proper palmar digital artery (see dotted area in illustration above, right).

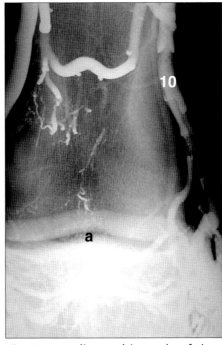

Contrast radiographic study of the veins (venography) of the digit, dorsopalmar view (see the valves).
a Proximal interphalangeal joint.

Dissection 3: Annular Ligaments

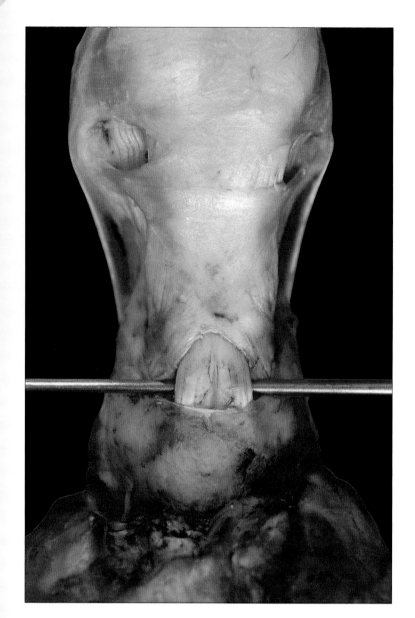

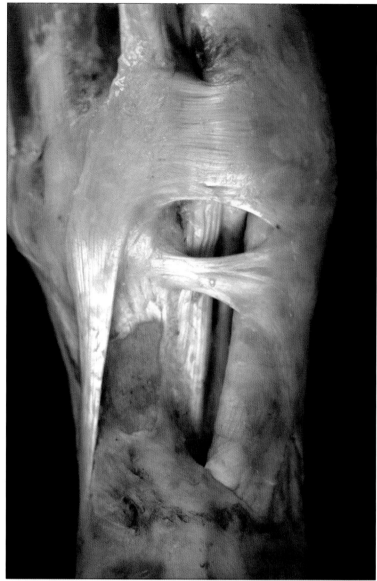

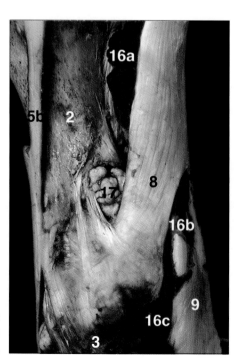

Palmarolateral aspect of the pastern after latex injection into the synovial cavities.

Dissection 3: Annular Ligaments

1 Third metacarpal bone
2 Proximal phalanx
  2a Palmar eminence
3 Middle phalanx
4 Collateral ligament of the metacarpophalangeal joint
5 Third interosseus muscle
  5a Distal branch
  5b Extensor branch
6 Oblique sesamoidean ligament
7 Straight sesamoidean ligament
8 Superficial digital flexor tendon (distal branch)
9 Deep digital flexor tendon
10 Palmar annular ligament
  10a Attachment to the proximal sesamoid bone
11 Proximal digital annular ligament
  11a Proximal attachment
  11b Distal attachment
12 Distal digital annular ligament
  12a Proximal attachment
13 Digital cushion
14 Ungular cartilage
15 Canulated probe
16 Digital sheath synovial cavity
  16a Collateral recess
  16b Palmar distal recess
  16c Dorsal distal recess
17 Palmar recess of the proximal interphalangeal joint

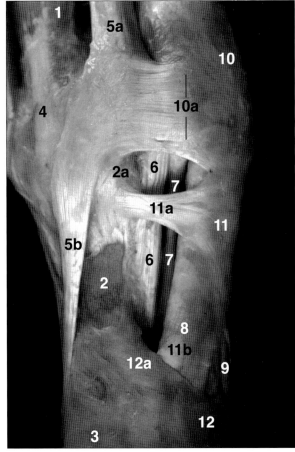

Palmarolateral aspect.

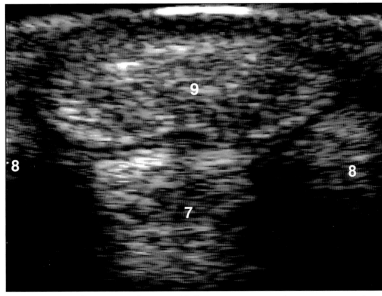

Transverse ultrasound scan of the pastern, palmar approach (see arrow on illustration at right).

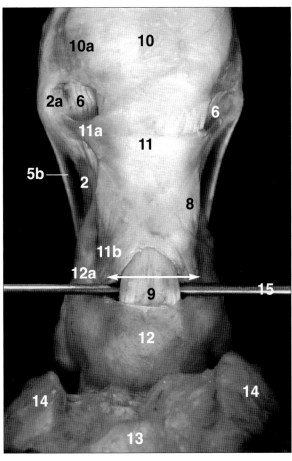

Palmar aspect.

135

Dissection 4: Flexor Tendons in the Digit – Palmar View
(With Annular Ligaments Removed)

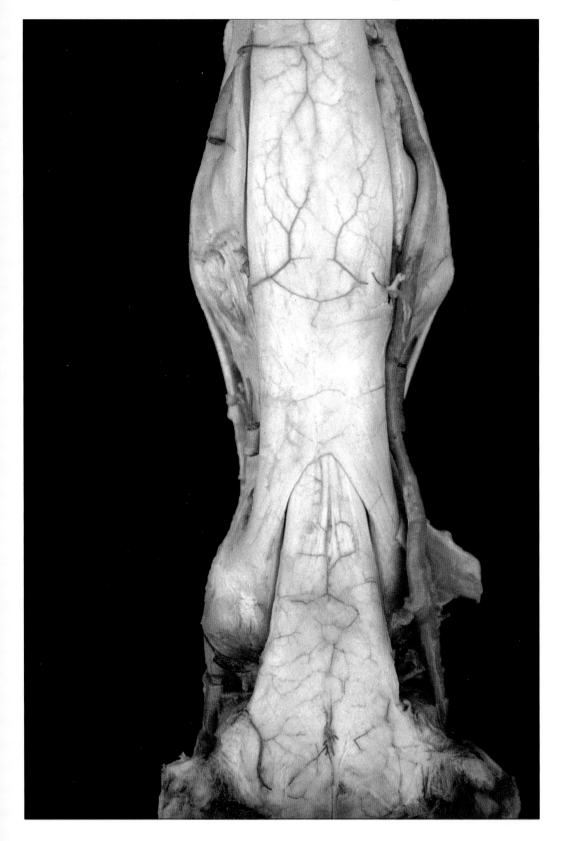

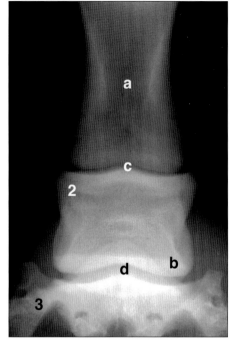

Dorsopalmar radiographic view of the digit.

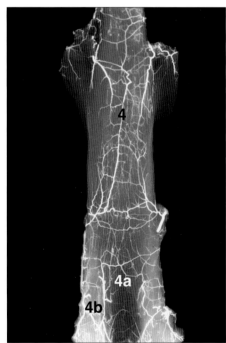

Contrast radiographic study of the arterial supply of the superficial digital flexor tendon, dorsopalmar view.

Dissection 4: Flexor Tendons in the Digit – Palmar View
(With Annular Ligaments Removed)

1 Proximal sesamoid bone (palmar border)
2 Middle phalanx, P2 (flexor tuberosity)
3 Distal phalanx (palmar process)
4 Superficial digital flexor tendon
    4a Sagittal part
    4b Distal branch
5 Deep digital flexor tendon
    5a Distal attachment
6 Palmar annular ligament insertion
7 Distal digital annular ligament (proximal insertion, reflected)
8 Proper palmar digital artery
    8a Ergot ramus
    8b Ramus of the digital torus
    8c Dorsal ramus of the proximal phalanx
    8d Palmar ramus of P2
9 Third interosseus muscle
    9a Distal branch
    9b Extensor branch

Ultrasound scans A and B below, and radiograph on facing page:
a Proximal phalanx
b Distal sesamoid bone
c Proximal interphalangeal joint
d Distal interphalangeal joint
e Straight sesamoidean ligament
f Oblique sesamoidean ligament

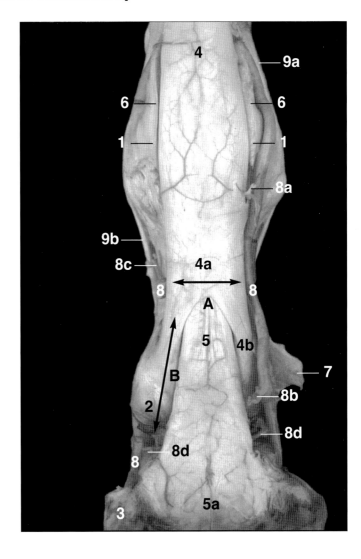

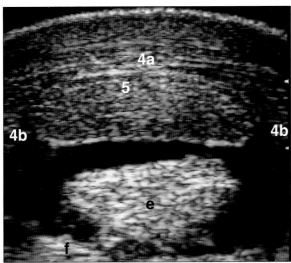

A Transverse ultrasound scan of the pastern, palmar approach (see arrow on illustration above, right).

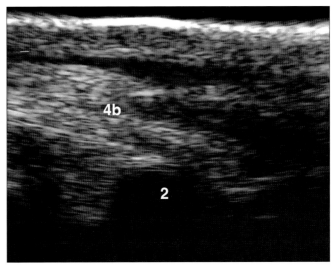

B Parasagittal ultrasound scan of the pastern, palmaro-lateral approach (see arrow on illustration above).

Dissection 5: Flexor Tendons in the Digit – Palmarolateral View
(With Annular Ligaments, Nerves and Major Part of Blood Vessels Removed)

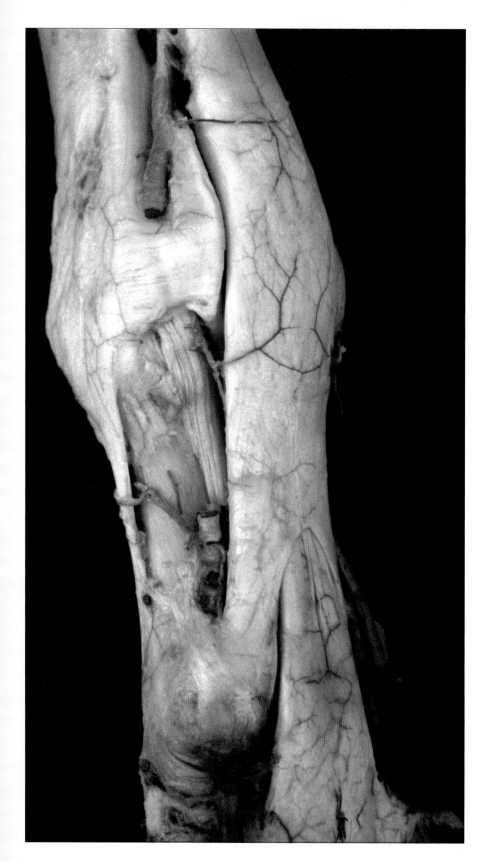

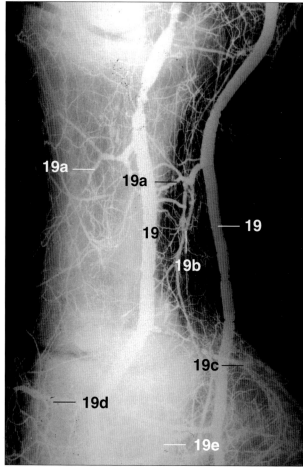

Contrast radiographic study of the arteries of the digit, oblique dorsolateral view.

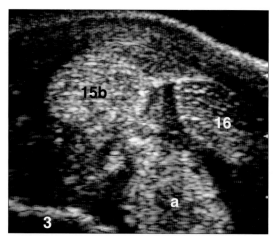

A Transverse ultrasound scan of the pastern, palmarolateral approach (see arrow on illustration on facing page).

(With Annular Ligaments, Nerves and Major Part of Blood Vessels Removed)

1 Third metacarpal bone
2 Proximal sesamoid bone (palmar border)
3 Proximal phalanx (P1)
4 Middle phalanx (P2)
   4a Flexor tuberosity
5 Distal phalanx (palmar process)
6 Metacarpophalangeal (MP) joint
7 Proximal interphalangeal (PIP) joint
   7a Middle scutum
8 Distal interphalangeal joint
9 Palmar (intersesamoidean) ligament
10 Collateral sesamoidean ligament
11 Oblique sesamoidean ligament
12 Collateral ligament of the MP joint
13 Collateral ligament of the PIP joint
14 Abaxial palmar ligament of the PIP joint
15 Superficial digital flexor tendon
   15a Manica flexoria
   15b Distal branch
16 Deep digital flexor tendon
17 Digital synovial sheath
   17a Proximal dorsal recess
   17b Collateral recess
   17c Dorsal distal recess
18 Third interosseus muscle
   18a Distal branch
   18b Extensor branch
19 Proper palmar digital artery
   19a Dorsal ramus of P1
   19b Palmar ramus of P1
   19c Ramus of the digital torus
   19d Dorsal ramus of P2
   19e Palmar ramus of P2
  a Straight sesamoidean ligament

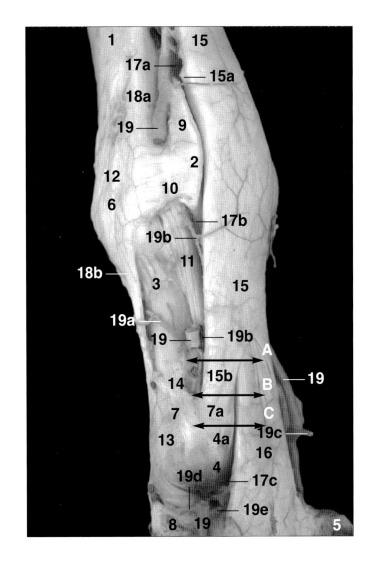

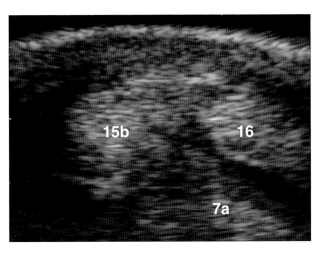

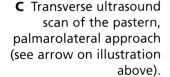

B Transverse ultrasound scan of the pastern, palmarolateral approach (see arrow on illustration at top right).

C Transverse ultrasound scan of the pastern, palmarolateral approach (see arrow on illustration above).

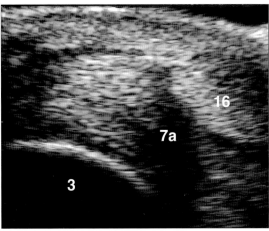

Dissection 6: Isolated Flexor Tendons – Dorsal View

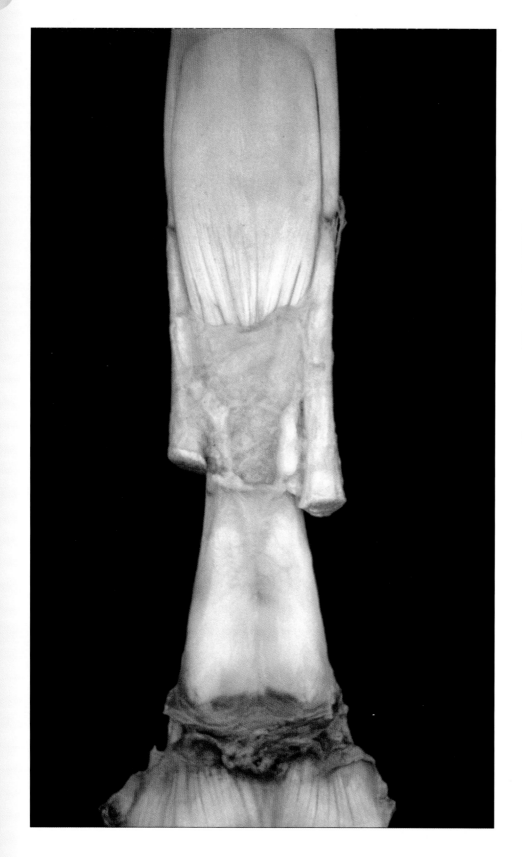

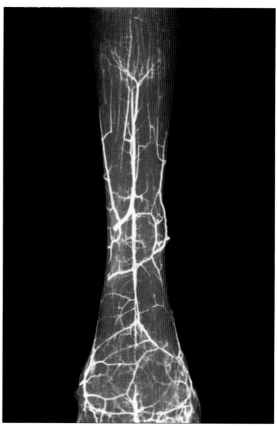

Contrast radiographic study of the arterial supply of the digital part of the DDFT, dorsopalmar view.

Dissection 6: Isolated Flexor Tendons – Dorsal View

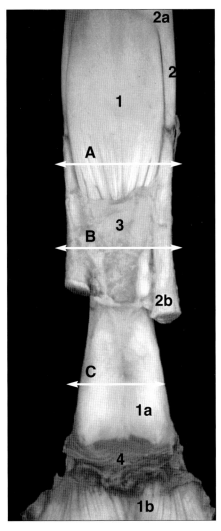

Fetlock

Pastern

Distal sesamoid
bone

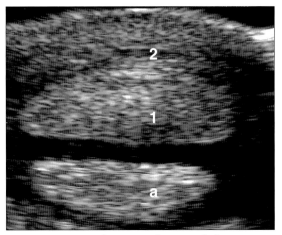

A Transverse ultrasound scan of the digital flexor tendons, palmar approach (see arrow at left).

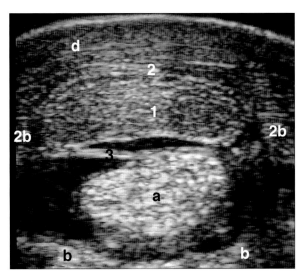

B Transverse ultrasound scan of the digital flexor tendons, palmar approach (see arrow on illustration above, left).

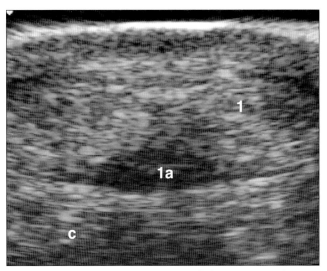

C Transverse ultrasound scan of the DDFT, palmar approach (see arrow on illustration above, left).

1 Deep digital flexor tendon (DDFT)
 1a Phalangeal fibrocartilaginous part in contact with the flexor tuberosity of the middle phalanx
 1b Distal part in contact with the distal sesamoid bone
2 Superficial digital flexor tendon (SDFT)
 2a Manica flexoria
 2b Distal branch
3 Synovial fold between the 2 SDFT distal branches
4 Synovial membranes of the digital sheath and podotrochlear bursa inserted on the DDFT

Ultrasound scans A, B and C:
 a Straight sesamoidean ligament
 b Oblique sesamoidean ligament
 c Middle scutum
 d Proximal digital annular ligament

Dissection 7: Digital Sheath

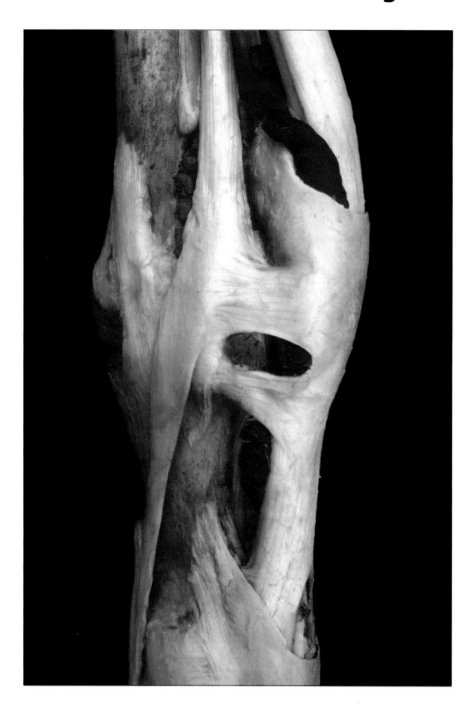

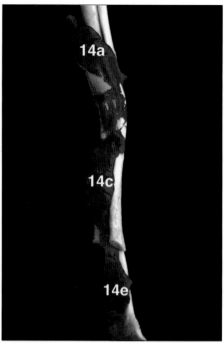

Isolated digital flexor tendons with latex injected into the digital sheath cavity, dorsolateral view.

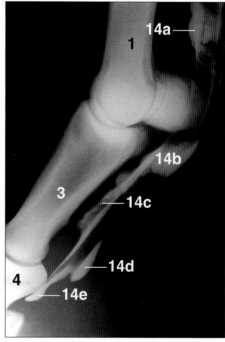

Contrast radiographic study of the digital sheath (tenography), lateromedial view.

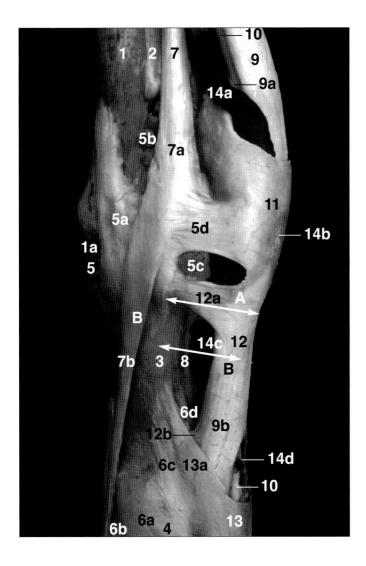

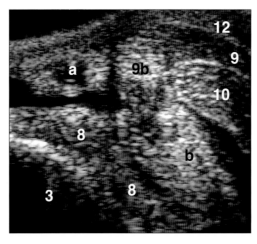

A Transverse ultrasound scan of the pastern, palmarolateral approach (see arrow on illustration at left).

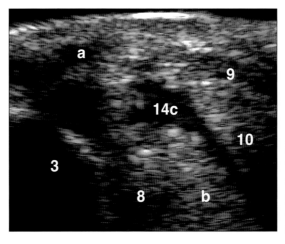

B Transverse ultrasound scan of the pastern palmarolateral approach (see arrow on illustration at left).

1 Third metacarpal bone
  1a Metacarpal condyle
2 Fourth metacarpal bone
3 Proximal phalanx
4 Middle phalanx
5 Metacarpophalangeal joint
  5a Collateral ligament
  5b Proximopalmar recess
  5c Collateral recess
  5d Collateral sesamoidean ligament
6 Proximal interphalangeal joint
  6a Collateral ligament
  6b Collateral sesamoidean ligament
  6c Abaxial palmar ligament
  6d Axial palmar ligament
7 Third interosseus muscle
  7a Distal branch
  7b Extensor branch
8 Oblique sesamoidean ligament
9 Superficial digital flexor tendon

  9a Manica flexoria
  9b Distal branch
10 Deep digital flexor tendon
11 Palmar annular ligament
12 Proximal digital annular ligament
  12a Proximal attachment
  12b Distal attachment
13 Distal digital annular ligament
  13a Proximal attachment
14 Digital sheath
  14a Dorsal proximal recess
  14b Palmar proximal recess
  14c Collateral recess
  14d Palmar distal recess
  14e Dorsal distal recess

Ultrasound scans A and B:
  a Proper palmar digital artery
  b Straight sesamoidean ligament

Dissection 8: Digital Sheath

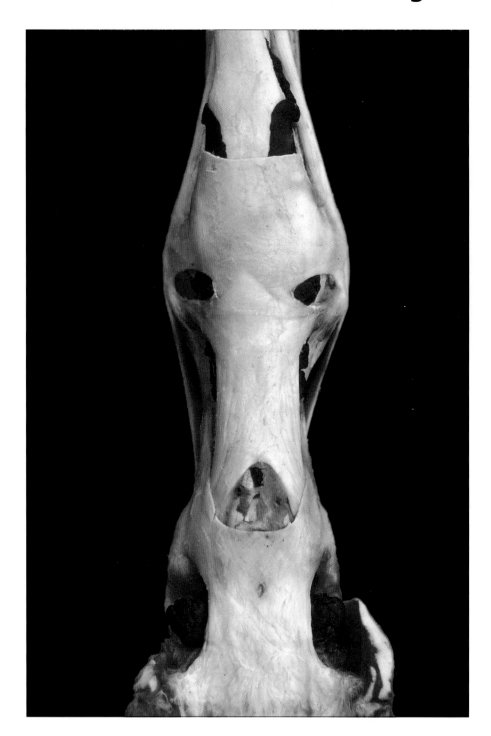

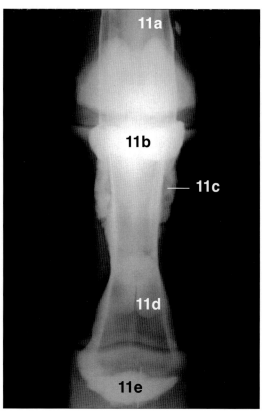

Contrast radiographic study of the digital sheath (tenography), dorsopalmar view.

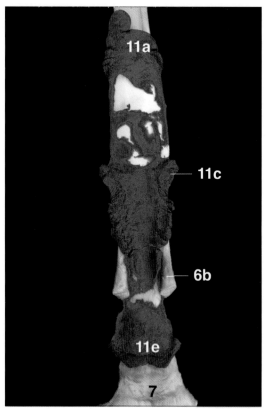

Isolated digital flexor tendons with latex injected into the digital sheath cavity, dorsal aspect.

Dissection 8: Digital Sheath

1 Third metacarpal bone
2 Proximal phalanx
3 Middle phalanx
4 Distal phalanx (palmar process)
5 Third interosseus muscle
   5a Distal branch
   5b Extensor branch
6 Superficial digital flexor tendon
   6a Digital sagittal part
   6b Distal branch
7 Deep digital flexor tendon
8 Palmar annular ligament
9 Proximal digital annular ligament
10 Distal digital annular ligament
   10a Proximal attachment
11 Digital sheath
   11a Dorsal proximal recess
   11b Palmar proximal recess
   11c Collateral recess
   11d Palmar distal recess
   11e Dorsal distal recess
12 Ungular cartilage
13 Collateral recess of the metacarpophalangeal joint
14 Proximopalmar recess of the distal interphalangeal joint

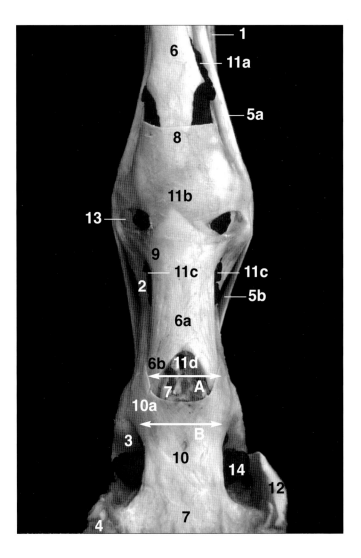

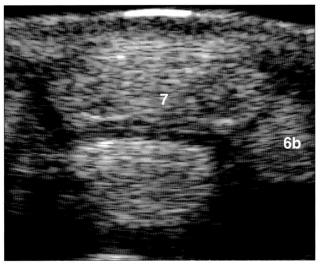

A Transverse ultrasound scan of the pastern, palmar approach (see arrow on illustration above right).

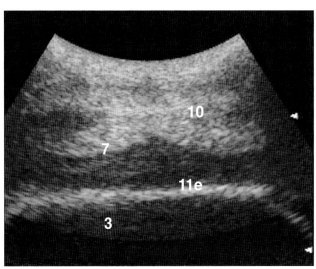

B Transverse ultrasound scan of the pastern, palmar approach (see arrow on illustration above).

Dissection 9: Palmar Aspect of the Pastern
(After Removal of the Flexor Tendons)

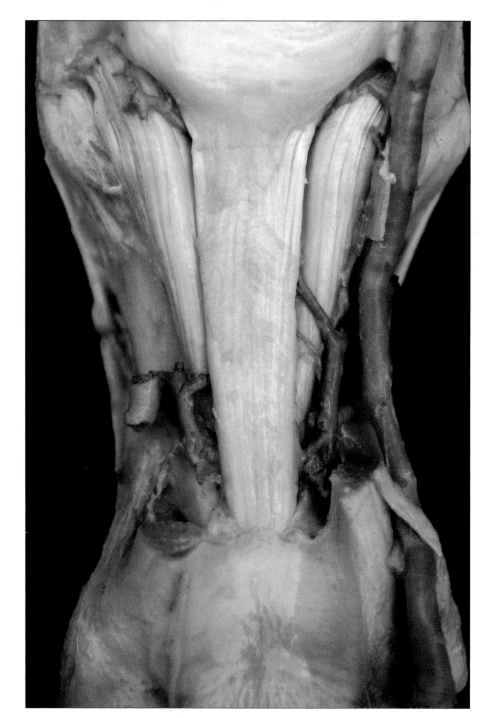

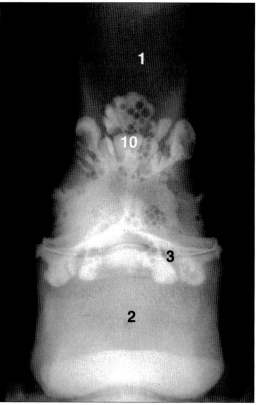

Contrast radiographic study of the PIP joint (arthrography), dorsopalmar view.

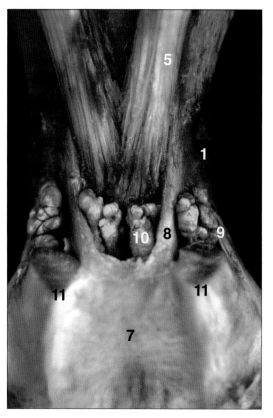

Dissected specimen after latex injection into the PIP joint, palmar view.

Dissection 9: Palmar Aspect of the Pastern
(After Removal of the Flexor Tendons)

1 Proximal phalanx (P1)
  1a Palmar eminence
2 Middle phalanx
  2a Flexor tuberosity
3 Proximal interphalangeal (PIP) joint
4 Palmar (intersesamoidean) ligament
5 Oblique sesamoidean ligament
6 Straight sesamoidean ligament
7 Middle scutum
8 Axial palmar ligament of the PIP joint
9 Abaxial palmar ligament of the PIP joint
10 Palmar recess of the PIP joint
11 Superficial digital flexor tendon (distal branch)
12 Proximal digital annular ligament (proximal attachment)
13 Proper palmar digital artery
  13a Palmar ramus of P1
  13b Dorsal ramus of P1
  13c Ramus of the digital torus
14 Proper palmar digital vein
  14a Palmar ramus of P1
15 Ergot ligament
16 Extensor branch of the third interosseus muscle

Ultrasound scans A and B:
  a Deep digital flexor tendon
  5a Sagittal part of the oblique sesamoidean ligament

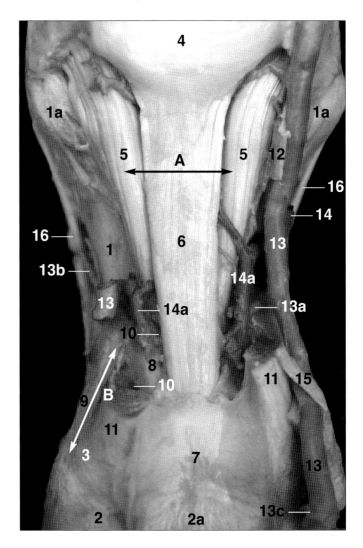

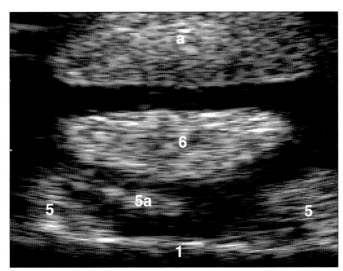

A Transverse ultrasound scan of the pastern, palmar approach (see arrow on illustration above, right).

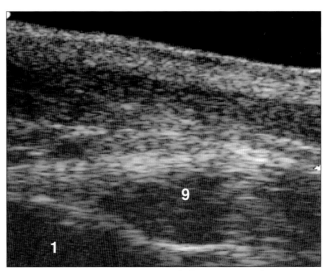

B Frontal ultrasound scan of the pastern (see arrow on illustration above).

Dissection 10: Palmarolateral View of the Pastern
(After Removal of the Flexor Tendons)

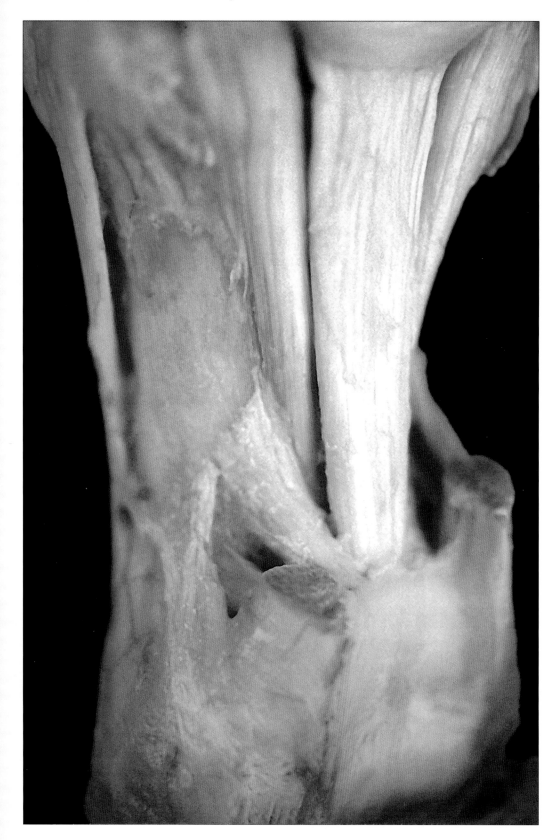

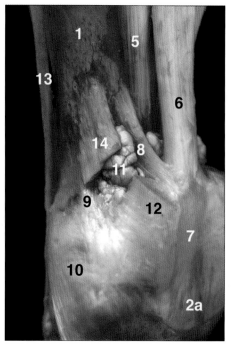

Dissected specimen after latex injection in the PIP joint, palmarolateral view.

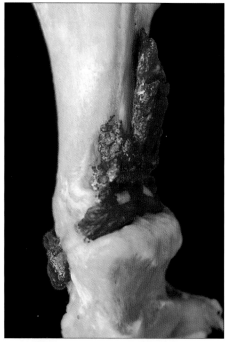

Anatomical specimen with casting preparation of the proximal interphalangeal joint cavity, palmarolateral view.

Dissection 10: Palmarolateral View of the Pastern
(After Removal of the Flexor Tendons)

1 Proximal phalanx (P1)
2 Middle phalanx
   2a Flexor tuberosity
3 Proximal interphalangeal (PIP) joint
4 Palmar (intersesamoidean) ligament
5 Oblique sesamoidean ligament
6 Straight sesamoidean ligament
7 Middle scutum
   7a Insertion on P1
8 Axial palmar ligament of the PIP joint
9 Abaxial palmar ligament of the PIP joint
10 Collateral ligament of the PIP joint
11 Palmar recess of the PIP joint
12 Superficial digital flexor tendon (distal branch)
13 Extensor branch of the third interosseus muscle
14 Proximal attachment of the distal digital annular ligament and digital cushion (on the dissected specimen, facing page)

Ultrasound scan A:
  a Proper palmar digital artery

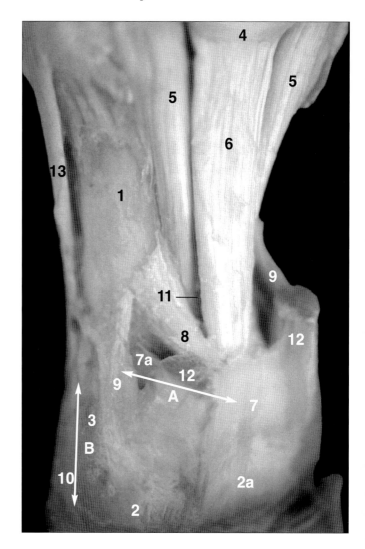

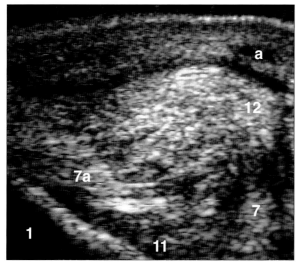

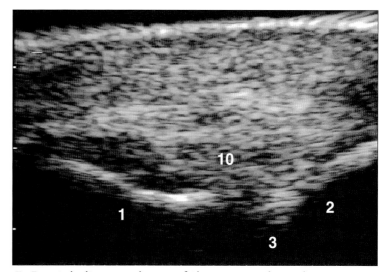

A Transverse ultrasound scan of the pastern, oblique palmarolateral approach (see arrow on illustration, above right).

B Frontal ultrasound scan of the pastern, lateral approach (see arrow on illustration above).

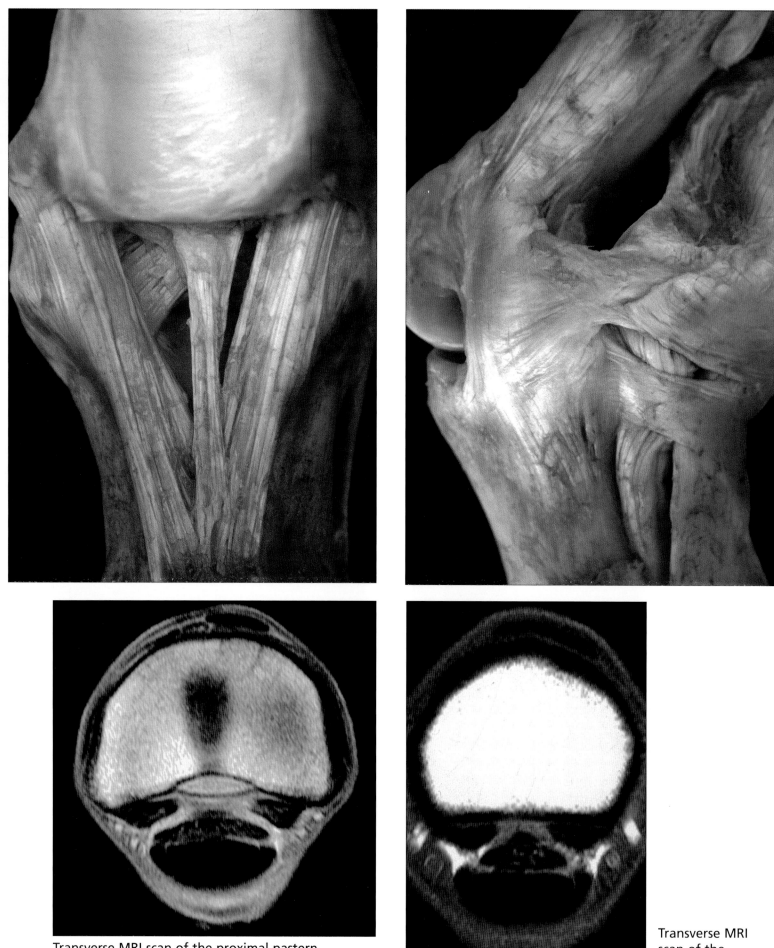

Transverse MRI scan of the proximal pastern showing the cruciate sesamoidean ligaments

Transverse MRI scan of the pastern.

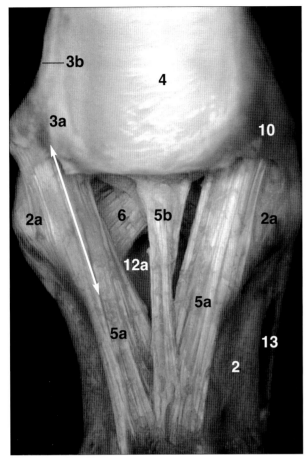

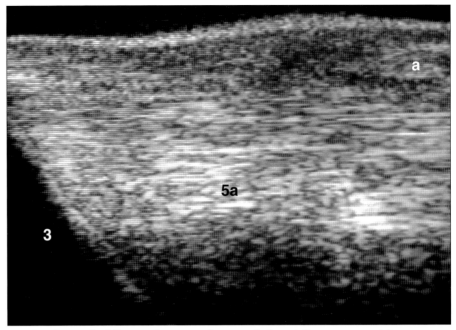

Sagittofrontal oblique ultrasound scan of the oblique sesamoidean ligament (see arrow on illustration at left). **a** Proximal attachment of the proximal digital annular ligament.

Palmar aspect.

1 Third metacarpal bone
   1a Metacarpal condyle
2 Proximal phalanx
   2a Palmar eminence
3 Proximal sesamoid bone
   3a Palmar border
   3b Interosseus face
4 Palmar (intersesamoidean) ligament
5 Oblique sesamoidean ligament
   5a Collateral (main) part
   5b Sagittal part
6 Cruciate sesamoidean ligament
7 Superficial digital flexor tendon
8 Palmar annular ligament
9 Proximal digital annular ligament (proximal attachment)
10 Collateral sesamoidean ligament
11 Collateral ligament of the metacarpophalangeal joint
12 Recesses of the metacarpophalangeal joint
   12a Distopalmar recess
   12b Proximopalmar recess
13 Extensor branch of the third interosseus muscle

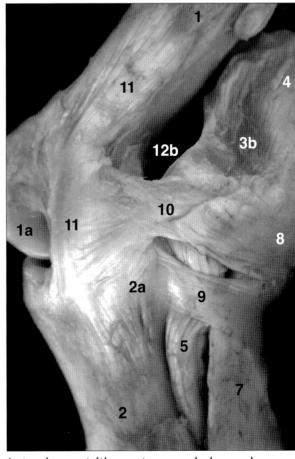

Lateral aspect (the metacarpophalangeal joint is flexed).

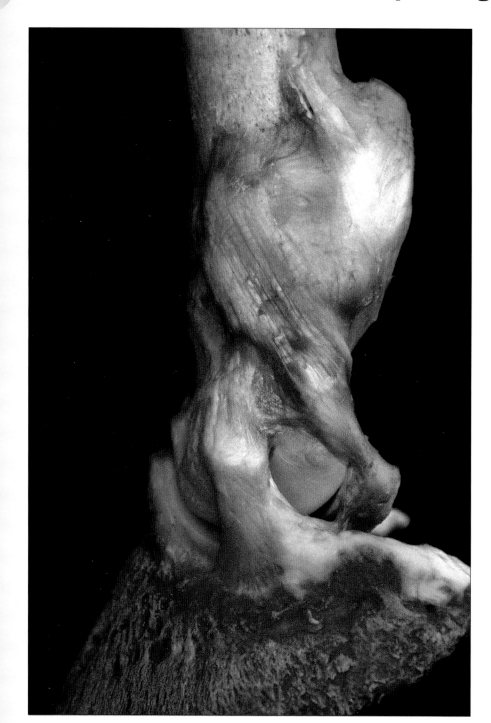

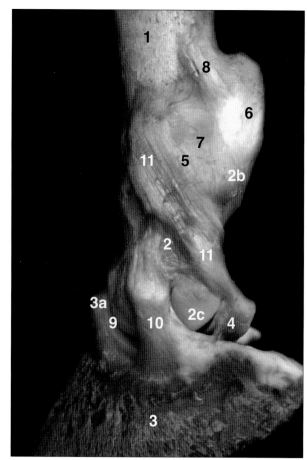

Extended joints.

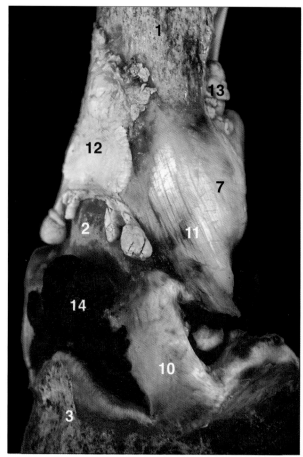

Dissected specimen after injection of coloured latex in the interphalangeal joints, dorsolateral view.

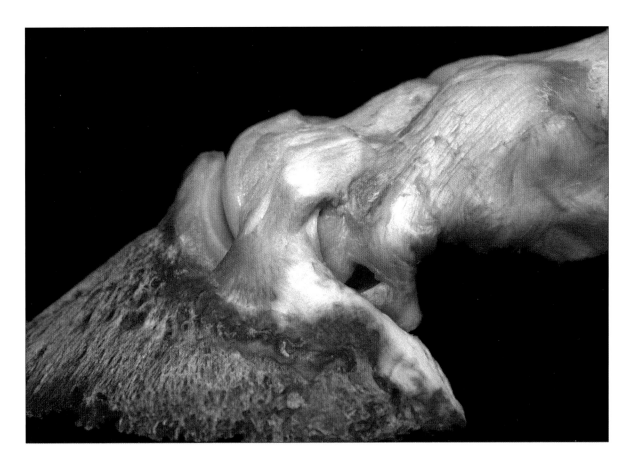

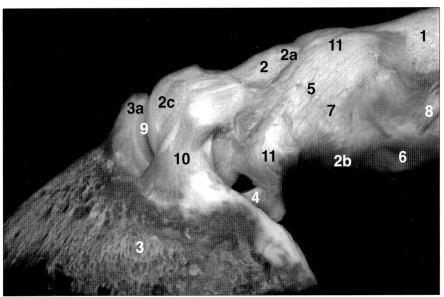

Flexed joints.

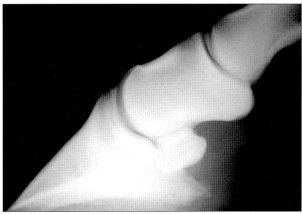

Angulation of the interphalangeal joints on a isolated limb under compression (pressure on the radius = 10 000 N).

1 Proximal phalanx
2 Middle phalanx
    2a Extensor process
    2b Flexor tuberosity
    2c Distal condyle
3 Distal phalanx
    3a Extensor process
4 Distal sesamoid bone
5 Proximal interphalangeal (PIP) joint

6 Middle scutum
7 Collateral ligament of the PIP joint
8 Abaxial palmar ligament of the PIP joint
9 Distal interphalangeal (DIP) joint
10 Collateral ligament of the DIP joint
11 Collateral sesamoidean ligament
12 Dorsal recess of the PIP joint
13 Palmar recess of the PIP joint
14 Dorsal recess of the DIP joint

Dissection 13: Recesses of the Proximal Interphalangeal Joint – Dorsal View

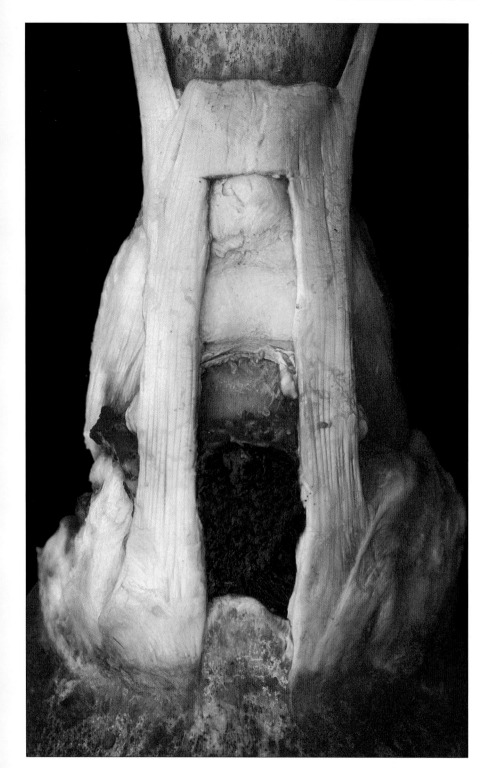

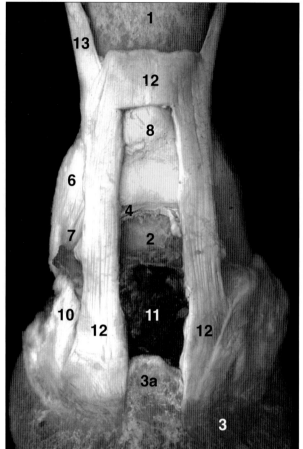

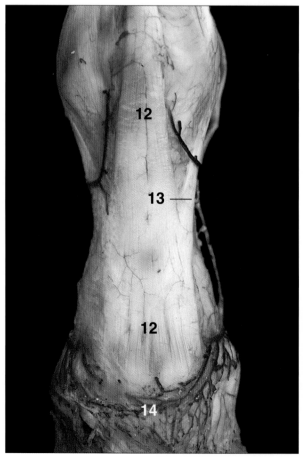

Dissected digit,
dorsal view.

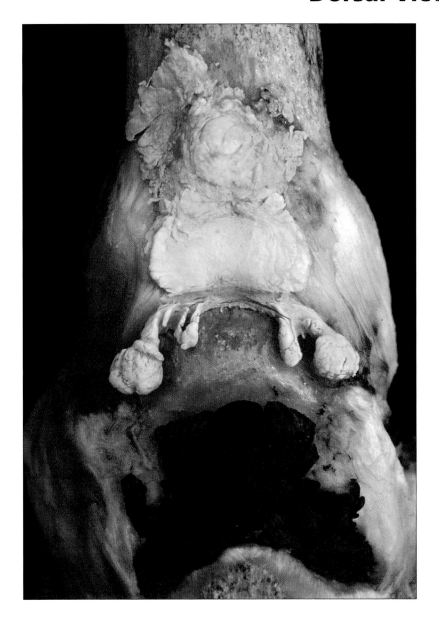

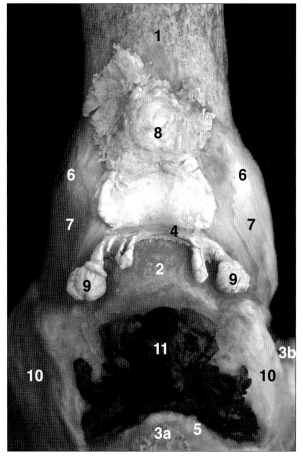

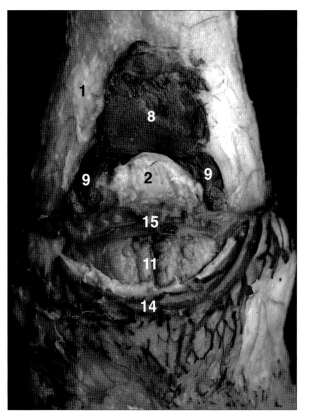

1 Proximal phalanx
2 Middle phalanx (P2)
3 Distal phalanx
   3a Extensor process
   3b Palmar process
4 Proximal interphalangeal (PIP) joint
5 Distal interphalangeal (DIP) joint
6 Collateral ligament of the PIP joint
7 Collateral sesamoidean ligament
8 Dorsal recess of the PIP joint
9 Distodorsocollateral recess of the PIP joint
10 Collateral ligament of the DIP joint
11 Dorsal recess of the DIP joint
12 Dorsal digital extensor tendon
13 Third interosseus muscle extensor branch
14 Coronal artery and vein
15 Dorsal rami (artery and vein) of P2

Anatomical relationships between the dorsal recesses and vessels.

Sagittal and Parasagittal Sections of the Equine Pastern

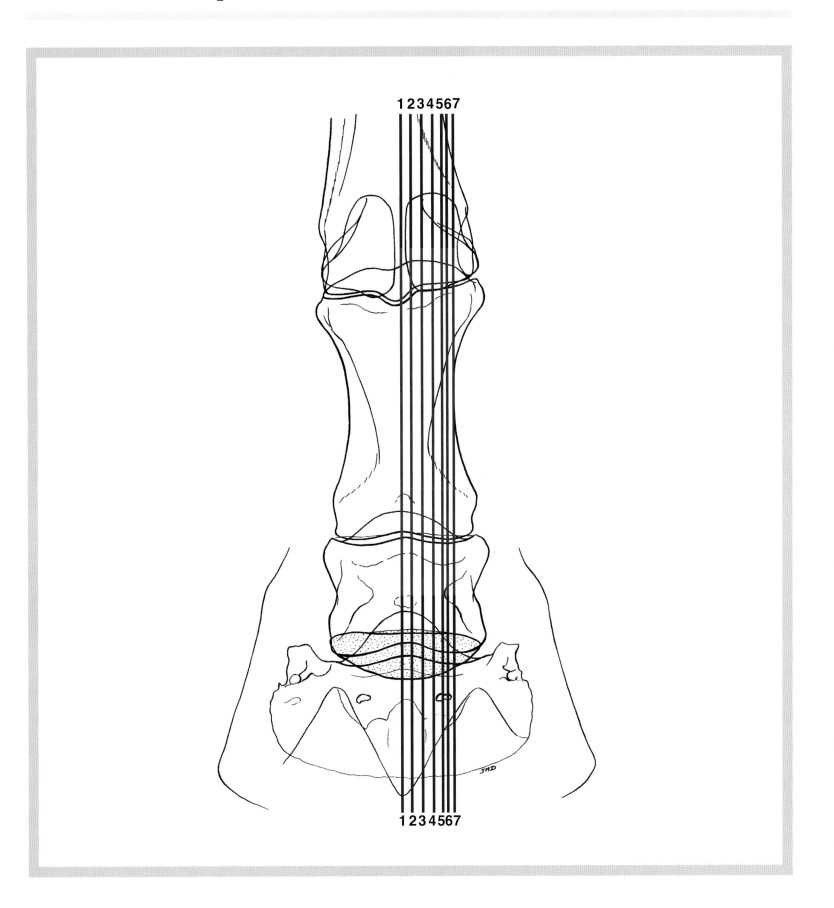

S1a: Sagittal Section of the Pastern

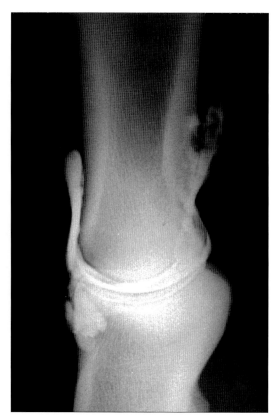

Double contrast radiographic study of the PIP joint (arthrography), lateromedial view.

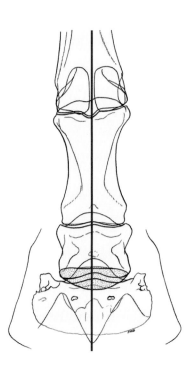

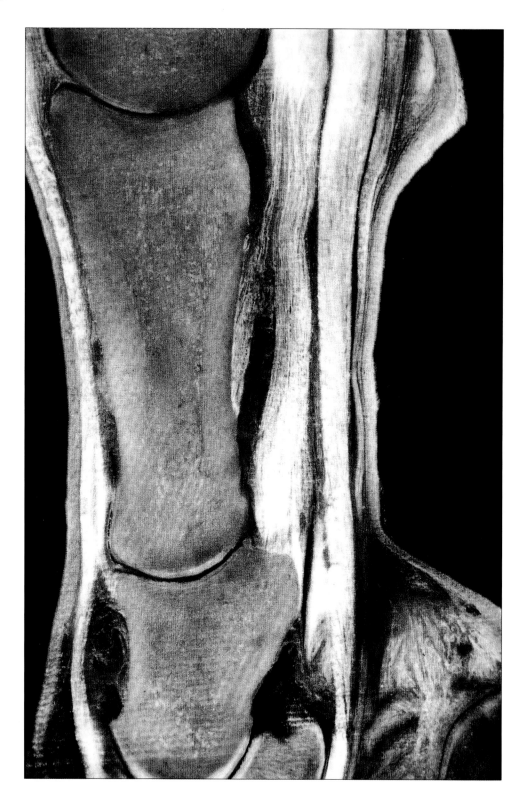

1 Metacarpal condyle
 1a Sagittal ridge
2 Proximal phalanx (P1)
 2a Proximal sagittal groove
 2b Distal sagittal groove
3 Middle phalanx (P2)
 3a Sagittal ridge
 3b Flexor tuberosity
4 Distal phalanx, P3 (extensor process)
5 Distal sesamoid bone
6 Metacarpophalangeal (MP) joint
7 Dorsal articular capsule
8 Palmar (intersesamoidean) ligament
9 Cruciate sesamoidean ligament
10 Oblique sesamoidean ligament
11 Straight sesamoidean ligament
12 Distopalmar recess of the MP joint
13 Proximal interphalangeal (PIP) joint
14 Middle scutum
15 Palmar recess of the PIP joint
16 Dorsal recess of the PIP joint
17 Distal interphalangeal (DIP) joint
18 Collateral sesamoidean ligament
19 Proximopalmar recess of the DIP joint
20 Dorsal recess of the DIP joint
21 Dorsal digital extensor tendon
 21a Insertion on P1
 21b Insertion on the extensor process of P2
 21c Insertion on the extensor process of P3
22 Superficial digital flexor tendon
23 Deep digital flexor tendon
 23a MP fibrocartilaginous part
 23b Phalangeal fibrocartilaginous part
24 Palmar annular ligament
25 Proximal digital annular ligament
26 Distal digital annular ligament
27 Digital sheath cavity
 27a Synovial fold
 27b Palmar distal recess
 27c Dorsal distal recess
28 Proximal recess of the podotrochlear bursa
29 Palmar rami (artery and vein) of P1
30 Dorsal ramus (artery) of P1
31 Dorsal rami (artery and vein) of P2
32 Digital cushion
33 Ergot
34 Skin

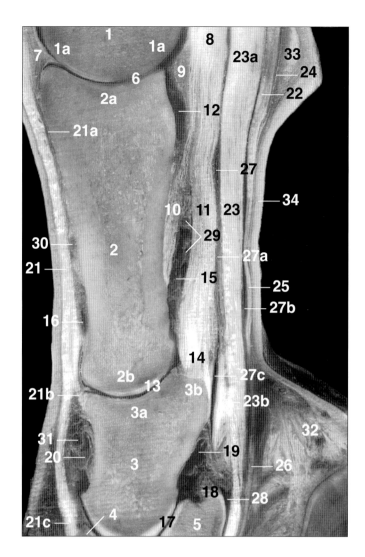

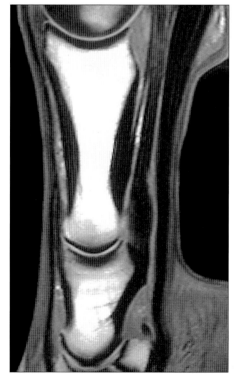

Sagittal MRI scan of the pastern after injection of latex into the arteries and fat material into the veins.

S1b: Sagittal Section of the Palmar Pastern – Proximal Part

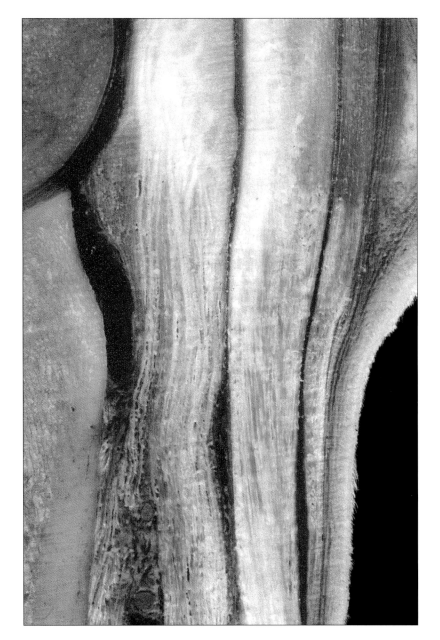

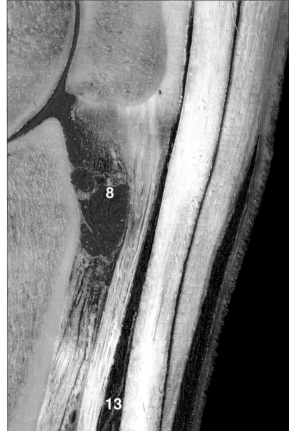

Section of the proximal pastern after latex injection in the MP joint and digital sheath cavities.

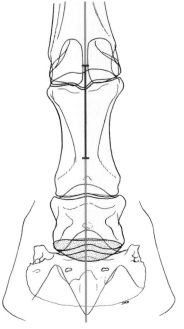

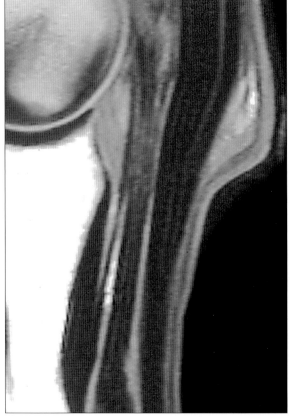

Sagittal MRI scan of the pastern.

1 Metacarpal condyle
   1a Sagittal ridge
2 Proximal phalanx
   2a Proximal sagittal groove
3 Metacarpophalangeal (MP) joint
4 Palmar (intersesamoidean) ligament
5 Cruciate sesamoidean ligament
6 Oblique sesamoidean ligament
   6a Sagittal part
   6b Collateral part
7 Straight sesamoidean ligament
8 Distopalmar recess of the MP joint
9 Superficial digital flexor tendon
10 Deep digital flexor tendon
   10a MP fibrocartilaginous part
11 Palmar annular ligament
12 Proximal digital annular ligament
13 Digital sheath cavity
   13a Synovial fold
14 Palmar ramus (vein) of P1
15 Ergot cushion
16 Skin

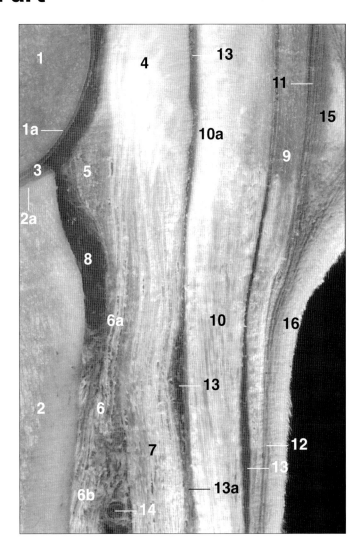

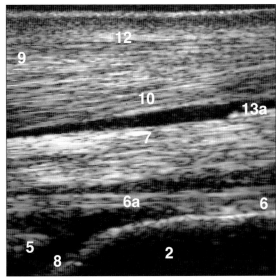

Sagittal ultrasound scan of the proximal pastern, palmar approach (7.5 MHz linear probe).

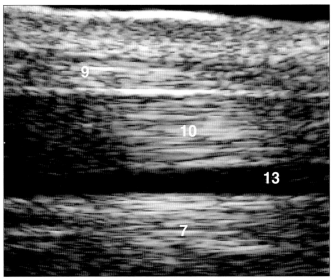

Sagittal ultrasound scan of the proximal pastern, palmar approach (10 MHz sector probe).

S1c: Sagittal Section of the Palmar Pastern – Proximal Part

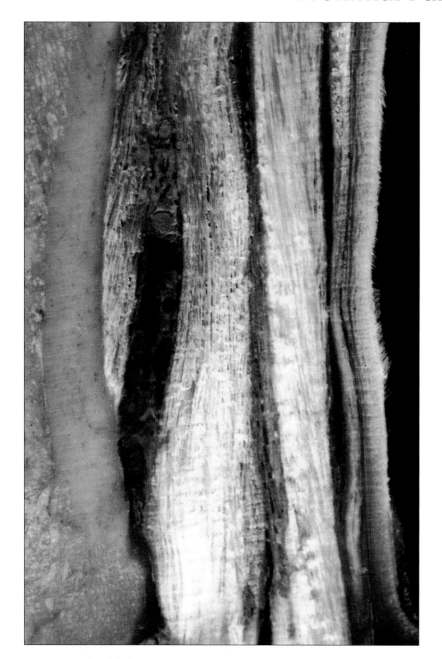

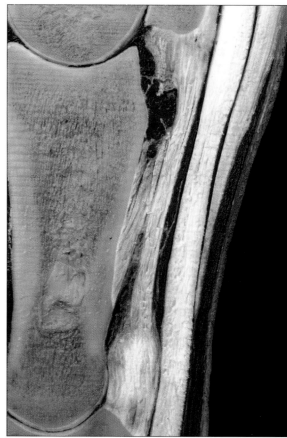

Section of the middle pastern after latex injection into the joints and digital sheath cavities.

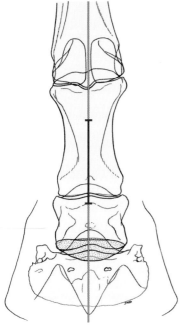

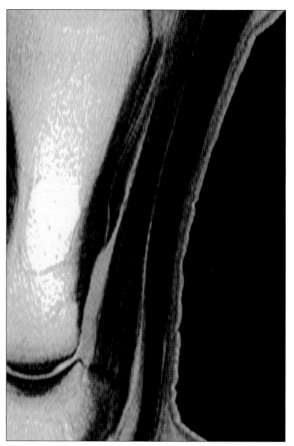

Sagittal MRI scan of the pastern.

S1c: Sagittal Section of the Palmar Pastern – Middle Part

1 Proximal phalanx (P1)
  1a Distal condyle
  1b Trigone of P1
2 Oblique sesamoidean ligament
3 Straight sesamoidean ligament
4 Middle scutum
5 Proximal interphalangeal (PIP) joint
6 Palmar recess of the PIP joint
7 Superficial digital flexor tendon
8 Deep digital flexor tendon
9 Proximal digital annular ligament
10 Distal digital annular ligament
11 Digital sheath cavity
  11a Dorsal distal recess
  11b Palmar distal recess
12 Synovial fold
13 Palmar rami (artery and vein) of P1
14 Skin

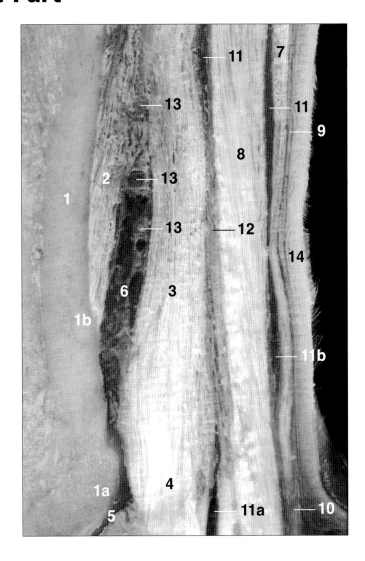

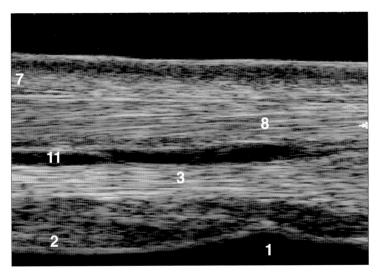

Sagittal ultrasound scan of the middle pastern, palmar approach (7.5 MHz linear probe).

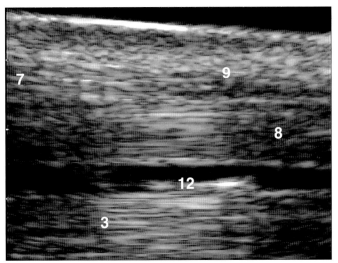

Sagittal ultrasound scan of the middle pastern, palmar approach (10 MHz sector probe).

S1d: Sagittal Section of the Palmar Pastern – Distal Part

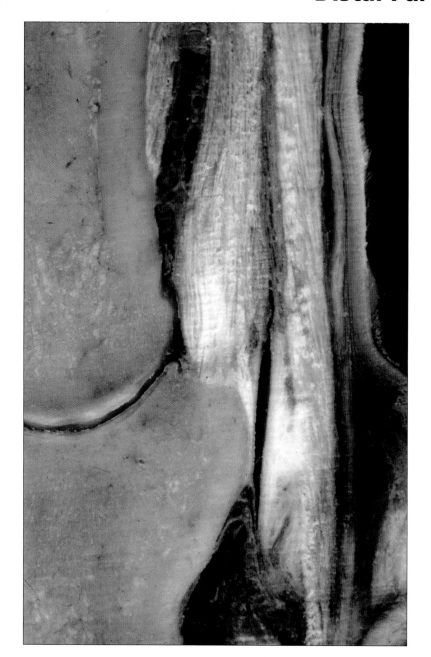

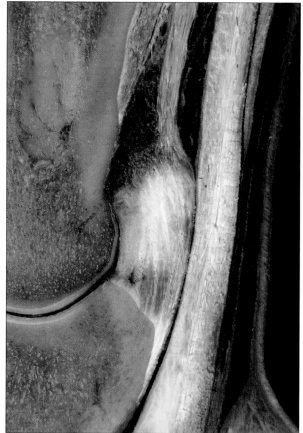

Section of the distal pastern after latex injection into the digital sheath and PIP joint cavities.

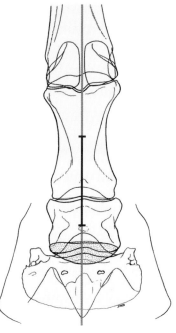

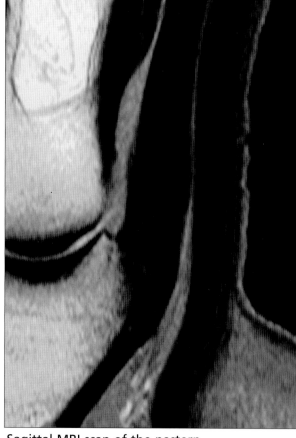

Sagittal MRI scan of the pastern.

S1d: Sagittal Section of the Palmar Pastern – Distal Part

1 Proximal phalanx (P1)
   1a Distal sagittal groove
   1b Trigone of P1
2 Middle phalanx
   2a Sagittal ridge
   2b Flexor tuberosity
3 Collateral sesamoidean ligament
4 Oblique sesamoidean ligament
5 Straight sesamoidean ligament
6 Middle scutum
7 Proximal interphalangeal (PIP) joint
8 Palmar recess of the PIP joint
9 Proximopalmar recess of the distal interphalangeal joint
10 Superficial digital flexor tendon
11 Deep digital flexor tendon
   11a Phalangeal fibrocartilaginous part
12 Proximal digital annular ligament
13 Distal digital annular ligament
14 Digital sheath cavity
   14a Dorsal distal recess
   14b Palmar distal recess
15 Proximal recess of the podotrochlear bursa
16 Palmar rami (artery and vein) of P1
17 Digital cushion (toric part)
18 Skin

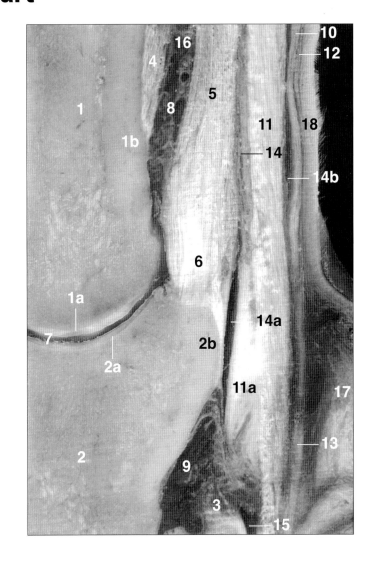

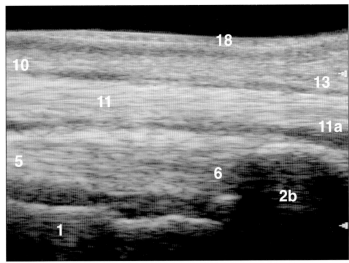

Sagittal ultrasound scan of the distal pastern, palmar approach (7.5 MHz linear probe).

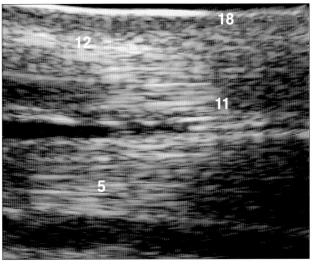

Sagittal ultrasound scan of the distal pastern, palmar approach (10 MHz sector probe).

S1e: Sagittal Section of the Dorsal Pastern – Middle Part

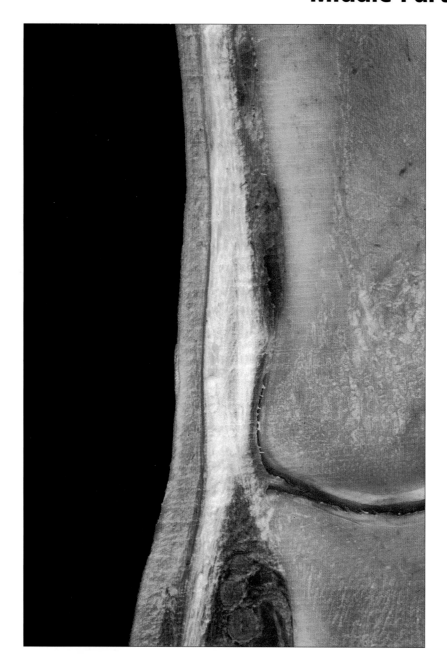

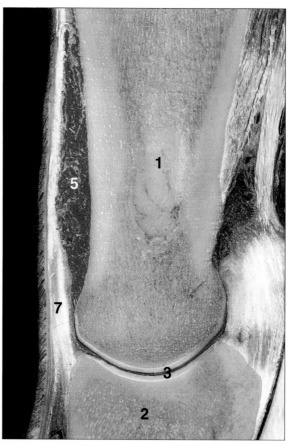

Section of the pastern after latex injection into the dorsal recess of the PIP joint.

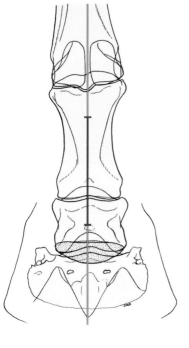

Dissected specimen after latex injection into the recesses of the interphalangeal joints.

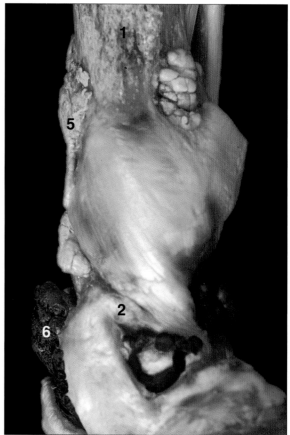

S1e: Sagittal Section of the Dorsal Pastern – Middle Part

1 Proximal phalanx
   1a Distal sagittal groove
2 Middle phalanx (P2)
   2a Sagittal ridge
   2b Extensor process
3 Proximal interphalangeal (PIP) joint
4 Synovial membrane
   4a Synovial plica
5 Dorsal recess of the PIP joint
6 Dorsal recess of the distal interphalangeal joint
7 Dorsal digital extensor tendon
   7a Insertion on the extensor process of P2
8 Dorsal ramus (artery) of P1
9 Dorsal rami (artery and vein) of P2
10 Skin

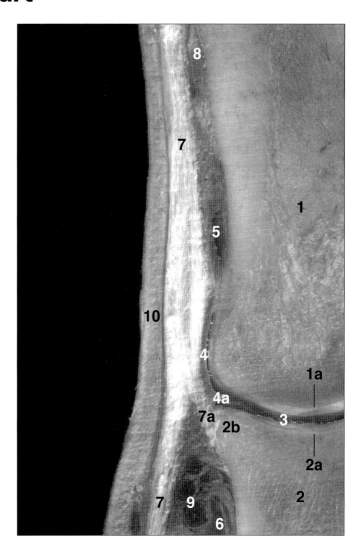

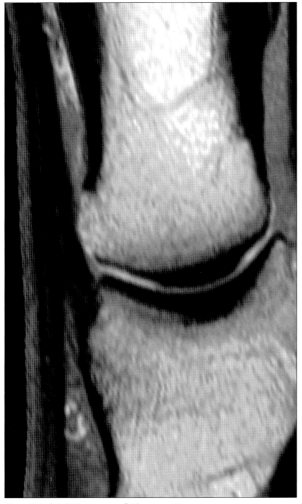

Sagittal MRI scan of the pastern.

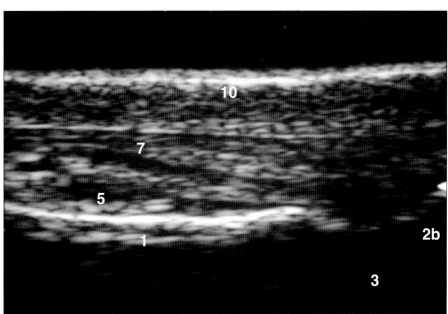

Sagittal ultrasound scan of the pastern, dorsal approach.

S1f: Sagittal Section of the Dorsal Pastern – Distal Part

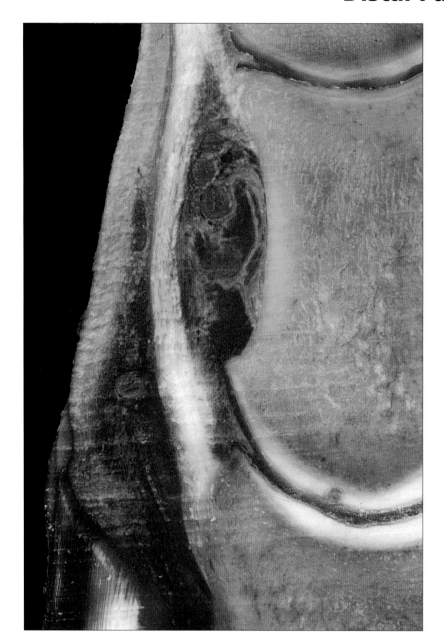

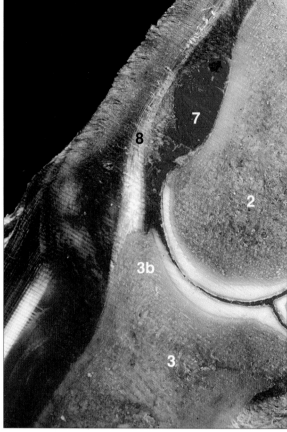

Sagittal section of the coronet after latex injection into the DIP joint.

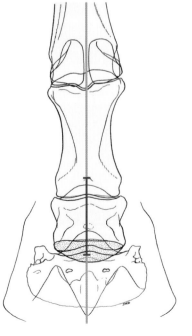

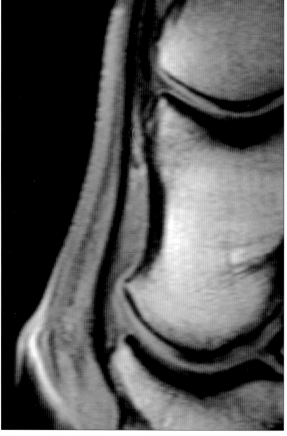

Parasagittal MRI scan of the pastern.

1 Proximal phalanx (P1)
  1a Distal sagittal groove
2 Middle phalanx (P2)
  2a Sagittal ridge
  2b Extensor process
  2c Sagittal groove
  2d Dorsal margin of the distal articular surface
3 Distal phalanx (P3)
  3a Sagittal ridge
  3b Extensor process
  3c Parietal surface
4 Proximal interphalangeal (PIP) joint
5 Distal interphalangeal (DIP) joint
6 Synovial membrane
  6a Synovial plica
7 Dorsal recess of the DIP joint
8 Dorsal digital extensor tendon
  8a Insertion on the extensor process of P2
  8b Insertion on the extensor process of P3
9 Dorsal rami (artery and vein) of P2
10 Coronal artery and vein
11 Pulvinus coronae
12 Corium limbi
13 Corium coronae
14 Corium parietis
15 Periople
16 Hoof wall
17 Skin

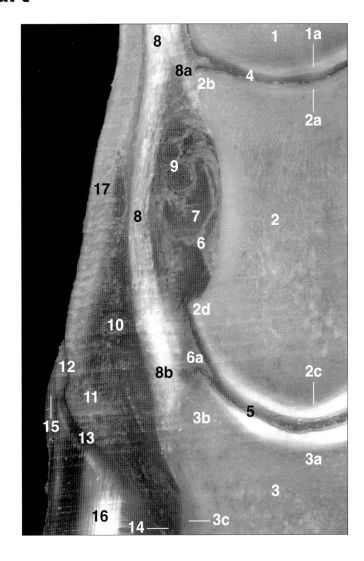

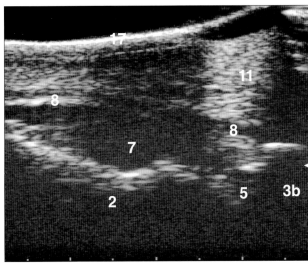

Sagittal ultrasound scan of the distal pastern and coronet, dorsal approach (7.5 MHz linear probe).

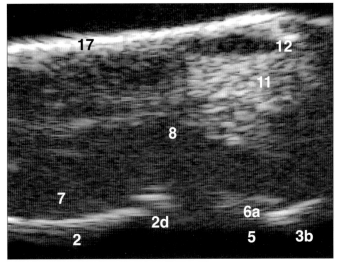

Sagittal ultrasound scan of the distal pastern and coronet, dorsal approach (10 MHz sector probe).

S2: Parasagittal Section of the Pastern

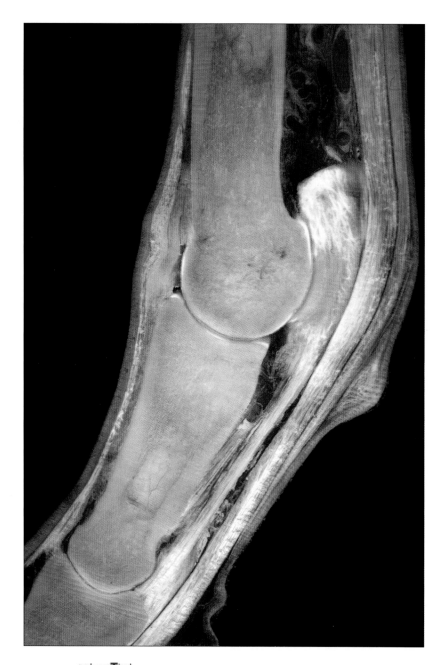

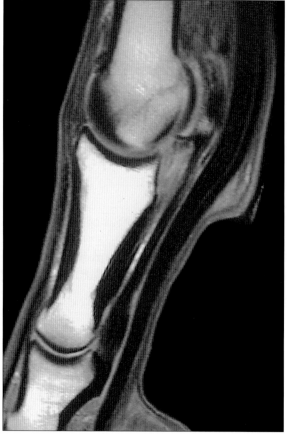

Parasagittal MRI scan of the pastern after injection of latex into the arteries and fat material into the veins.

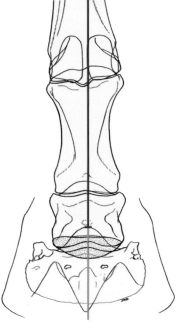

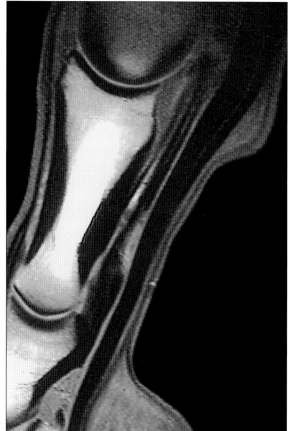

Parasagittal MRI scan of the pastern after injection of latex into the arteries and veins.

1 Metacarpal bone
   1a Metacarpal condyle
2 Proximal phalanx (P1)
   2a Proximal sagittal groove
   2b Distal sagittal groove
3 Middle phalanx (P2)
   3a Sagittal ridge
   3b Flexor tuberosity
4 Proximal sesamoid bone
5 Metacarpophalangeal (MP) joint
6 Dorsal articular capsule
7 Palmar (intersesamoidean) ligament
8 Cruciate sesamoidean ligament
9 Oblique sesamoidean ligament
10 Straight sesamoidean ligament
11 Proximopalmar recess of the MP joint
12 Distopalmar recess of the MP joint
13 Dorsal recess of the MP joint
14 Proximal interphalangeal (PIP) joint
15 Middle scutum
16 Palmar recess of the PIP joint
17 Dorsal recess of the PIP joint
18 Dorsal digital extensor tendon
   18a Insertion on P1
   18b Insertion on the extensor process of P2
19 Superficial digital flexor tendon
20 Deep digital flexor tendon
21 Palmar annular ligament
22 Proximal digital annular ligament
23 Digital sheath
   23a Synovial membrane
24 Common palmar digital artery
25 Common palmar digital vein
26 Palmar metacarpal arteries
27 Palmar metacarpal veins
28 Ergot
29 Skin

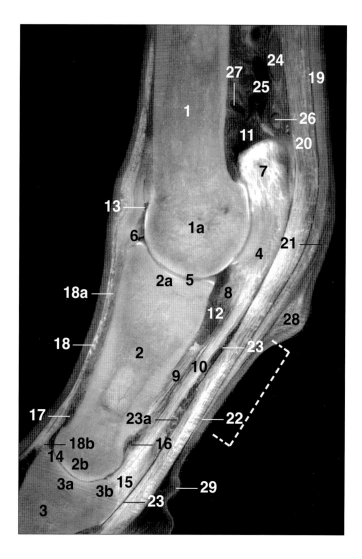

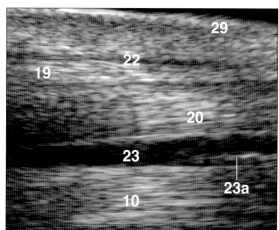

Parasagittal ultrasound scan of the pastern, palmar approach (see dotted area in illustration above).

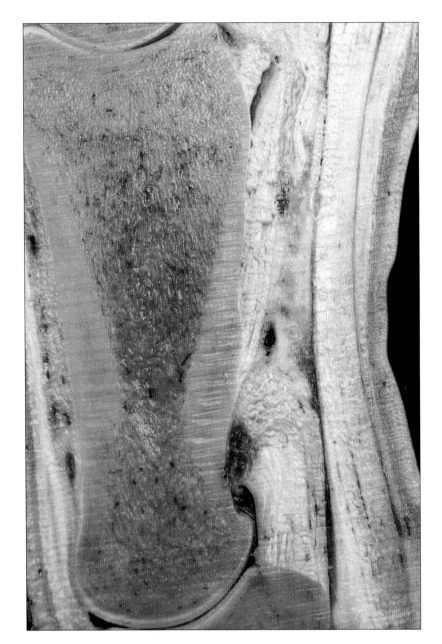

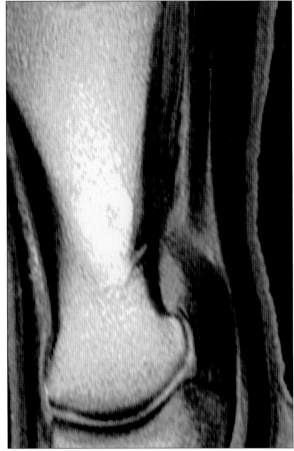

Parasagittal MRI scan of the pastern.

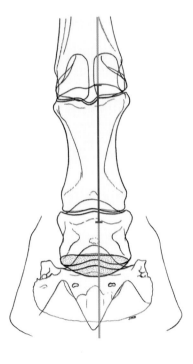

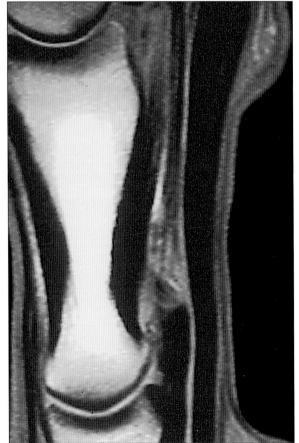

Parasagittal MRI scan of the pastern after injection of latex into the arteries and veins.

1 Metacarpal condyle (medial part)
2 Proximal phalanx (P1)
    2a Medial glenoid cavity
    2b Medial condyle
    2c Trigone of P1
3 Middle phalanx (flexor tuberosity)
4 Metacarpophalangeal joint (MP joint)
5 Cruciate sesamoidean ligament
6 Oblique sesamoidean ligament
7 Straight sesamoidean ligament
8 Distopalmar recess of the MP joint
9 Proximal interphalangeal (PIP) joint
10 Middle scutum
11 Axial palmar ligament of the PIP joint
12 Palmar recess of the PIP joint
13 Dorsal recess of the PIP joint
14 Dorsal digital extensor tendon
15 Superficial digital flexor tendon
16 Deep digital flexor tendon
    16a Phalangeal fibrocartilaginous part
17 Palmar annular ligament
18 Proximal digital annular ligament
19 Digital sheath
20 Synovial fold
21 Connective tissue
22 Palmar rami (artery and vein) of P1
23 Dorsal rami (artery and vein) of P1
24 Skin

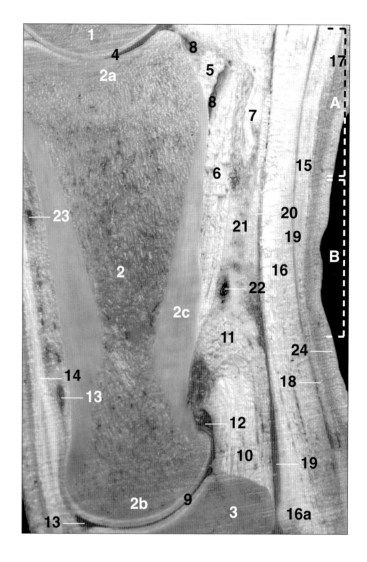

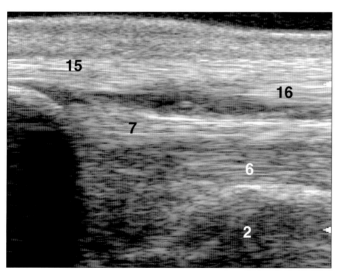

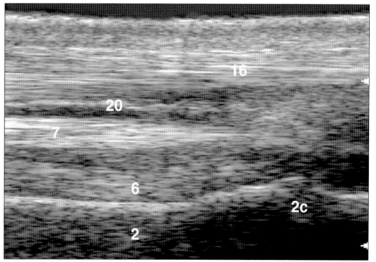

A Parasagittal ultrasound scan of the proximal pastern, palmar approach (see dotted area in illustration above, right).

B Parasagittal ultrasound scan of the middle pastern, palmar approach (see dotted area in illustration above).

S4: Parasagittal Section of the Pastern

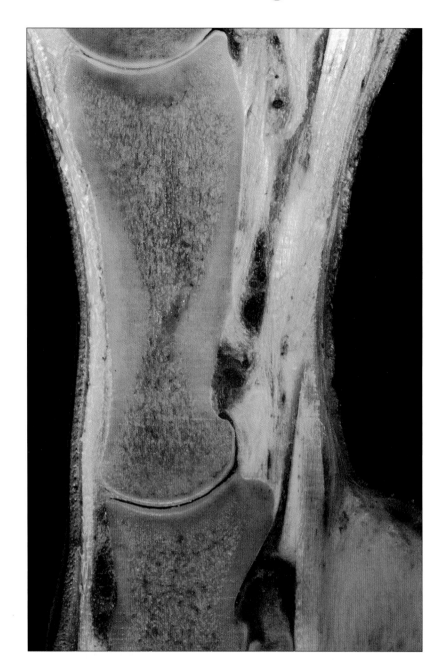

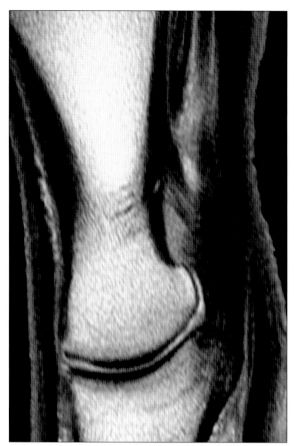

Parasagittal MRI scan of the pastern.

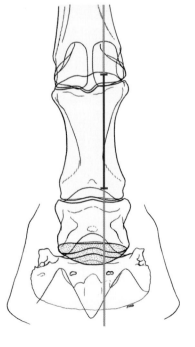

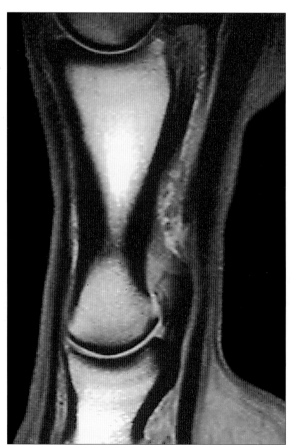

Parasagittal MRI scan of the pastern after injection of latex into the arteries and veins.

1 Metacarpal condyle (medial part)
2 Proximal phalanx (P1)
   2a Medial glenoid cavity
   2b Medial condyle
   2c Trigone of P1
3 Middle phalanx (P2)
   3a Flexor tuberosity
4 Metacarpophalangeal (MP) joint
5 Cruciate sesamoidean ligament
6 Oblique sesamoidean ligament
7 Straight sesamoidean ligament
8 Distopalmar recess of the MP joint
9 Proximal interphalangeal (PIP) joint
10 Middle scutum
11 Axial palmar ligament of the PIP joint
12 Palmar recess of the PIP joint
13 Distal interphalangeal (DIP) joint, proximopalmar recess
14 Collateral sesamoidean ligament
15 Proximopalmar recess of the DIP joint
16 Dorsal digital extensor tendon
17 Superficial digital flexor tendon
   17a Distal branch
18 Deep digital flexor tendon
19 Palmar annular ligament
20 Proximal digital annular ligament
21 Digital sheath
   21a Collateral recess
   21b Dorsal distal recess
22 Proximal recess of the podotrochlear bursa
23 Palmar rami (artery and vein) of P1
24 Dorsal rami (artery and vein) of P2
25 Digital cushion (pars torica)
26 Skin

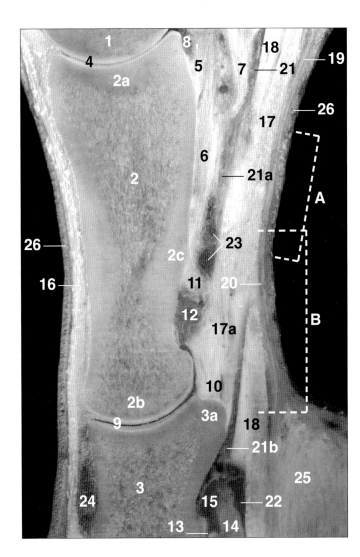

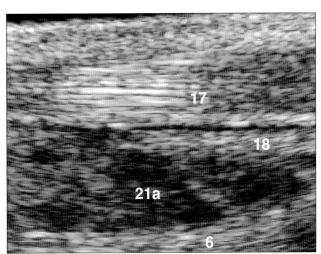

A Parasagittal ultrasound scan of the pastern, palmar approach (see dotted area in illustration above).

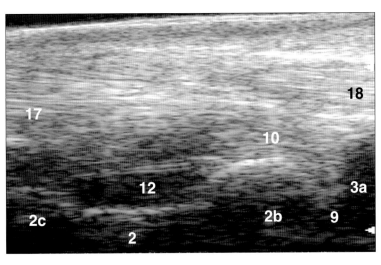

B Parasagittal ultrasound scan of the pastern, palmar approach (see dotted area in illustration above, right).

S5: Parasagittal Section of the Pastern

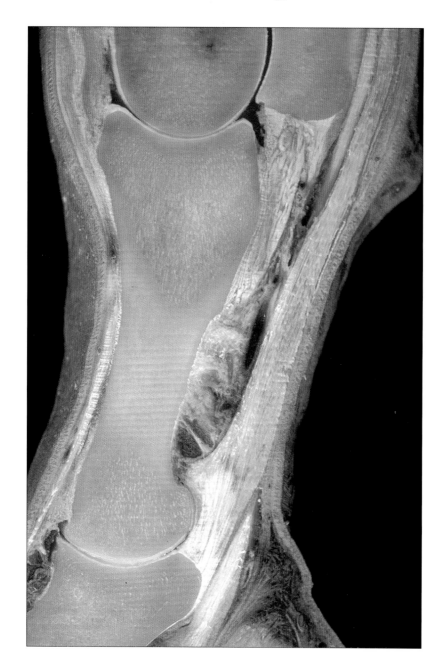

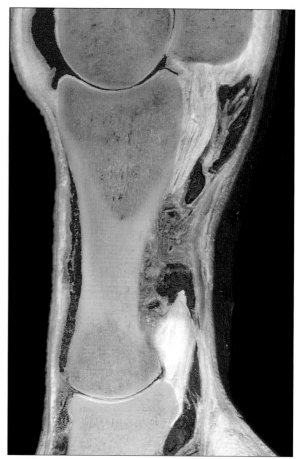

Parasagittal section of the pastern after injection of coloured latex into the synovial cavities.

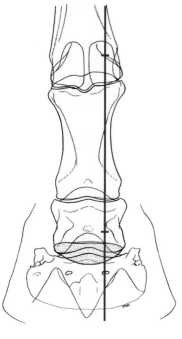

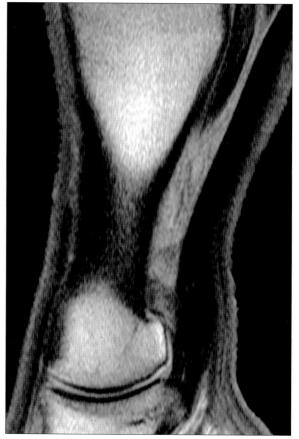

Parasagittal MRI scan of the pastern.

1 Metacarpal condyle
   1a Medial part
2 Proximal phalanx (P1)
   2a Medial glenoid cavity
   2b Medial condyle
   2c Trigone of P1
3 Middle phalanx (P2)
   3a Medial glenoid cavity
   3b Flexor tuberosity
4 Medial proximal sesamoid bone
5 Metacarpophalangeal (MP) joint
6 Dorsal articular capsule
7 Cruciate sesamoidean ligament
8 Oblique sesamoidean ligament
9 Straight sesamoidean ligament
10 Dorsal recess of the MP joint
11 Distopalmar recess of the MP joint
12 Proximal interphalangeal (PIP) joint
13 Middle scutum
   13a Insertion on P1
14 Palmar recess of the PIP joint
15 Distodorsocollateral recess of the PIP joint
16 Dorsal digital extensor tendon
17 Superficial digital flexor tendon
   17a Distal branch
18 Deep digital flexor tendon
19 Palmar annular ligament
20 Proximal digital annular ligament
21 Distal digital annular ligament
22 Digital sheath
   22a Collateral recess
   22b Palmar distal recess
23 Palmar ramus (artery) of P1
24 Dorsal ramus (artery) of P1
25 Proper palmar digital vein
26 Digital cushion (toric part)
27 Ergot
28 Skin

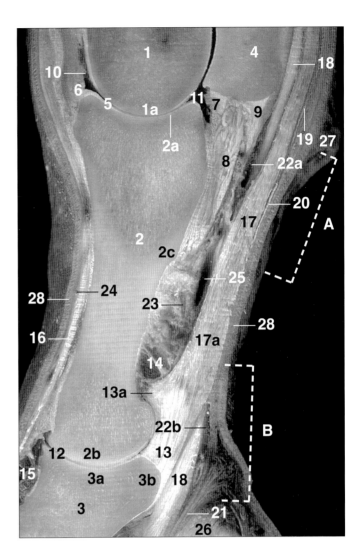

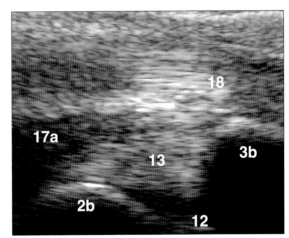

B Parasagittal ultrasound scan of the pastern, palmar approach (see dotted area in illustration above).

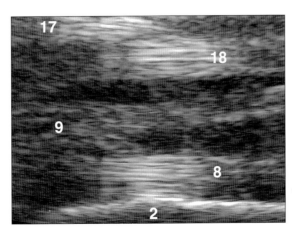

A Parasagittal ultrasound scan of the pastern, palmar approach (see dotted area in illustration above, right).

S6: Parasagittal Section of the Pastern

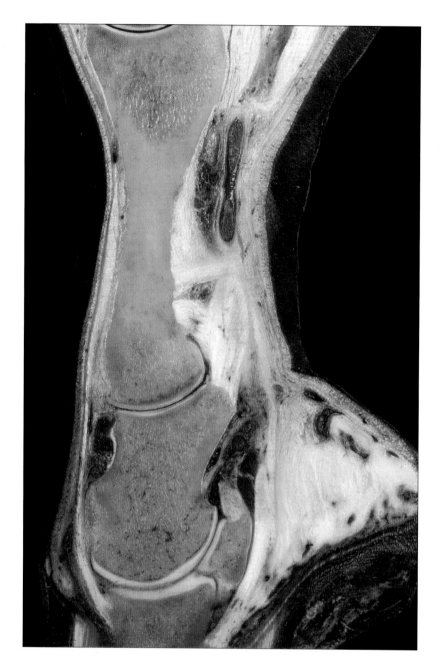

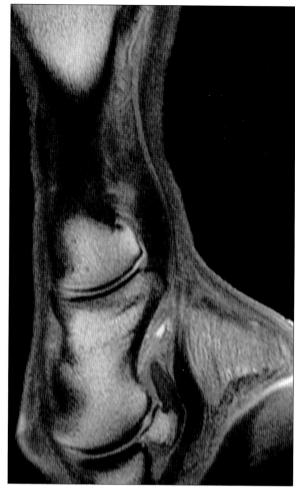

Parasagittal MRI scan of the pastern.

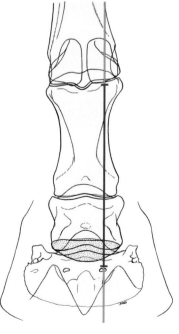

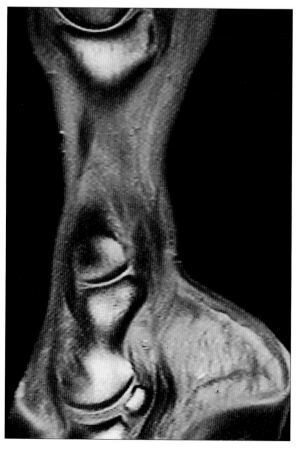

Parasagittal MRI scan of the
pastern after injection of latex
into the arteries and veins.

1 Metacarpal condyle (medial part)
2 Proximal phalanx (P1)
   2a Medial glenoid cavity
   2b Medial condyle
3 Middle phalanx (P2)
   3a Medial glenoid cavity
   3b Medial condyle
   3c Flexor tuberosity
4 Distal phalanx (P3)
   4a Medial glenoid cavity
5 Distal sesamoid bone
6 Metacarpophalangeal joint
7 Proximal interphalangeal (PIP) joint
8 Distal interphalangeal (DIP) joint
9 Oblique sesamoidean ligament
10 Middle scutum
   10a Insertion on P1
11 Recesses of the PIP joint
   11a Distodorsocollateral recess
   11b Palmar recess
12 Collateral sesamoidean ligament
13 Impar distal sesamoidean ligament
14 Proximopalmar recess of the DIP joint
15 Dorsal digital extensor tendon
16 Deep digital flexor tendon
17 Superficial digital flexor tendon
   17a Distal branch
18 Palmar annular ligament
19 Proximal digital annular ligament
   19a Distal insertion
20 Distal digital annular ligament
   20a Proximal attachment
21 Digital sheath
   21a Collateral recess
   21b Dorsal distal recess
22 Podotrochlear bursa (proximal recess)
23 Proper palmar digital artery
24 Dorsal rami (artery and vein) of P1
25 Palmar rami (artery and vein) of P1
26 Ramus of the digital torus
27 Dorsal rami (artery and vein) of P2
28 Palmar rami (artery and vein) of P2
29 Digital cushion
30 Ungular cartilage
31 Skin

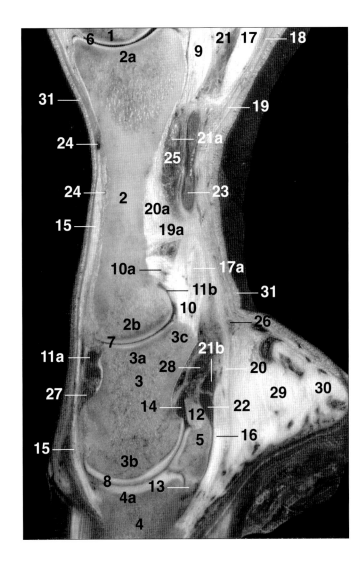

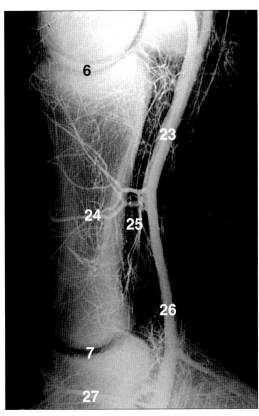

Contrast radiographic study of
the arteries (arteriography) of
the digit, lateromedial view.

S7: Parasagittal Section of the Pastern

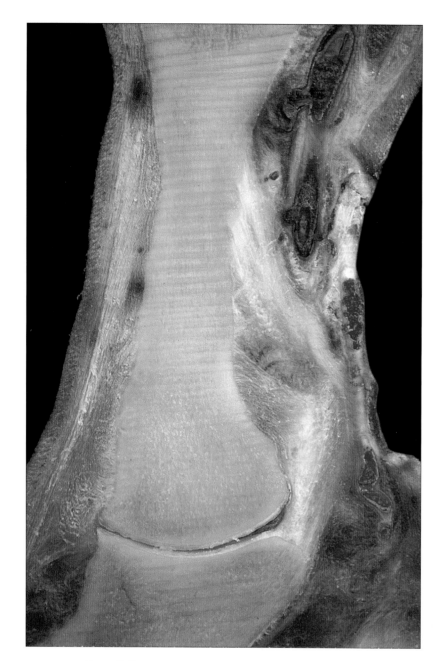

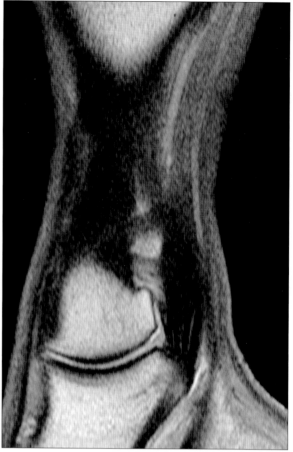

Parasagittal MRI scan of the pastern after injection of latex into the arteries and fat material into the veins.

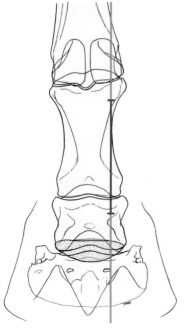

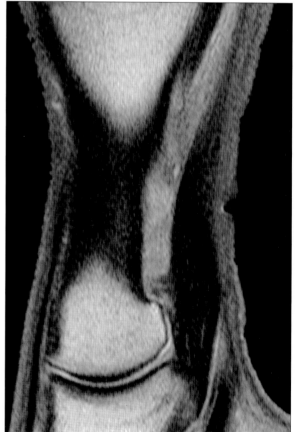

Parasagittal MRI scan of the pastern.

1 Proximal phalanx (P1)
   1a Medial condyle
2 Middle phalanx
   2a Medial glenoid cavity
   2b Flexor tuberosity
3 Proximal interphalangeal joint
   3a Distodorsocollateral recess
   3b Abaxial palmar ligament
4 Middle scutum
5 Collateral sesamoidean ligament (of the distal interphalangeal joint)
6 Dorsal digital extensor tendon
7 Extensor branch of the third interosseus muscle
8 Distal digital annular ligament (proximal attachment)
9 Proper palmar digital artery
10 Proper palmar digital vein
11 Dorsal ramus (vein) of P1
12 Palmar ramus (artery) of P1
13 Palmar ramus (vein) of P1
14 Dorsal rami (artery and vein) of P2
15 Ramus of the digital torus
16 Proper palmar digital nerve
17 Digital cushion
18 Skin

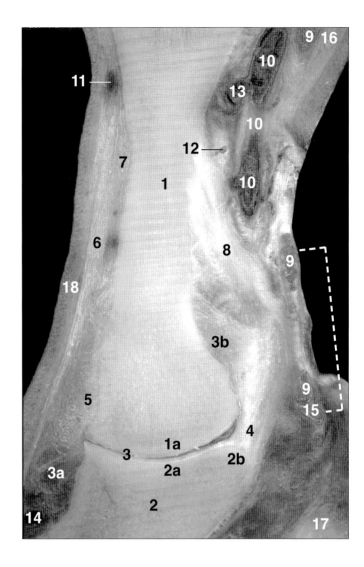

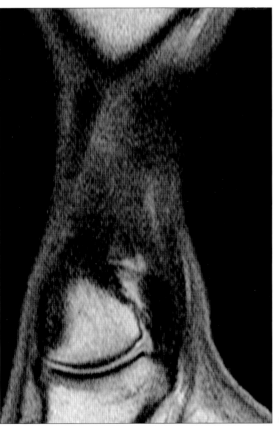

Parasagittal MRI scan of the pastern.

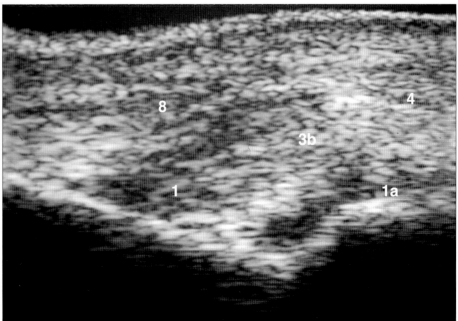

Parasagittal ultrasound scan of the pastern, palmar approach (see dotted area in illustration above).

Transverse Sections of the Equine Pastern

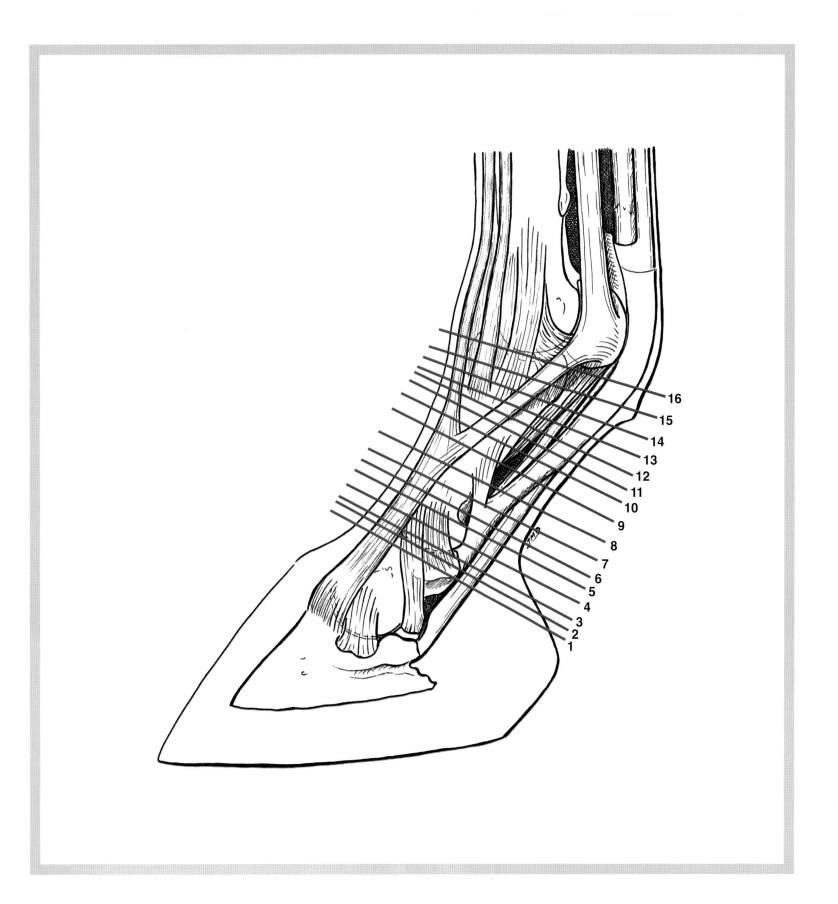

T1: Transverse Section of the Pastern

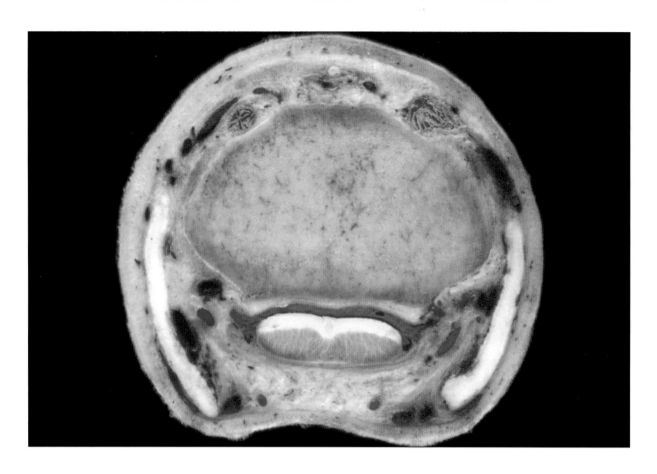

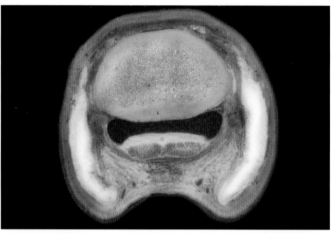

Transverse
anatomical section
after latex
injection into the
digital sheath
cavity and arteries.

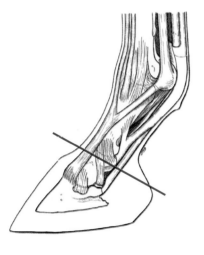

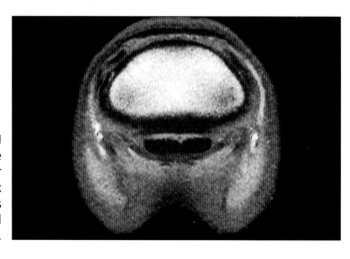

Transverse MRI
scan of the
pastern after
injection of latex
into the arteries
and fat material
into the veins.

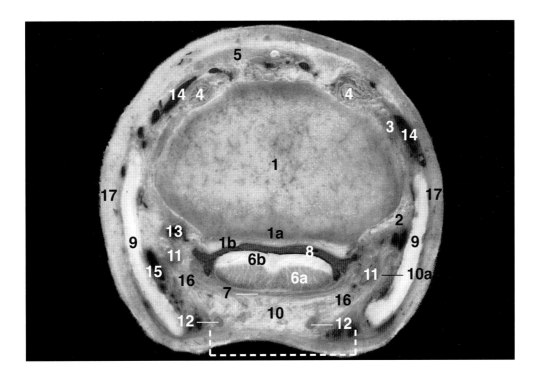

1 Middle phalanx (P2)
  1a Flexor tuberosity
  1b Fibrocartilaginous surface
2 Collateral ligament of the proximal interphalangeal (PIP) joint
3 Collateral sesamoidean ligament
4 Distodorsocollateral recess of the PIP joint
5 Dorsal digital extensor tendon
6 Deep digital flexor tendon
  6a Fibrous part
  6b Phalangeal fibrocartilaginous part
7 Distal digital annular ligament

8 Digital sheath (dorsal distal recess)
9 Ungular cartilage
10 Digital cushion
  10a Proximal attachment
11 Proper palmar digital artery
12 Ramus of digital torus
13 Proper palmar digital vein
14 Dorsal ramus (vein) of P2
15 Deep ungular plexus
16 Proper palmar digital nerve
17 Skin

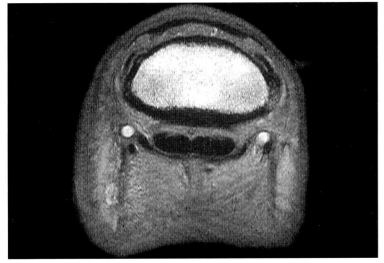

Transverse MRI scan of the pastern after injection of fat material into the arteries and latex into the veins.

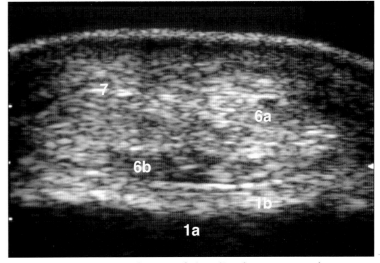

Transverse ultrasound scan of the distal pastern, palmar approach (see dotted area in illustration at top of page).

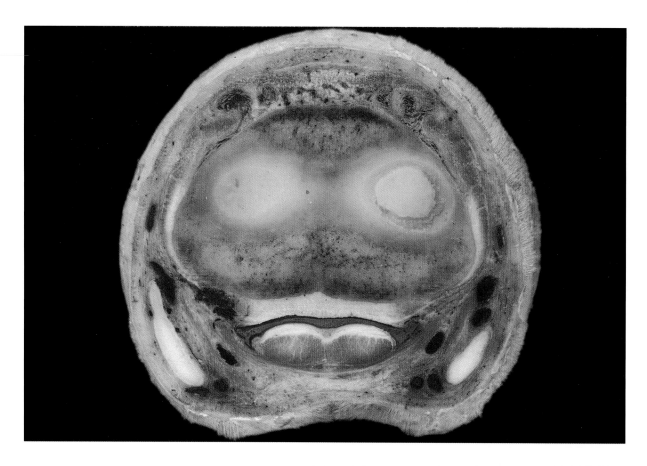

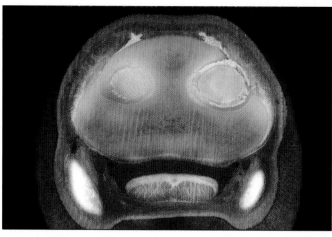

Transverse
anatomical
section after
latex injection
into the
synovial cavities
and arteries.

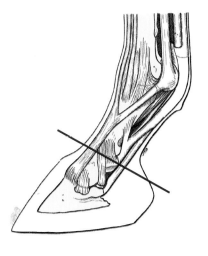

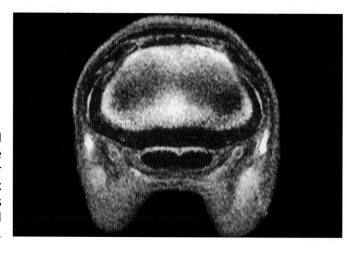

Transverse MRI
scan of the
pastern after
injection of latex
into the arteries
and fat material
into the veins.

T2a: Transverse Section of the Pastern

1 Middle phalanx (P2)
  1a Extensor process
  1b Articular cartilage of the proximal interphalangeal (PIP) joint
  1c Flexor tuberosity
2 Articular cartilage of the proximal phalanx
3 Proximal interphalangeal (PIP) joint space
4 Middle scutum
5 Distodorsocollateral recess of the PIP joint
6 Collateral ligament of the PIP joint
7 Collateral sesamoidean ligament
8 Dorsal digital extensor tendon
9 Deep digital flexor tendon
  9a Fibrous part
  9b Phalangeal fibrocartilaginous part
10 Distal digital annular ligament
11 Dorsal distal recess of the digital sheath
12 Digital cushion
  12a Proximal attachment
13 Ungular cartilage
14 Proper palmar digital artery
15 Proper palmar digital vein
16 Ungular plexus
17 Dorsal ramus (vein) of P2
18 Proper palmar digital nerve
19 Skin

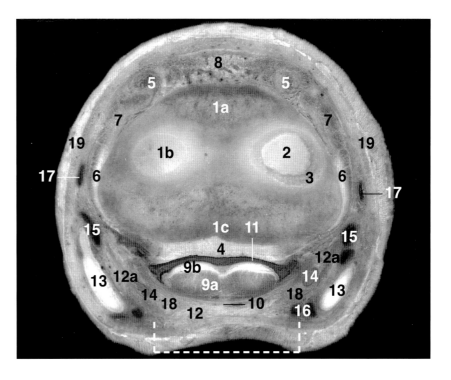

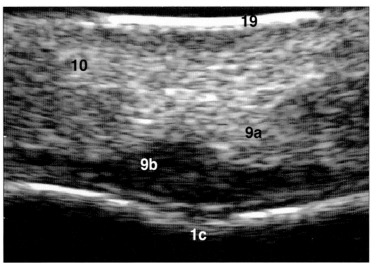

Transverse ultrasound scan of the pastern, palmar approach (see dotted area in illustration above).

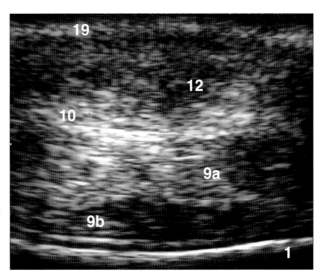

Transverse ultrasound scan of the pastern, palmar approach (see dotted area in illustration at top of page).

T2b: Transverse Section of the Pastern

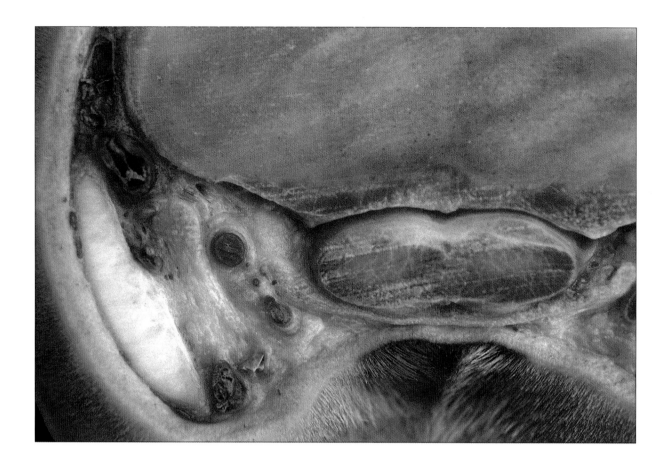

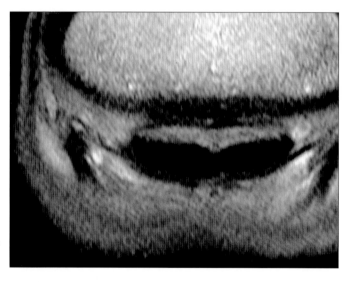

Transverse MRI scan of the pastern.

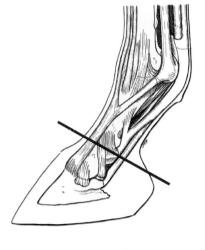

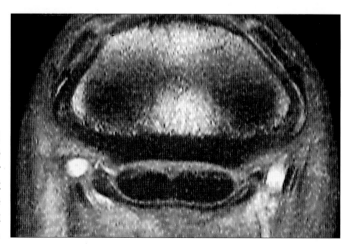

Transverse MRI scan of the pastern after injection of fat material into the arteries and latex into the veins.

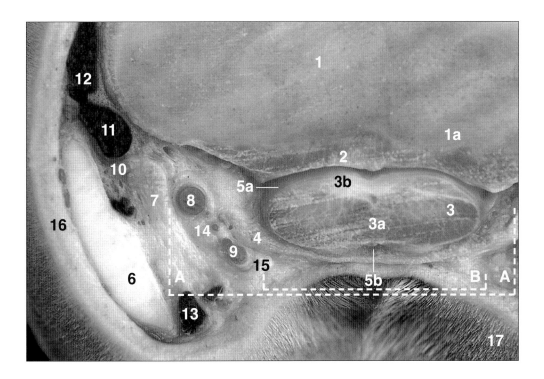

1 Middle phalanx (P2)	**7** Proximal attachment of the digital cushion
1a Flexor tuberosity	**8** Proper palmar digital artery
2 Middle scutum	**9** Ramus of the digital torus
3 Deep digital flexor tendon	**10** Coronal artery
3a Fibrous part	**11** Proper palmar digital vein
3b Phalangeal fibrocartilaginous part	**12** Coronal vein and dorsal ramus of P2
4 Distal digital annular ligament	**13** Ungular plexus
5 Digital sheath	**14** Proper palmar digital nerve
5a Dorsal distal recess	**15** Ramus of the digital torus
5b Mesotendon	**16** Skin
6 Ungular cartilage	**17** Heel

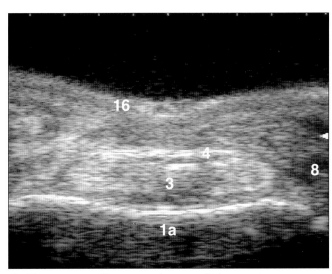

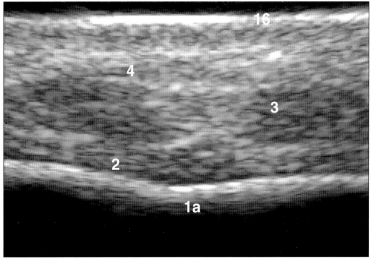

A Transverse ulltrasound scan of the pastern, palmar approach (see dotted area in illustration above).

B Transverse ulltrasound scan of the pastern, palmar approach (see dotted line in illustration above).

T3: Transverse Section of the Pastern

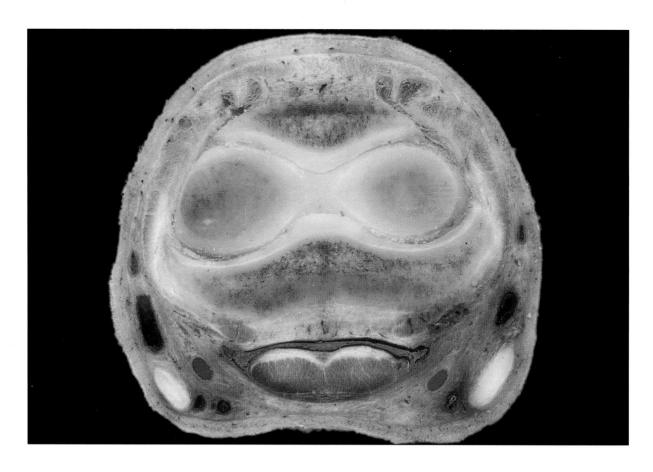

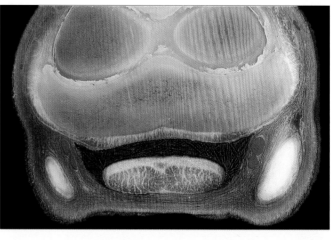

Transverse anatomical section after latex injection into the synovial cavities and arteries.

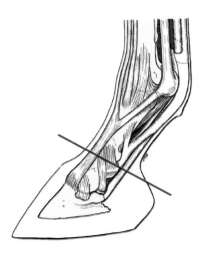

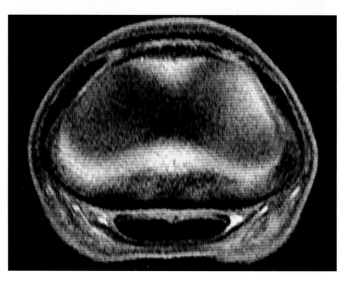

Transverse MRI scan of the pastern.

T3: Transverse Section of the Pastern

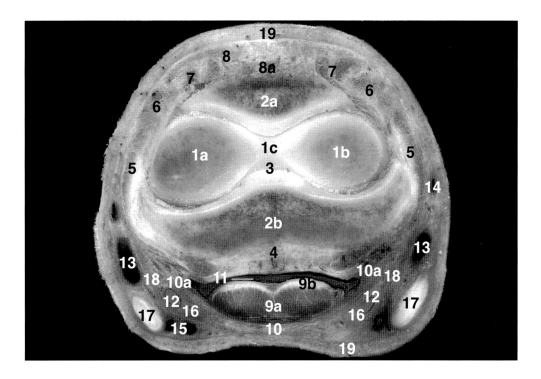

1 Proximal phalanx (distal extremity)
  1a Medial condyle
  1b Lateral condyle
  1c Distal sagittal groove
2 Middle phalanx (P2)
  2a Extensor process
  2b Flexor tuberosity
3 Proximal interphalangeal (PIP) joint
4 Middle scutum
5 Collateral ligament of the PIP joint
6 Collateral sesamoidean ligament
7 Distodorsocollateral recess of the PIP joint
8 Dorsal digital extensor tendon
  8a Insertion on the extensor process of P2
9 Deep digital flexor tendon
  9a Fibrous part
  9b Phalangeal fibrocartilaginous part
10 Distal digital annular ligament
  10a Proximal attachment
11 Digital sheath
12 Proper palmar digital artery
13 Proper palmar digital vein
14 Dorsal ramus (vein) of P2
15 Ungular plexus
16 Proper palmar digital nerve
17 Ungular cartilage
18 Proximal attachment of the digital cushion
19 Skin

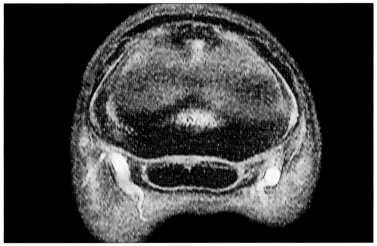

Transverse MRI scan of the pastern after injection of fat material into the arteries and latex into the veins.

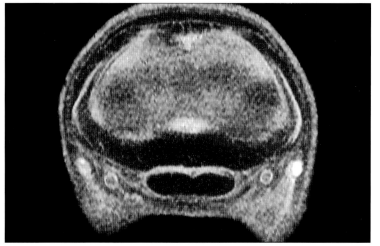

Transverse MRI scan of the pastern after injection of latex into the arteries and fat material into the veins.

T4: Transverse Section of the Pastern

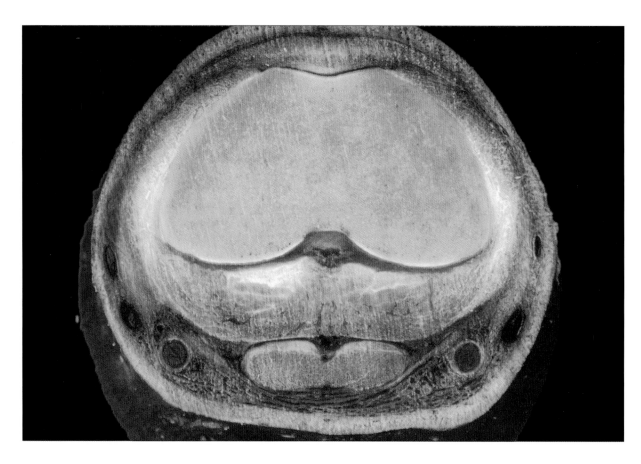

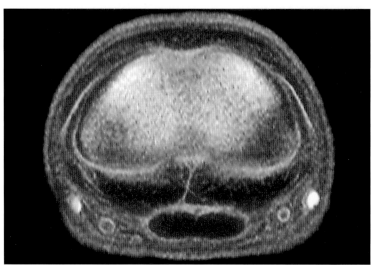

Transverse MRI scan of the pastern after injection of latex into the arteries and fat material into the veins.

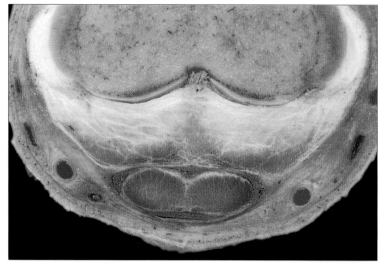

Transverse anatomical section after latex injection into the synovial cavities and vessels.

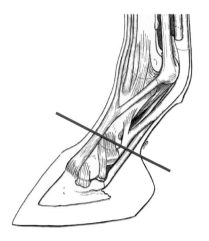

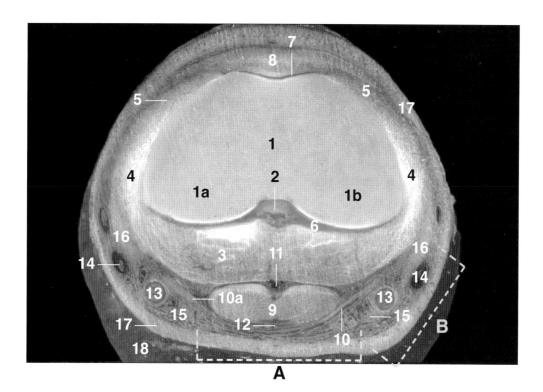

A

1 **Proximal phalanx**
   1a Medial condyle
   1b Lateral condyle
2 Proximal interphalangeal (PIP) joint
3 Middle scutum
4 Collateral ligament of the PIP joint
5 Collateral sesamoidean ligament
6 Palmar recess of the PIP joint
7 Dorsal recess of the PIP joint
8 Dorsal digital extensor tendon
9 Deep digital flexor tendon

10 Distal digital annular ligament
   10a Proximal attachment
11 Digital sheath cavity
12 Mesotendon
13 Proper palmar digital artery
14 Proper palmar digital vein
15 Proper palmar digital nerve
16 Proximal attachment of the digital cushion
17 Skin
18 Heel

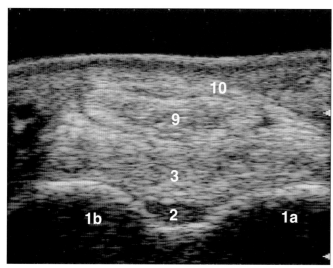

A Transverse ultrasound scan of the pastern, palmar approach (see dotted area in illustration above).

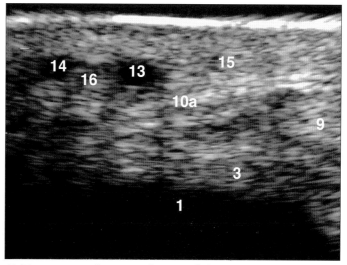

B Transverse ultrasound scan of the pastern, palmarolateral approach (see dotted area in illustration above).

T5: Transverse Section of the Pastern

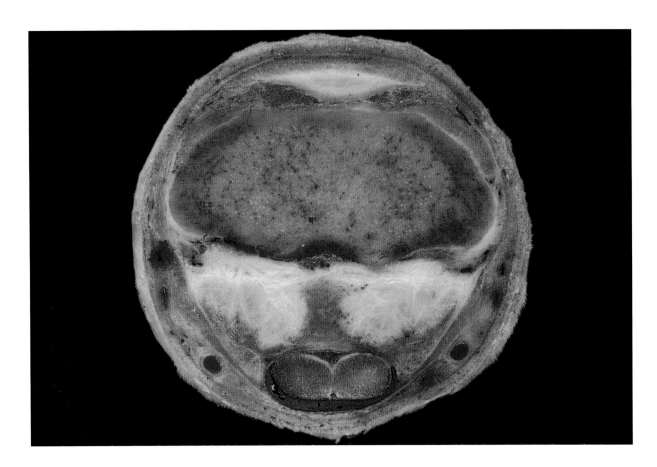

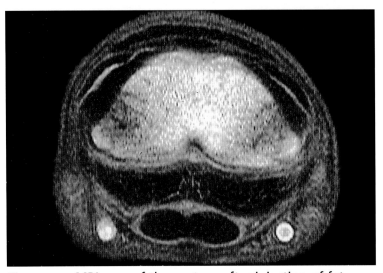

Transverse MRI scan of the pastern after injection of fat material into the arteries and latex into the veins.

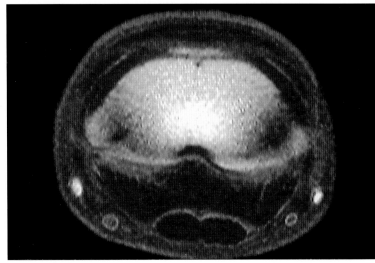

Transverse MRI scan of the pastern after injection of latex into the arteries and fat material into the veins.

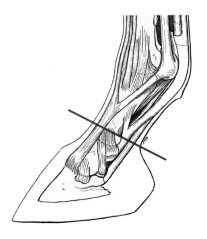

T5: Transverse Section of the Pastern

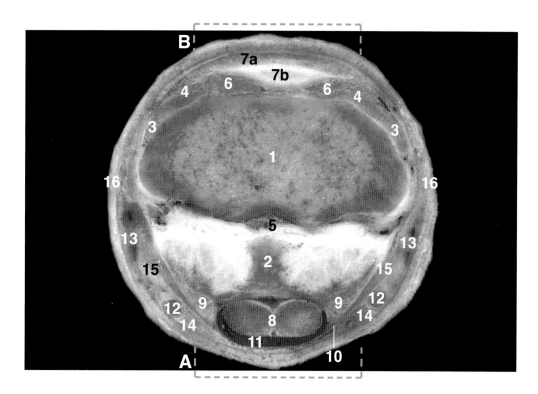

1 Proximal phalanx
2 Middle scutum
3 Collateral ligament of the proximal interphalangeal (PIP) joint
4 Collateral sesamoidean ligament
5 Palmar recess of the PIP joint
6 Dorsal recess of the PIP joint
7 Dorsal digital extensor tendon
   7a Fibrous part
   7b Fibrocartilaginous part
8 Deep digital flexor tendon

9 Superficial digital flexor tendon (distal branch)
10 Distal digital annular ligament
11 Digital sheath cavity (palmar distal recess)
12 Proper palmar digital artery
13 Proper palmar digital vein
14 Proper palmar digital nerve
15 Proximal attachment of the digital cushion and distal digital annular ligament
16 Skin

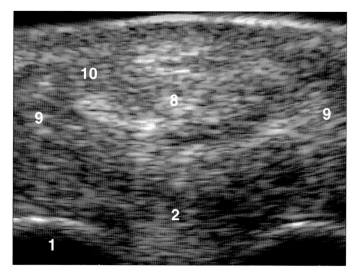

A Transverse ultrasound scan of the pastern, palmar approach (see dotted area in illustration above).

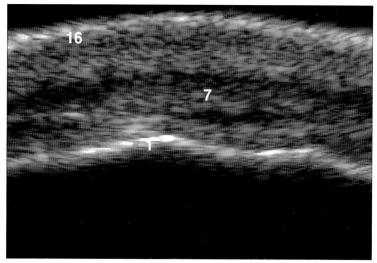

B Transverse ultrasound scan of the pastern, dorsal approach (see dotted area in illustration above).

T6: Transverse Section of the Pastern

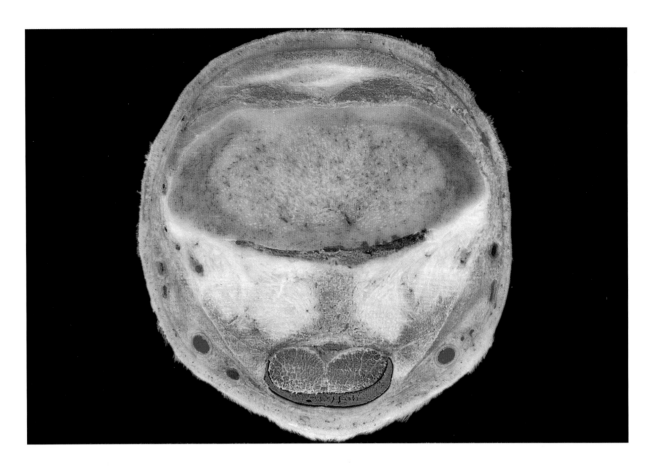

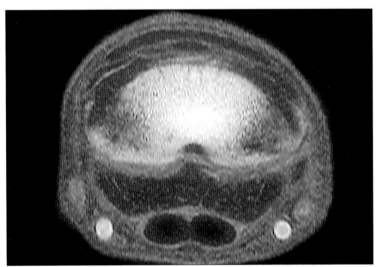

Transverse MRI scan of the pastern after injection of fat material into the arteries and latex into the veins.

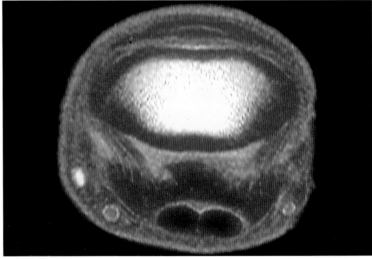

Transverse MRI scan of the pastern after injection of latex into the arteries and fat material into the veins.

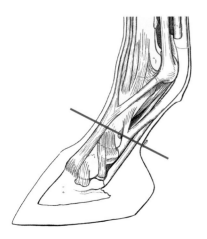

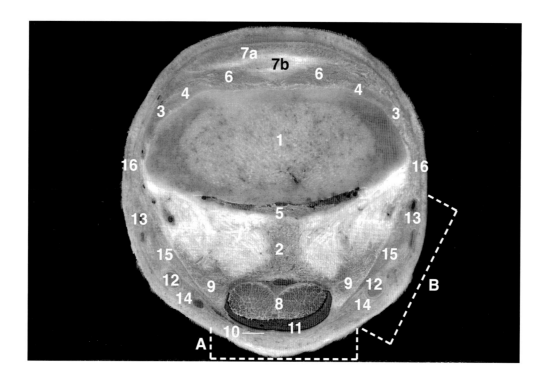

1 Proximal phalanx
2 Middle scutum
3 Collateral ligament of the proximal interphalangeal (PIP) joint
4 Collateral sesamoidean ligament
5 Palmar recess of the PIP joint
6 Dorsal recess of the PIP joint
7 Dorsal digital extensor tendon
  7a Fibrous part
  7b Fibrocartilaginous part
8 Deep digital flexor tendon

9 Superficial digital flexor tendon (distal branch)
10 Distal digital annular ligament
11 Digital sheath cavity (palmar distal recess)
12 Proper palmar digital artery
13 Proper palmar digital vein
14 Proper palmar digital nerve
15 Proximal attachment of the digital cushion and distal digital annular ligament
16 Skin

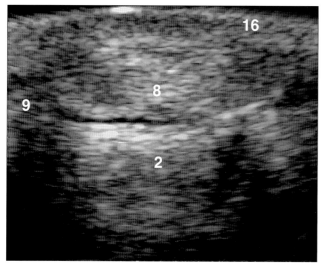

A Transverse ultrasound scan of the pastern, palmar approach (see dotted area in illustration above).

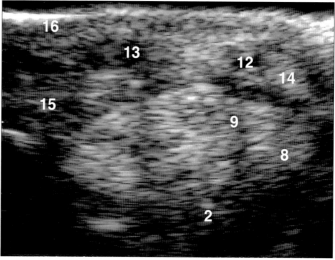

B Transverse ultrasound scan of the pastern, palmarolateral approach (see dotted area in illustration above).

T7: Transverse Section of the Pastern

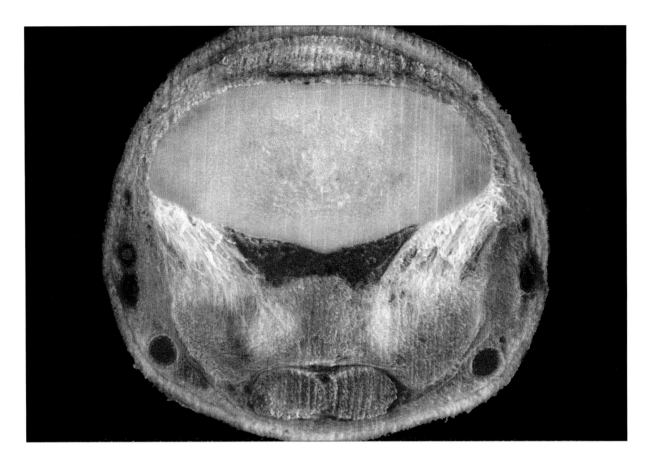

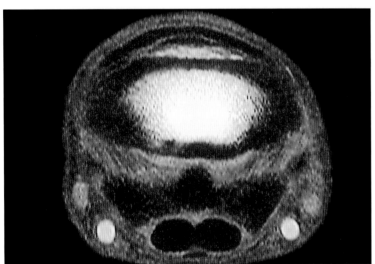

Transverse MRI scan of the pastern after injection of fat material into the arteries and latex into the veins.

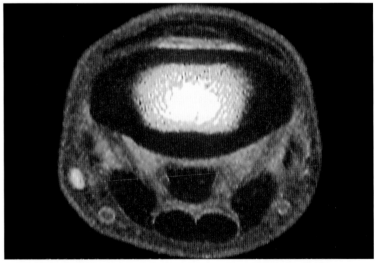

Transverse MRI scan of the pastern after injection of latex into the arteries and fat material into the veins.

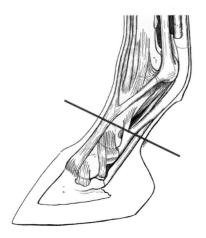

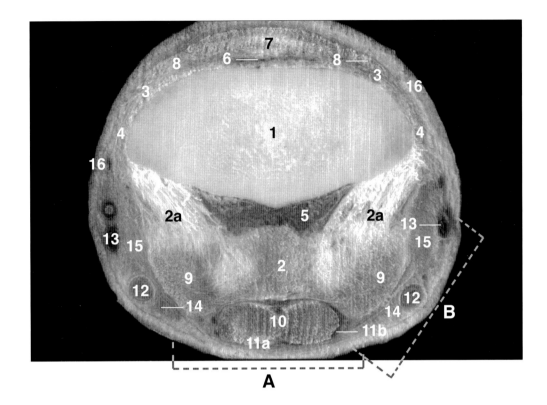

1 Proximal phalanx (P1)
2 Middle scutum
   2a Insertion on P1
3 Collateral sesamoidean ligament
4 Collateral ligament of the proximal
   interphalangeal (PIP) joint
5 Palmar recess of the PIP joint
6 Dorsal recess of the PIP joint
7 Dorsal digital extensor tendon
8 Extensor branch of the third interosseus muscle
9 Superficial digital flexor tendon (distal branch)

10 Deep digital flexor tendon
11 Digital sheath
   11a Wall
   11b Cavity
12 Proper palmar digital artery
13 Proper palmar digital vein
14 Proper palmar digital nerve
15 Abaxial palmar ligament of the PIP joint,
   proximal attachment of the digital cushion
   and distal digital annular ligament
16 Skin

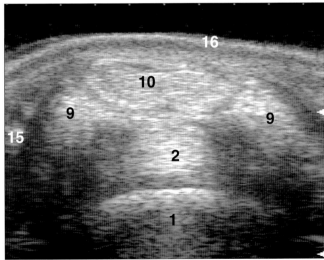

A Transverse ultrasound scan of the pastern, palmar approach (see dotted area in illustration above).

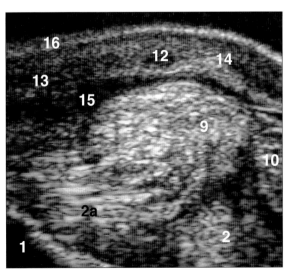

B Transverse ultrasound scan of the pastern, palmarolateral approach (see dotted area in illustration above).

T8: Transverse Section of the Pastern

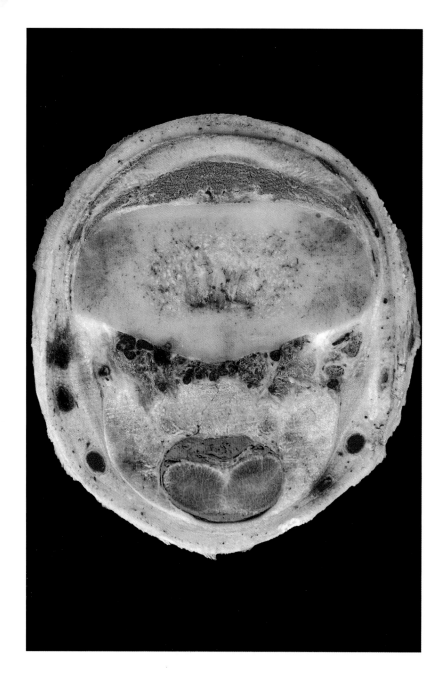

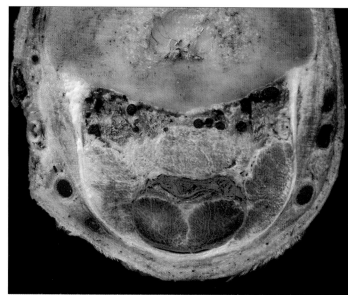

Transverse anatomical section after latex injection into the synovial cavities and vessels.

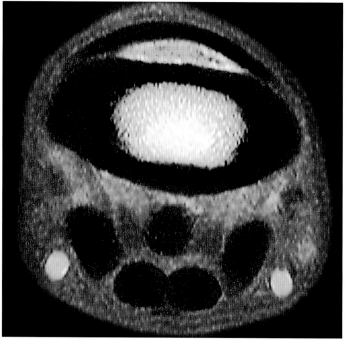

Transverse MRI scan of the pastern after injection of fat material into the arteries and latex into the veins.

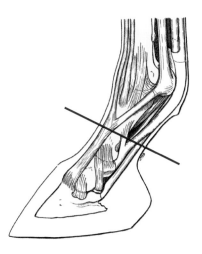

1 Proximal phalanx (P1)
2 Axial palmar ligament of the proximal interphalangeal (PIP) joint
3 Abaxial palmar ligament of the PIP joint
4 Sagittal palmar recess of the PIP joint
5 Collateral palmar recess of the PIP joint
6 Dorsal recess of the PIP joint
7 Straight sesamoidean ligament
8 Dorsal digital extensor tendon
9 Extensor branch of the third interosseus muscle
10 Superficial digital flexor tendon (distal branch)
11 Deep digital flexor tendon
12 Digital sheath cavity
13 Proper palmar digital artery
14 Dorsal ramus of P1
15 Proper palmar digital vein
16 Dorsal ramus of P1
17 Palmar rami of P1
18 Proper palmar digital nerve
   18a Intermediate ramus
19 Ergot ligament
20 Proximal attachment of the digital cushion and distal digital annular ligament
21 Skin

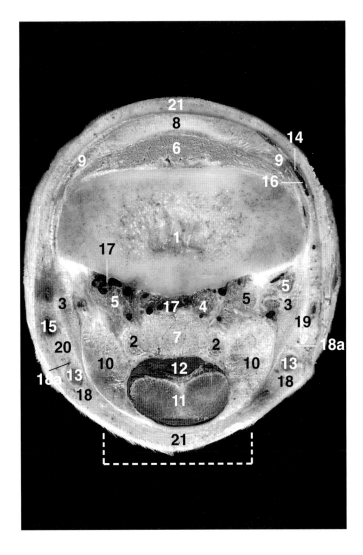

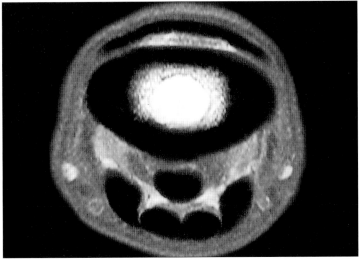

Transverse MRI scan of the pastern after injection of latex into the arteries and fat material into the veins.

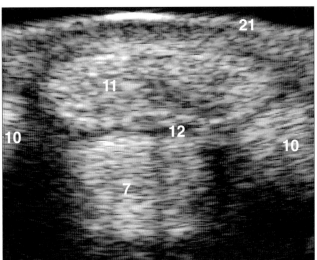

Transverse ultrasound scan of the pastern, palmar approach (see dotted area in illustration above).

T9: Transverse Section of the Pastern

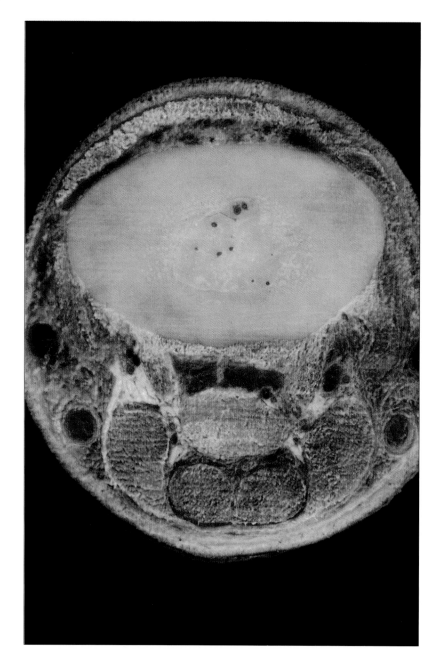

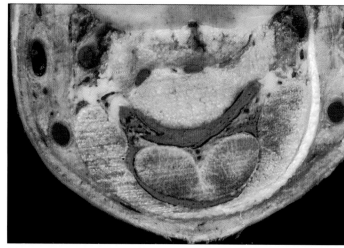

Transverse anatomical section after latex injection into the synovial cavities and vessels.

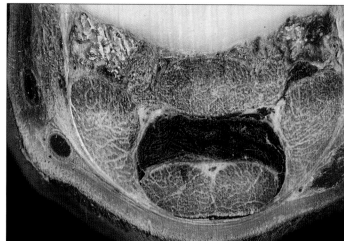

Transverse anatomical section after latex injection into the synovial cavities and arteries.

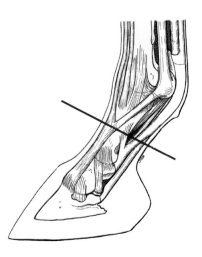

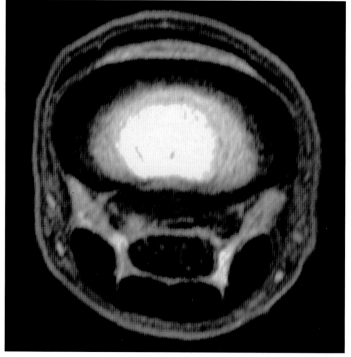

Transverse MRI scan of the pastern.

T9: Transverse Section of the Pastern

1 Proximal phalanx (P1)
2 Oblique sesamoidean ligament
3 Straight sesamoidean ligament
4 Axial palmar ligament of the proximal interphalangeal (PIP) joint
5 Abaxial palmar ligament of the PIP joint
6 Sagittal palmar recess of the PIP joint
7 Dorsal digital extensor tendon
8 Extensor branch of the third interosseus muscle
9 Superficial digital flexor tendon (distal branch)
10 Deep digital flexor tendon
11 Proximal digital annular ligament
12 Digital sheath
    12a Wall
    12b Cavity
13 Proper palmar digital artery
14 Dorsal ramus of P1
15 Palmar ramus of P1
16 Proper palmar digital vein
17 Dorsal ramus of P1
18 Palmar ramus of P1
19 Proper palmar digital nerve
    19a Intermediate ramus
20 Proximal attachment of the digital cushion and distal digital annular ligament
21 Skin

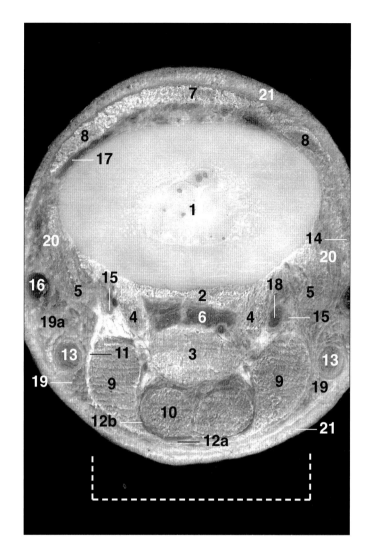

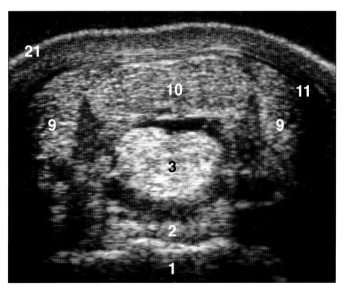

Transverse ultrasound scan of the pastern, palmar approach (see dotted area in illustration above, right).

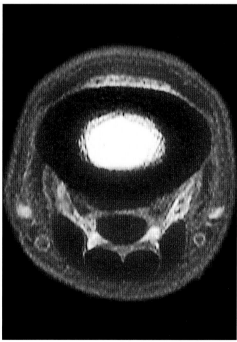

Transverse MRI scan of the pastern after injection of latex into the arteries and fat material into the veins.

T10: Transverse Section of the Pastern

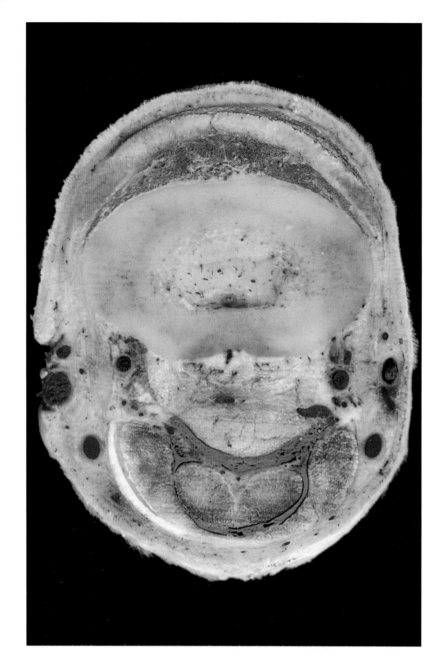

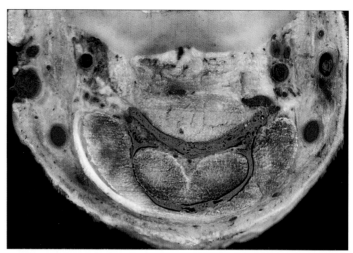

Transverse anatomical section after latex injection into the synovial cavities and vessels.

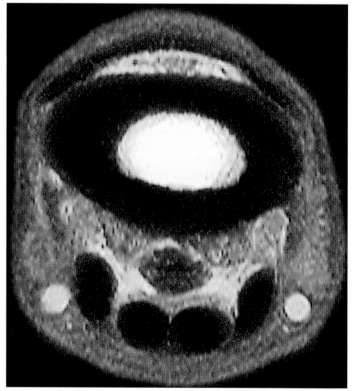

Transverse MRI scan of the pastern after injection of fat material into the arteries and latex into the veins.

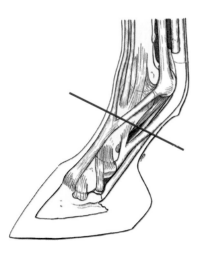

1 Proximal phalanx (P1)
2 Oblique sesamoidean ligament
3 Straight sesamoidean ligament
4 Axial palmar ligament of the proximal interphalangeal (PIP) joint
5 Abaxial palmar ligament of the PIP joint
6 Dorsal recess of the PIP joint
7 Sagittal palmar recess of the PIP joint
8 Dorsal digital extensor tendon
9 Extensor branch of the third interosseus muscle
10 Superficial digital flexor tendon
    10a Distal branch
    10b Sagittal part
11 Deep digital flexor tendon
12 Proximal digital annular ligament
13 Digital sheath
    13a Cavity
    13b Synovial fold (mesotendon)
14 Proper palmar digital artery
15 Palmar ramus of P1
16 Proper palmar digital vein
17 Palmar ramus of P1
18 Proper palmar digital nerve
    18a Intermediate ramus
19 Proximal attachment of the digital cushion and distal digital annular ligament
20 Skin
21 Artefact: subcutaneous reflux of latex

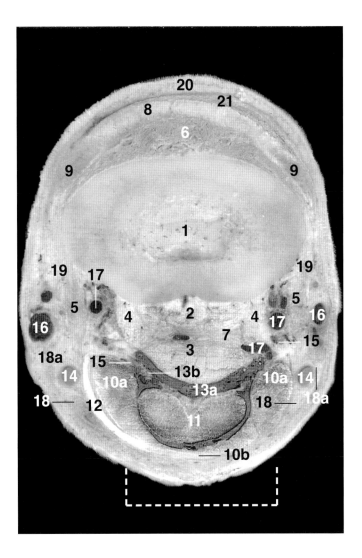

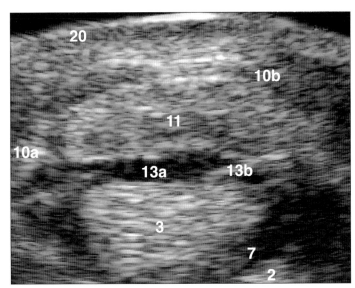

Transverse ultrasound scan of the pastern, palmar approach (see dotted area in illustration above, right).

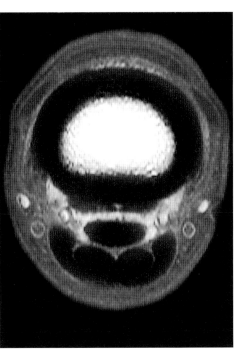

Transverse MRI scan of the pastern after injection of latex into the arteries and fat material into the veins.

T11: Transverse Section of the Pastern

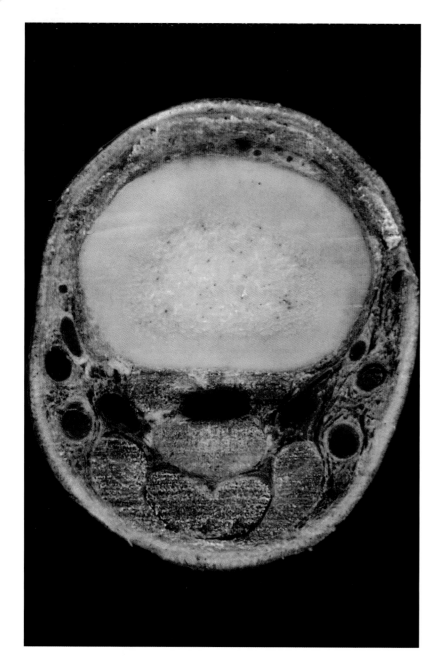

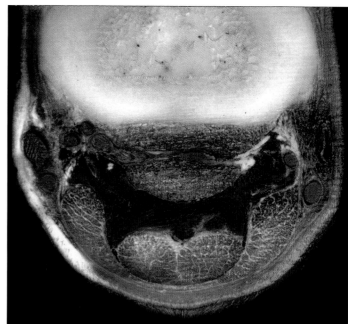

Transverse anatomical section after latex injection into the synovial cavities and vessels.

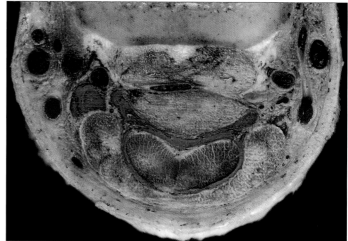

Transverse anatomical section after latex injection into the synovial cavities and vessels.

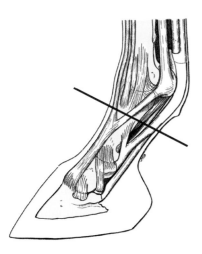

1 Proximal phalanx (P1)
2 Oblique sesamoidean ligament
3 Straight sesamoidean ligament
4 Abaxial palmar ligament of the proximal interphalangeal joint
5 Dorsal digital extensor tendon
6 Extensor branch of the third interosseus muscle
7 Superficial digital flexor tendon
  7a Distal branch
  7b Sagittal part
8 Deep digital flexor tendon
9 Proximal digital annular ligament
10 Digital sheath cavity
11 Proper palmar digital artery
12 Dorsal ramus (artery) of P1
13 Proper palmar digital vein
14 Palmar ramus (vein) of P1
15 Proper palmar digital nerve
16 Skin

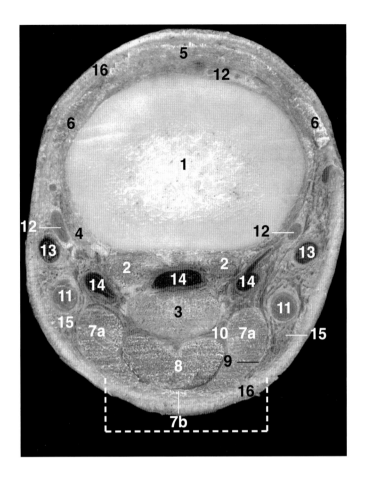

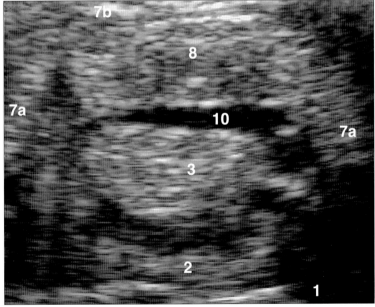

Transverse ultrasound scan of the pastern, palmar approach (see dotted area in illustration above, right).

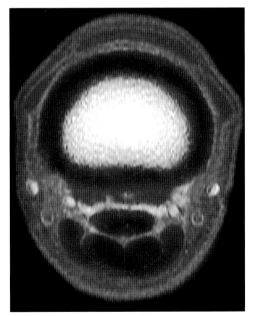

Transverse MRI scan of the pastern after injection of latex into the arteries and fat material into the veins.

T12: Transverse Section of the Pastern

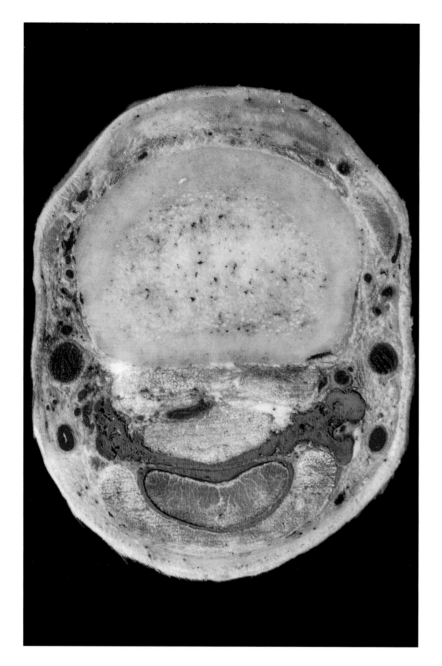

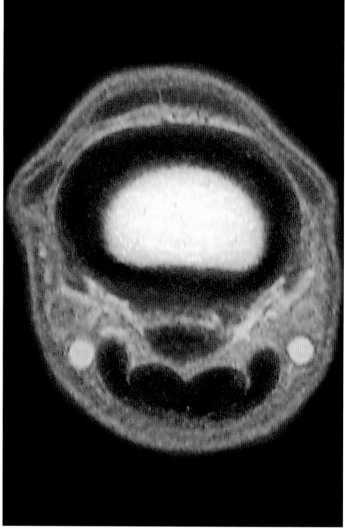

Transverse MRI scan of the pastern after injection of fat material into the arteries and latex into the veins.

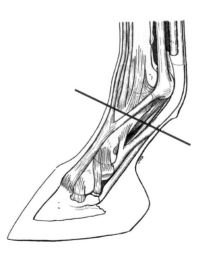

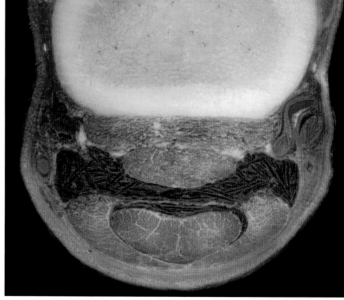

Transverse anatomical section after latex injection into the synovial cavities and vessels.

1 Proximal phalanx (P1)
2 Oblique sesamoidean ligament
3 Straight sesamoidean ligament
4 Dorsal recess of the proximal interphalangeal joint
5 Dorsal digital extensor tendon
6 Extensor branch of the third interosseus muscle
7 Superficial digital flexor tendon
  7a Distal branch
  7b Sagittal part
8 Deep digital flexor tendon
9 Proximal digital annular ligament
10 Digital sheath
  10a Cavity (collateral recess)
  10b Synovial fold
11 Proper palmar digital artery
12 Dorsal ramus (artery) of P1
13 Proper palmar digital vein
14 Dorsal ramus (vein) of P1
15 Palmar ramus (vein) of P1
16 Proper palmar digital nerve
17 Skin

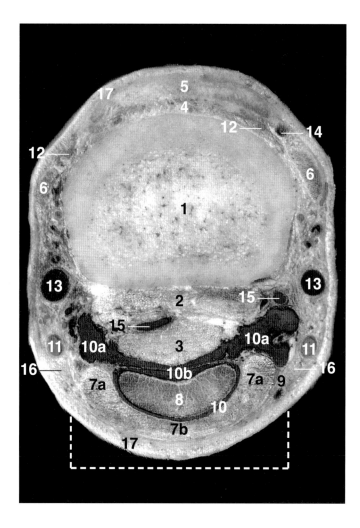

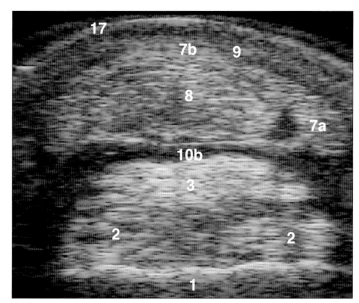

Transverse ultrasound scan of the pastern, palmar approach (see dotted area in illustration above, right).

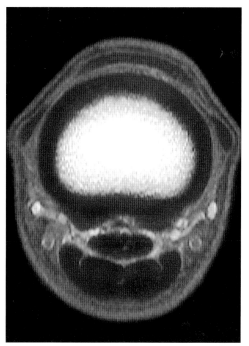

Transverse MRI scan of the pastern after injection of latex into the arteries and fat material into the veins.

T13: Transverse Section of the Pastern

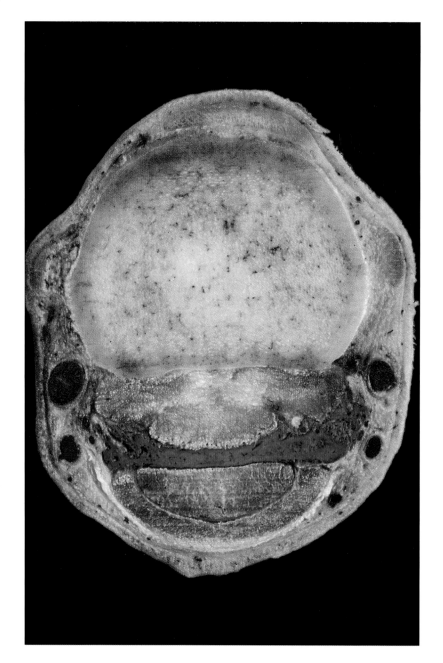

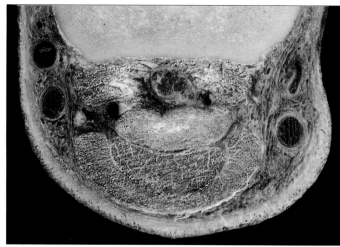

Transverse anatomical section after injection of latex into the arteries.

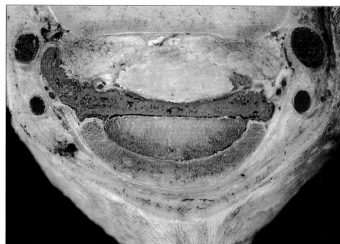

Transverse anatomical section after latex injection into the synovial cavities and vessels.

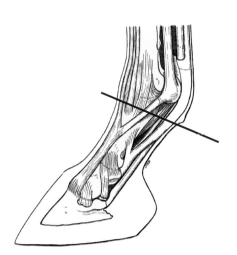

Transverse MRI scan of the pastern.

1 Proximal phalanx (P1)
2 Oblique sesamoidean ligament
  2a Sagittal part
3 Straight sesamoidean ligament
4 Distal insertion of the collateral ligament of the metacarpophalangeal joint
5 Dorsal digital extensor tendon
6 Extensor branch of the third interosseus muscle
7 Superficial digital flexor tendon
8 Deep digital flexor tendon
9 Proximal digital annular ligament
10 Digital sheath cavity
  10a Collateral recess
  10b Synovial fold
11 Proper palmar digital artery
12 Dorsal ramus (artery) of P1
13 Palmar ramus (artery) of P1
14 Proper palmar digital vein
15 Palmar ramus (vein) of P1
16 Proper palmar digital nerve
17 Skin

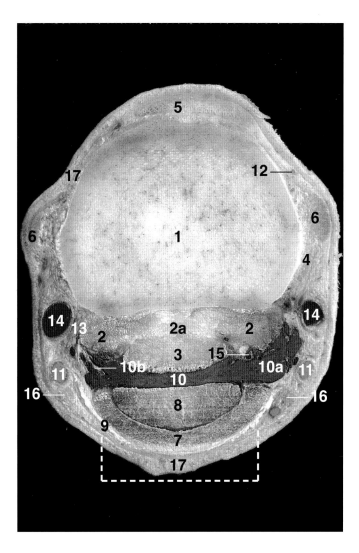

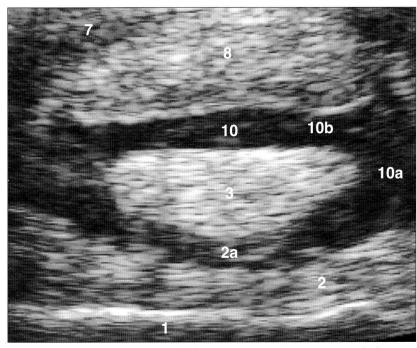

Transverse ultrasound scan of the pastern, palmar approach (see dotted area in illustration above, right).

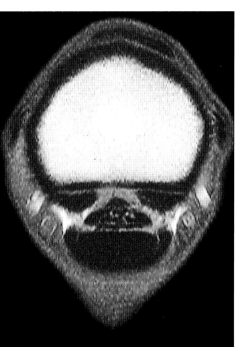

Transverse MRI scan of the pastern after injection of latex into the arteries and fat material into the veins.

T14: Transverse Section of the Pastern

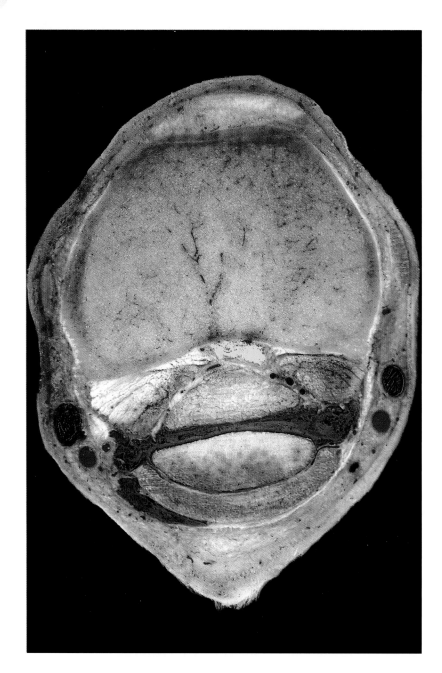

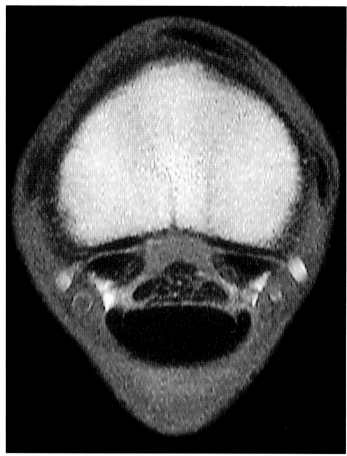

Transverse MRI scan of the pastern after injection of latex into the arteries and fat material into the veins.

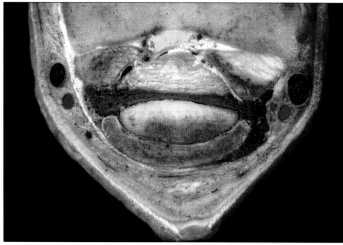

Transverse anatomical section after latex injection into the synovial cavities and vessels.

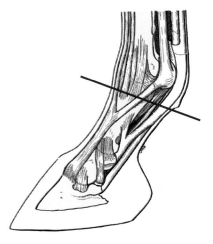

1 Proximal phalanx (P1)
2 Distal insertion of the collateral ligament of the metacarpophalangeal (MP) joint
3 Distal insertion of the dorsal articular capsule of the MP joint
4 Cruciate sesamoidean ligament
5 Oblique sesamoidean ligament
   5a Sagittal part
6 Straight sesamoidean ligament
7 Distopalmar recess of the MP joint
8 Dorsal digital extensor tendon
9 Extensor branch of the third interosseus muscle
10 Superficial digital flexor tendon
11 Deep digital flexor tendon
12 Proximal digital annular ligament
13 Digital sheath cavity
   13a Collateral recess
   13b Palmar middle recess
14 Proper palmar digital artery
15 Palmar ramus (artery) of P1
16 Proper palmar digital vein
17 Palmar ramus (vein) of P1
18 Proper palmar digital nerve
   18a Dorsal ramus
   18b Intermediate ramus
19 Ergot
   19a Ergot cushion
20 Skin

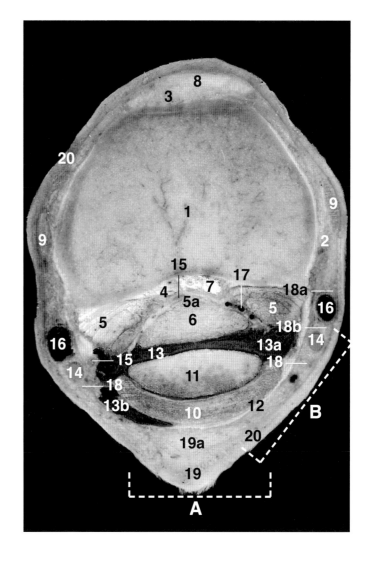

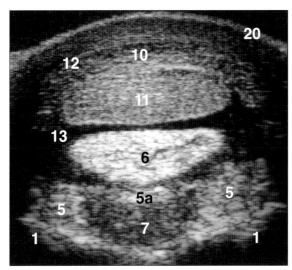

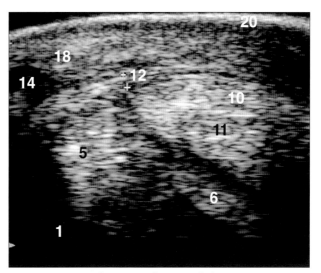

A Transverse ultrasound scan of the pastern, palmar approach (see dotted area in illustration above, right).

B Transverse ultrasound scan of the pastern, palmarolateral approach (see dotted area in illustration above).

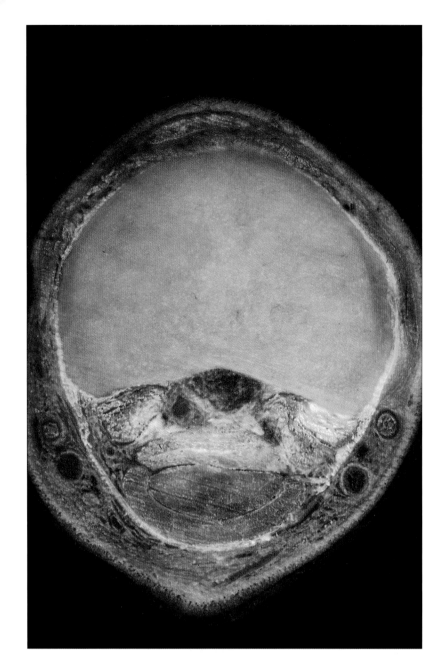

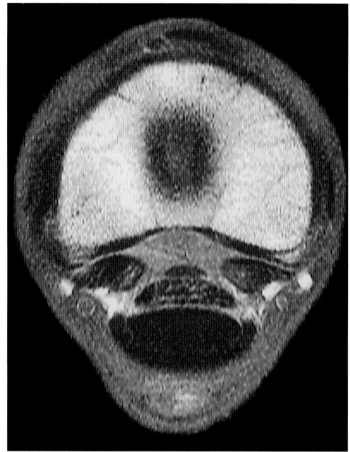

Transverse MRI scan of the pastern after injection of latex into the arteries and fat material into the veins.

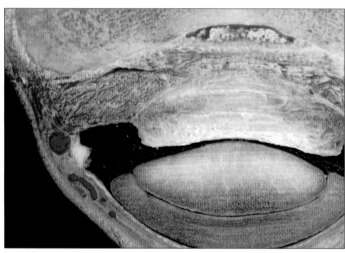

Transverse anatomical section after latex injection into the synovial cavities and vessels.

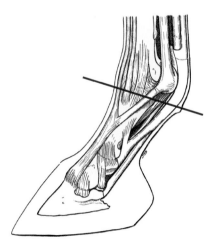

1 Proximal phalanx (P1)
2 Distal insertion of the collateral ligament of the metacarpophalangeal (MP) joint
3 Distal insertion of the dorsal articular capsule of the MP joint
4 Cruciate sesamoidean ligament
5 Oblique sesamoidean ligament
   5a Sagittal part
6 Straight sesamoidean ligament
7 Distopalmar recess of the MP joint
8 Dorsal digital extensor tendon
9 Extensor branch of the third interosseus muscle
10 Superficial digital flexor tendon
11 Deep digital flexor tendon
12 Proximal digital annular ligament
13 Digital sheath cavity
14 Proper palmar digital artery
15 Dorsal ramus (artery) of P1
16 Palmar ramus (artery) of P1
17 Ergot ramus
18 Proper palmar digital vein
19 Proper palmar digital nerve
20 Ergot cushion
21 Skin

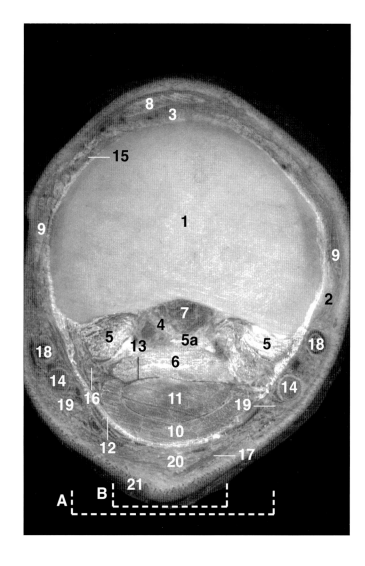

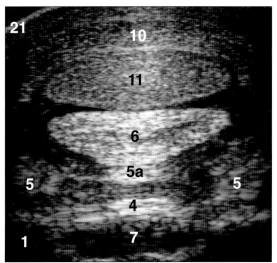

A Transverse ultrasound scan of the pastern, palmar approach (see dotted area in illustration above, right).

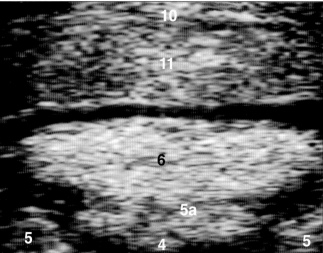

B Transverse ultrasound scan of the pastern, palmar approach (see dotted area in illustration above).

T16: Transverse Section of the Pastern

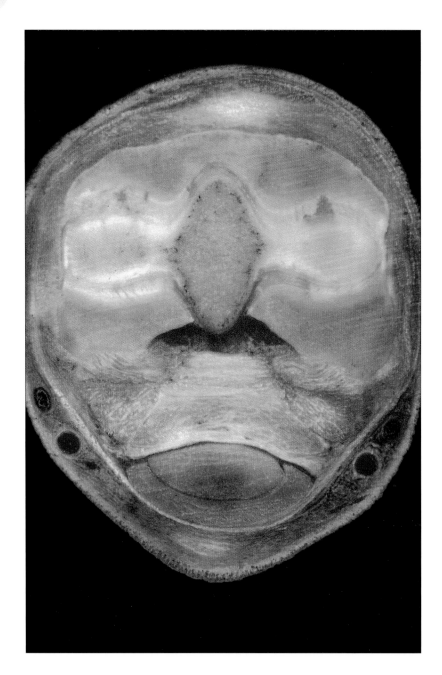

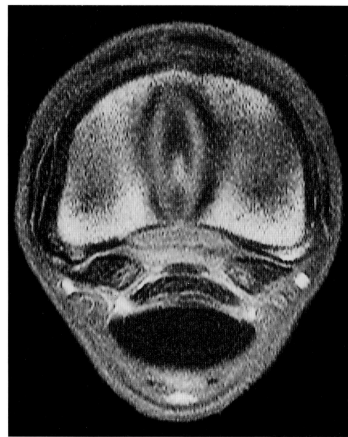

Transverse MRI scan of the pastern after injection of latex into the arteries and fat material into the veins.

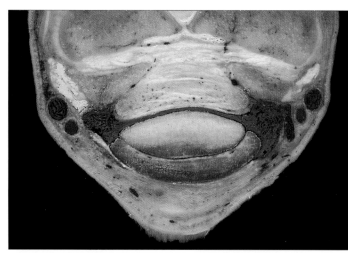

Transverse anatomical section after latex injection into the synovial cavities and vessels.

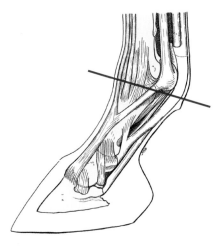

1 Metacarpal condyle
  1a Sagittal ridge
  1b Medial part
  1c Lateral part
2 Proximal phalanx
  2a Medial palmar eminence
  2b Lateral palmar eminence
3 Metacarpophalangeal (MP) joint
4 Dorsal articular capsule of the MP joint
5 Collateral ligament of the MP joint
6 Palmar (intersesamoidean) ligament
7 Cruciate sesamoidean ligament
8 Short sesamoidean ligament
9 Oblique sesamoidean ligament
10 Straight sesamoidean ligament
11 Distopalmar recess of the MP joint
12 Collateral recess of the MP joint
13 Dorsal digital extensor tendon
14 Lateral digital extensor tendon
15 Extensor branch of the third interosseus
  muscle
16 Superficial digital flexor tendon
17 Deep digital flexor tendon
18 Proximal digital annular ligament
19 Digital sheath cavity
20 Proper palmar digital artery
21 Ergot ramus
22 Proper palmar digital vein
23 Proper palmar digital nerve
24 Ergot cushion
25 Skin

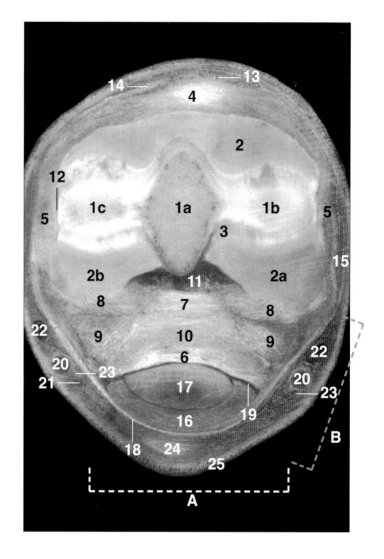

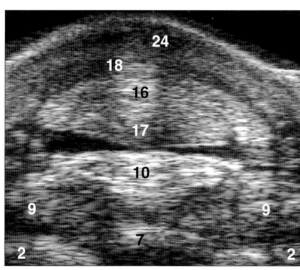

A Transverse ultrasound scan of the pastern, palmar approach (see dotted area in illustration above, right).

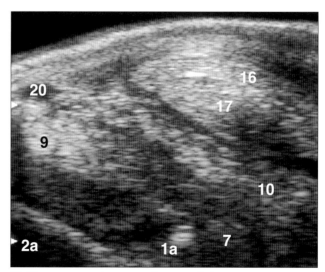

B Transverse ultrasound scan of the pastern, palmaromedial approach (see dotted area in illustration above).

Frontal Sections of the Equine Pastern

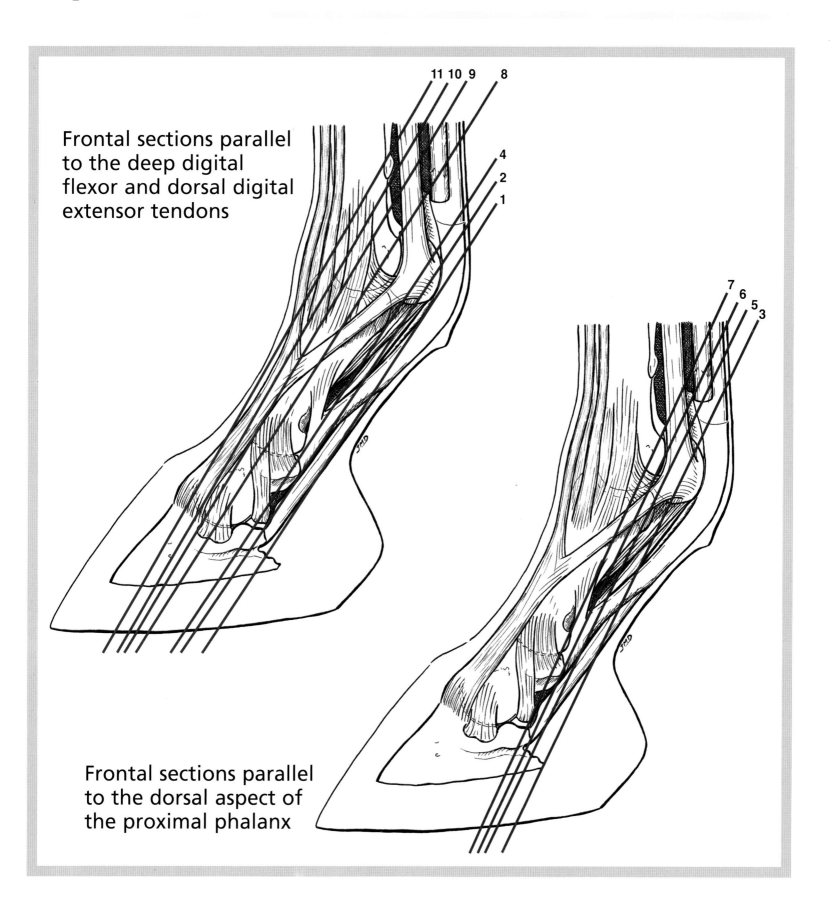

Frontal sections parallel to the deep digital flexor and dorsal digital extensor tendons

Frontal sections parallel to the dorsal aspect of the proximal phalanx

F1: Frontal Section of the Pastern

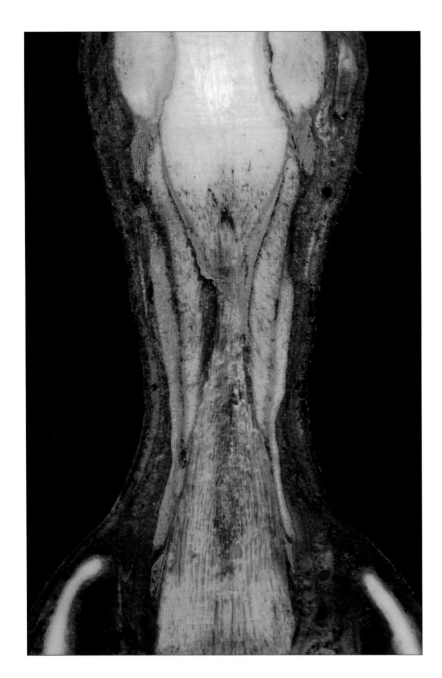

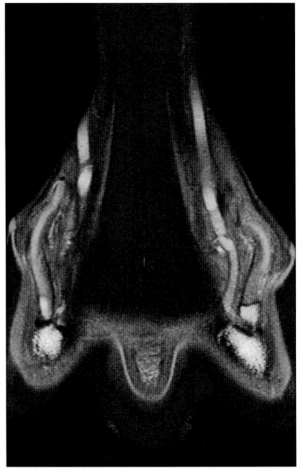

Frontal MRI scan of the pastern after injection of fat material into the arteries and latex into the veins.

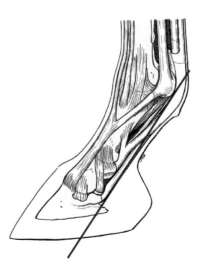

Frontal anatomical section of the pastern and foot after injection of coloured latex into the vessels.

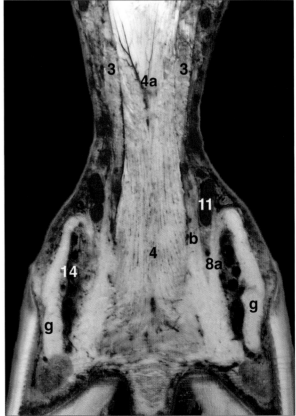

1 Lateral proximal sesamoid bone
2 Medial proximal sesamoid bone
3 Superficial digital flexor tendon
  3a Distal branch
4 Deep digital flexor tendon
  4a Vascular supply
5 Proximal digital annular ligament
6 Distal digital annular ligament
7 Digital sheath cavity
  7a Collateral recess
8 Digital cushion
  8a Proximal attachment
9 Ungular cartilage
10 Lateral proper palmar digital artery
11 Medial proper palmar digital artery
12 Ramus of the digital cushion
13 Ergot ramus (vein)
14 Deep ungular plexus
15 Lateral proper palmar digital nerve
16 Ergot ramus (nerve)
17 Skin

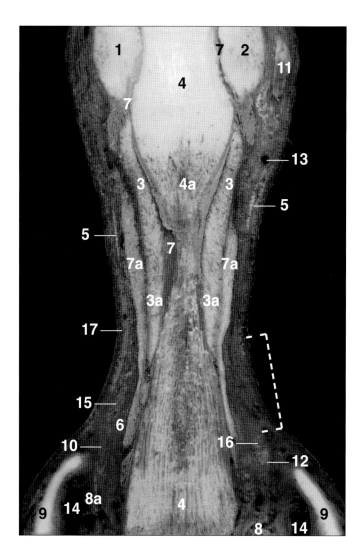

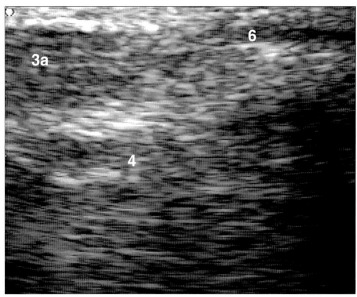

Frontal ultrasound scan of the deep digital flexor tendon, lateral approach (see dotted area in illustration above, right).

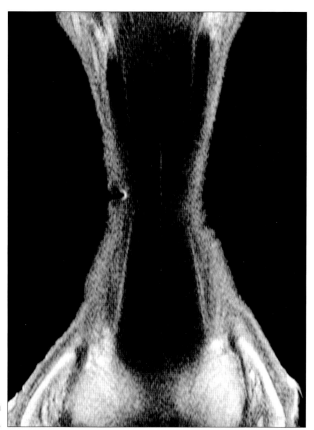

Frontal MRI scan of the pastern.

F2: Frontal Section of the Pastern

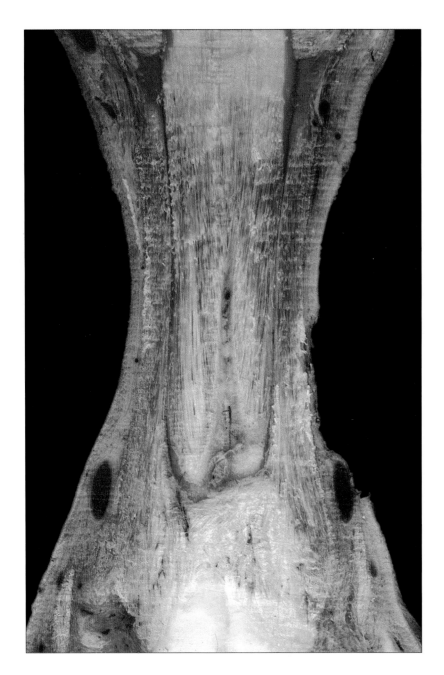

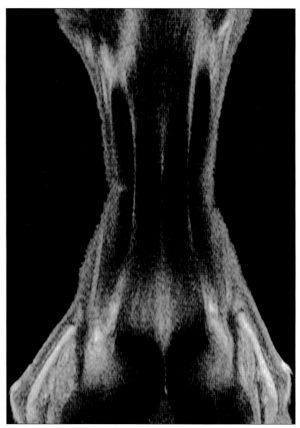

Frontal MRI scan of the pastern.

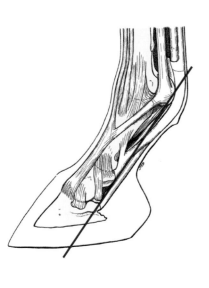

Frontal anatomical section
after injection of coloured
latex into the synovial
cavities and vessels.

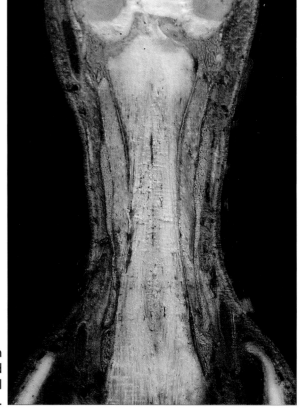

1 Palmar (intersesamoidean) ligament
2 Middle scutum
3 Superficial digital flexor tendon
   3a Distal branch
4 Deep digital flexor tendon
   4a Phalangeal fibrocartilaginous part
   4b Metacarpophalangeal fibrocartilaginous
      part
5 Digital sheath cavity
   5a Collateral recess
   5b Dorsal distal recess
6 Proper palmar digital artery
7 Ergot ramus (artery)
8 Ergot ramus (vein)
9 Proximal attachment of the digital cushion
10 Skin

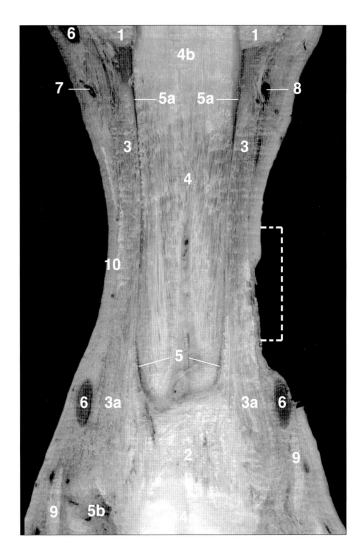

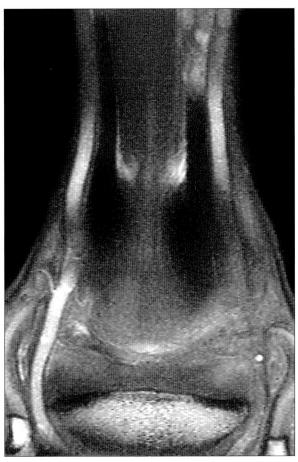

Frontal MRI scan of the pastern after injection of fat material into the arteries and latex into the veins.

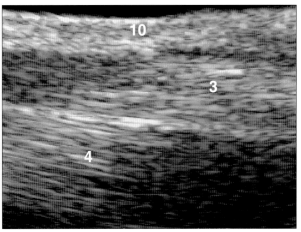

Frontal ultrasound scan of the digital flexor tendons, lateral approach (see dotted area in illustration above).

F3: Frontal Section of the Pastern

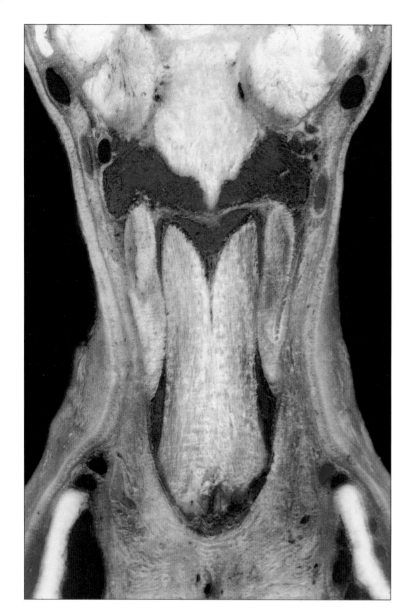

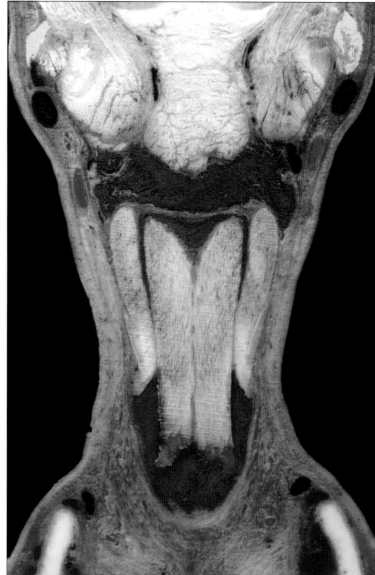

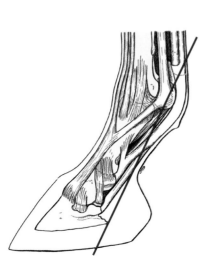

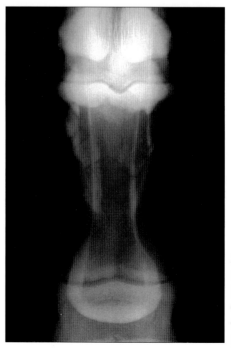

In vivo contrast radiographic study (tenography) of the digital sheath, dorsopalmar projection.

1 Palmar eminence of the proximal phalanx (P1)
2 Palmar (intersesamoidean) ligament
3 Oblique sesamoidean ligament
4 Straight sesamoidean ligament
5 Distocollateral recess of the metacarpophalangeal joint
6 Superficial digital flexor tendon (distal branches)
7 Deep digital flexor tendon
8 Proximal digital annular ligament
    8a Proximal insertion
    8b Distal insertion
9 Distal digital annular ligament
10 Digital sheath
    10a Collateral recess
    10b Synovial fold
    10c Palmar distal recess
11 Digital cushion (toric part)
    11a Proximal attachment
12 Ungular cartilage
13 Proper palmar digital artery
14 Ramus of the digital torus
15 Proper palmar digital vein
16 Palmar rami (artery and vein) of P1
17 Ungular plexus
    17a Deep ungular plexus
    17b Superficial ungular plexus
18 Proper palmar digital nerve
19 Skin

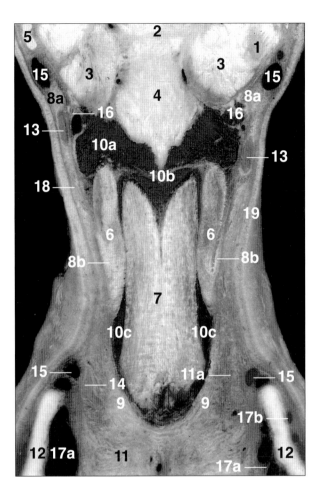

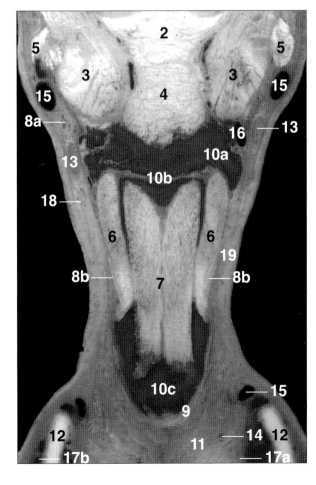

F4: Frontal Section of the Pastern

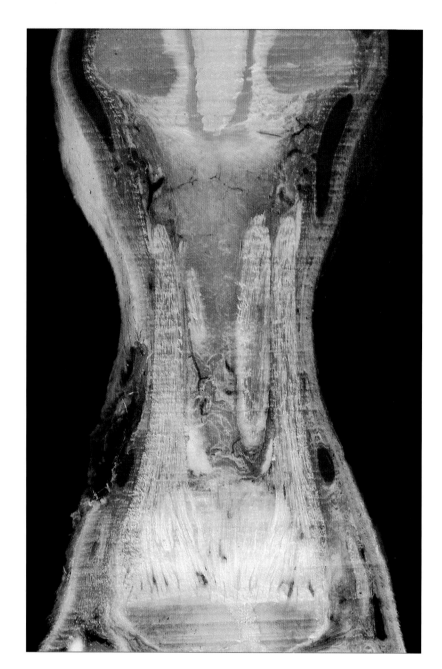

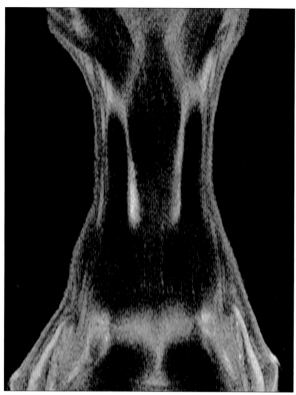

Frontal MRI scan of the pastern.

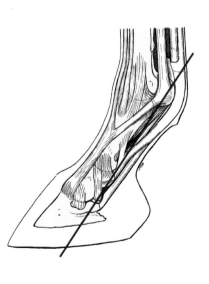

Frontal anatomical section after injection of coloured latex into the synovial cavities and vessels.

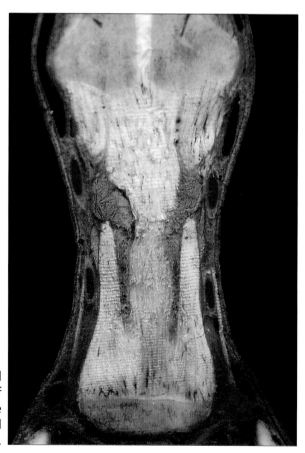

F4: Frontal Section of the Pastern

1 Lateral proximal sesamoid bone
2 Medial proximal sesamoid bone
3 Middle phalanx (flexor tuberosity)
4 Palmar (intersesamoidean) ligament
5 Oblique sesamoidean ligament
6 Straight sesamoidean ligament
7 Middle scutum
8 Deep digital flexor tendon
9 Superficial digital flexor tendon
  9a Distal branch
10 Proximal digital annular ligament
11 Digital sheath (synovial cavity)
12 Lateral proper digital artery
13 Medial proper digital artery
14 Medial proper palmar digital vein
15 Palmar ramus (vein) of the proximal phalanx
16 Proximal attachment of the digital cushion
17 Skin

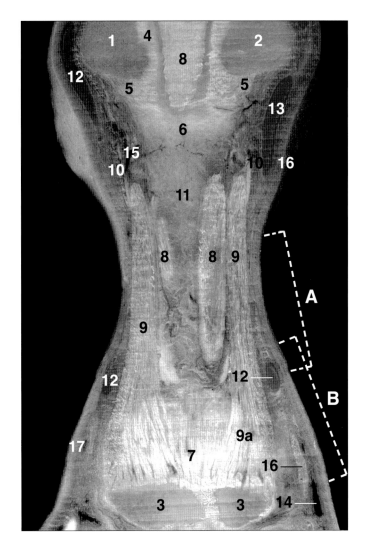

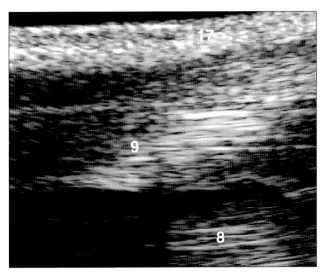

A Frontal ultrasound scan of the digital flexor tendons, lateral approach (see dotted area in illustration above, right).

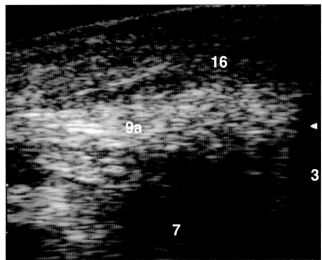

B Frontal ultrasound scan of the digital flexor tendons, lateral approach (see dotted area in illustration above).

F5: Frontal Section of the Pastern

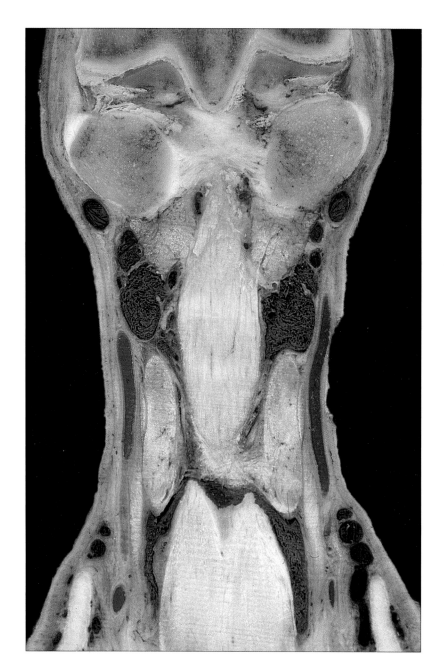

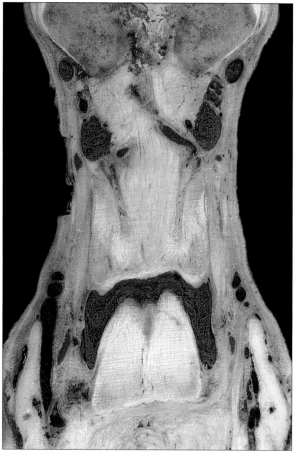

Frontal anatomical section after injection of coloured latex into the synovial cavities and vessels.

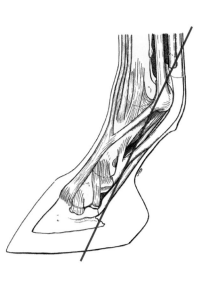

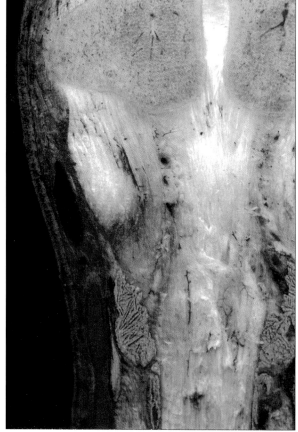

Frontal anatomical section after injection of coloured latex into the synovial cavities and vessels.

F5: Frontal Section of the Pastern

1 Metacarpal condyle
2 Proximal phalanx (P1)
   2a Lateral palmar eminence
   2b Medial palmar eminence
3 Lateral proximal sesamoid bone (base)
4 Medial proximal sesamoid bone (base)
5 Palmar (intersesamoidean) ligament
6 Cruciate sesamoidean ligament
7 Oblique sesamoidean ligament
8 Straight sesamoidean ligament
9 Collateral sesamoidean ligament of the metacarpophalangeal (MP) joint
10 Metacarpophalangeal joint cavity
11 Distopalmar recess of the MP joint
12 Collateral recess of the MP joint
13 Superficial digital flexor tendon (distal branch)
14 Deep digital flexor tendon
15 Proximal digital annular ligament
   15a Proximal attachment
   15b Distal attachment
16 Distal digital annular ligament (proximal attachment)
17 Digital sheath
   17a Collateral recess
   17b Dorsal distal recess
   17c Synovial fold
18 Proper palmar digital artery
19 Proper palmar digital vein
20 Palmar ramus (vein) of P1
21 Deep ungular plexus
22 Ungular cartilage
23 Proximal attachment of the digital cushion
24 Skin

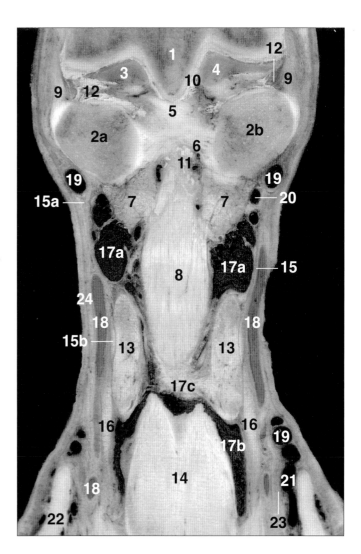

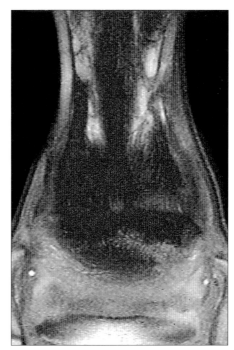

Frontal MRI scan of the pastern after injection of fat material into the arteries and latex into the veins.

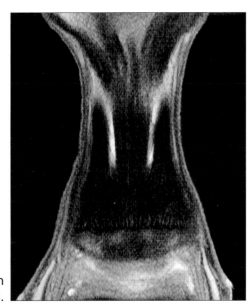

Frontal MRI scan of the pastern.

F6: Frontal Section of the Pastern

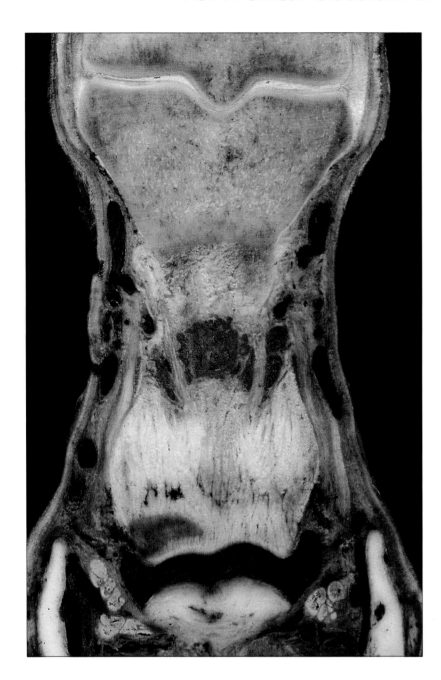

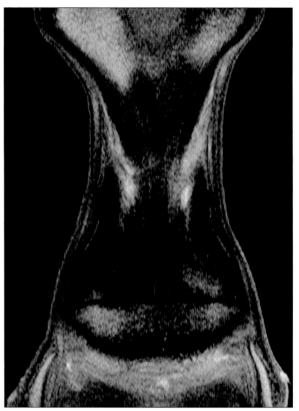

Frontal MRI scan of the pastern.

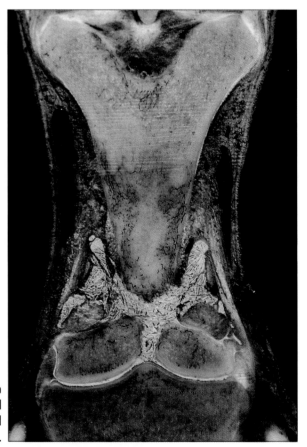

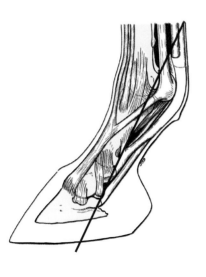

Frontal anatomical section after injection of coloured latex into the synovial cavities and vessels.

F6: Frontal Section of the Pastern

1 Metacarpal condyle
2 Proximal phalanx (P1)
3 Middle phalanx (P2) (flexor tuberosity)
4 Metacarpophalangeal (MP) joint
5 Collateral ligament of the MP joint
6 Oblique sesamoidean ligament
7 Straight sesamoidean ligament
8 Middle scutum
9 Axial palmar ligament of the PIP joint
10 Sagittal palmar recess of the proximal
   interphalangeal (PIP) joint
11 Collateral palmar recess of the PIP joint
12 Superficial digital flexor tendon
   (distal branches)
13 Deep digital flexor tendon
   13a Phalangeal fibrocartilaginous part
   13b Fibrous part
14 Proximal digital annular ligament
   14a Proximal attachment
   14b Distal attachment
15 Distal digital annular ligament
16 Digital sheath (dorsal distal recess)
17 Proximopalmar recess of the distal
   interphalangeal joint
18 Proximal recess of the podotrochlear bursa
19 Ungular cartilage
20 Proximal attachment of the digital cushion
21 Proper palmar digital artery
22 Dorsal ramus (artery) of P1
23 Dorsal ramus (artery) of P2
24 Palmar ramus (artery) of P2
25 Proper palmar digital vein
26 Palmar ramus (vein) of P1
27 Palmar ramus (vein) of P2
28 Deep ungular plexus
29 Skin

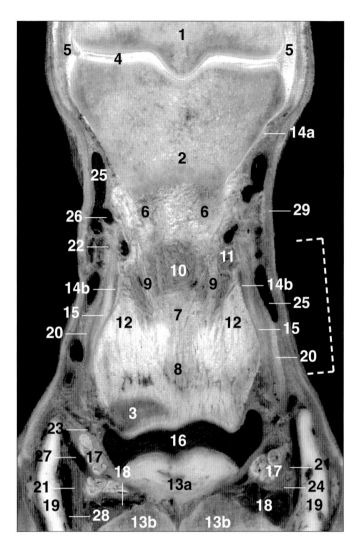

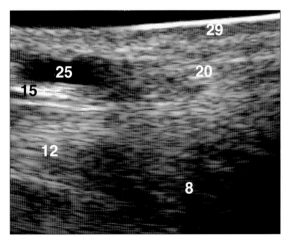

Frontal ultrasound scan of the pastern, lateral approach (see dotted area on illustration above, right).

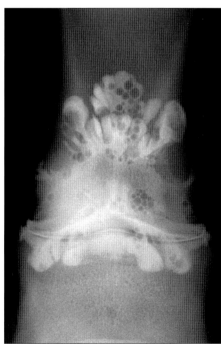

Contrast radiographic study (arthrography) of the PIP joint, dorsopalmar projection.

F7: Frontal Section of the Pastern

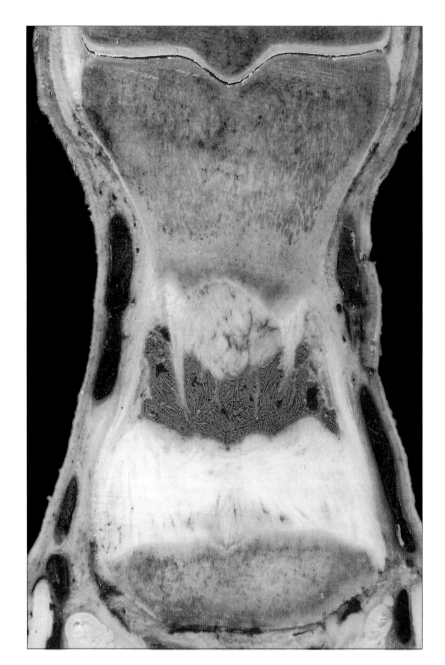

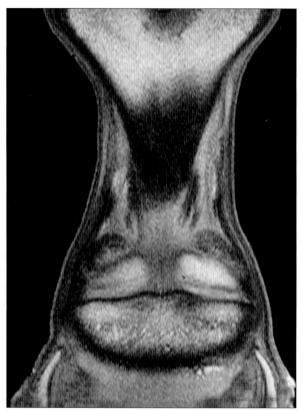

Frontal MRI scan of the pastern.

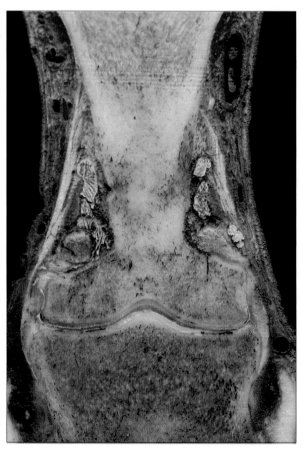

Frontal anatomical section after injection of coloured latex into the synovial cavities and vessels.

1 Metacarpal condyle
2 Proximal phalanx (P1)
3 Middle phalanx (P2) (flexor tuberosity)
4 Metacarpophalangeal (MP) joint
5 Collateral ligament of the MP joint
6 Oblique sesamoidean ligament
7 Middle scutum
8 Axial palmar ligament of the proximal interphalangeal (PIP) joint
9 Abaxial palmar ligament of the PIP joint
10 Sagittal palmar recess of the PIP joint
11 Collateral palmar recess of the PIP joint
12 Proximopalmar recess of the distal interphalangeal joint
13 Extensor branch of the third interosseus muscle
14 Dorsal distal recess of the digital sheath
15 Ungular cartilage
16 Proximal attachment of the digital cushion
17 Dorsal ramus (artery) of P1
18 Dorsal ramus (artery) of P2
19 Proper palmar digital vein
20 Deep ungular plexus
21 Skin

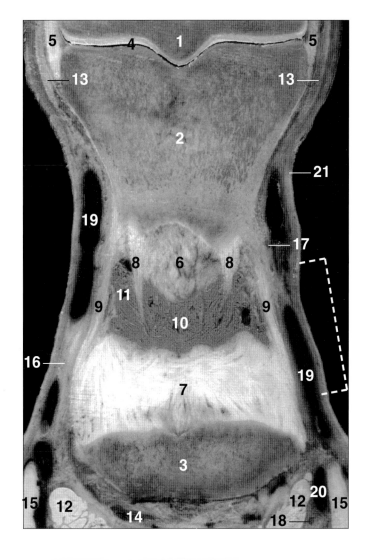

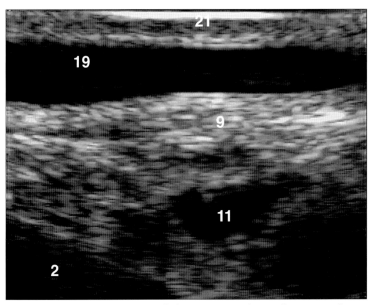

Frontal ultrasound scan of the pastern, lateral approach (see dotted area in illustration above, right).

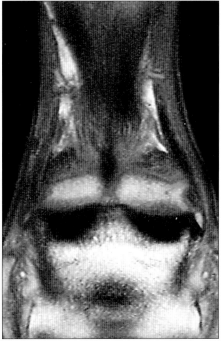

Frontal MRI scan of the pastern after injection of fat material into the arteries and latex into the veins.

F8: Frontal Section of the Pastern

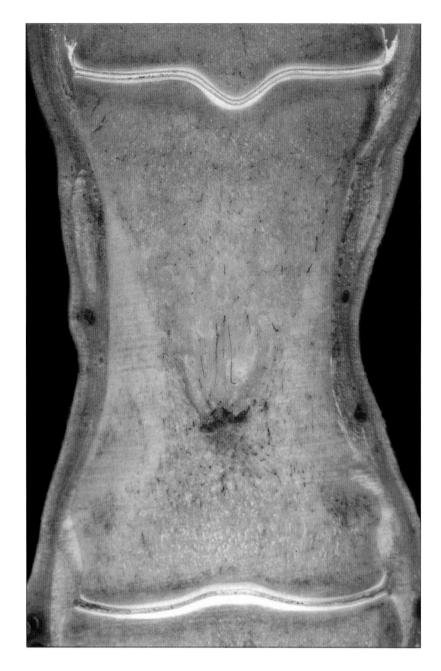

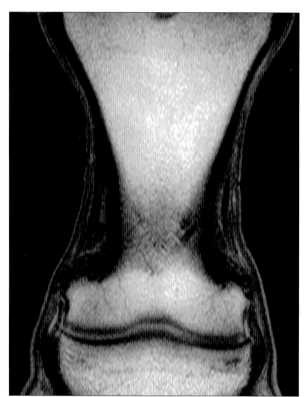

Frontal MRI scan of the pastern.

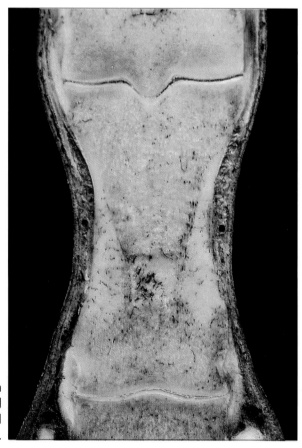

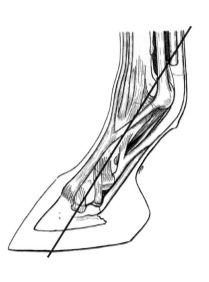

Frontal anatomical section after injection of coloured latex into the synovial cavities and vessels.

F8: Frontal Section of the Pastern

1 Metacarpal condyle
   1a Sagittal ridge
2 Proximal phalanx (P1)
   2a Proximal sagittal groove
   2b Medial glenoid cavity
   2c Lateral glenoid cavity
   2d Medial condyle
   2e Lateral condyle
   2f Distal sagittal groove
3 Middle phalanx
   3a Medial glenoid cavity
   3b Lateral glenoid cavity
4 Metacarpophalangeal (MP) joint
5 Collateral ligament of the MP joint
6 Proximal interphalangeal (PIP) joint
7 Collateral ligament of the PIP joint
8 Abaxial palmar ligament of the PIP joint
9 Extensor branch of the third interosseus muscle
10 Proximal attachment of the digital cushion and distal digital annular ligament
11 Dorsal ramus (artery) of P1
12 Dorsal ramus (vein) of P1
13 Coronal vein
14 Skin

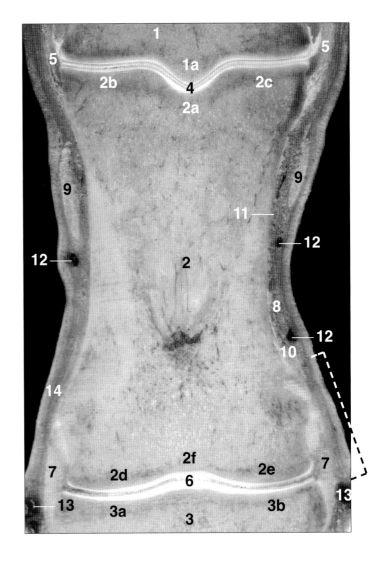

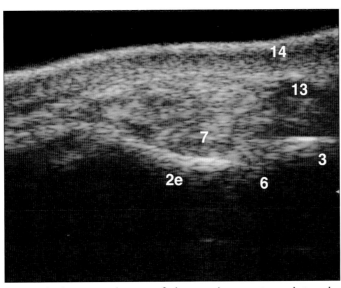

Frontal ultrasound scan of the equine pastern, lateral approach (see dotted area in illustration above, right).

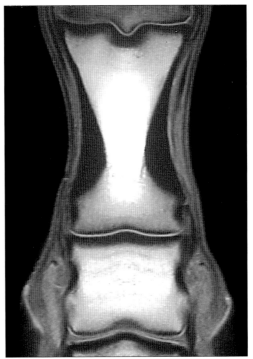

Frontal MRI scan of the pastern after injection of latex into the arteries and veins.

F9: Frontal Section of the Pastern

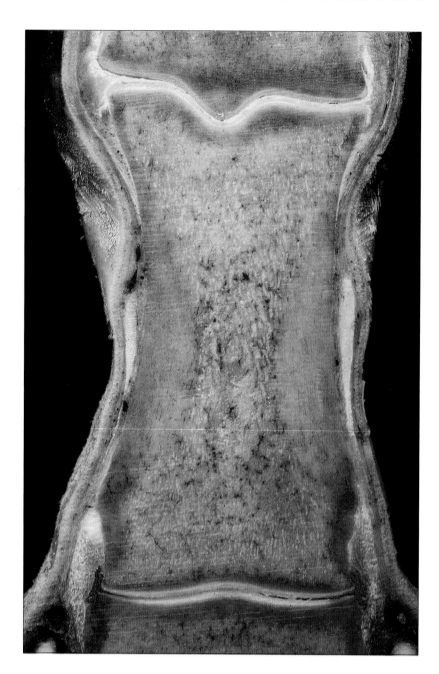

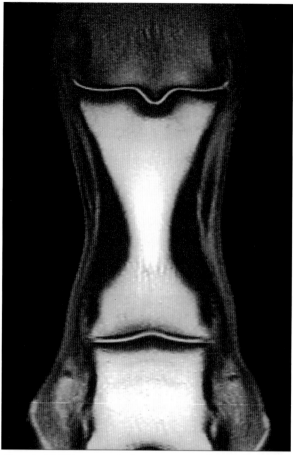

Frontal MRI scan of the pastern after injection of latex into the arteries and veins.

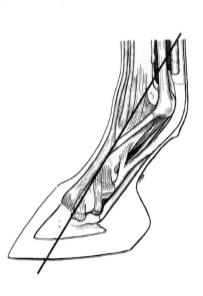

Frontal MRI scan of the pastern.

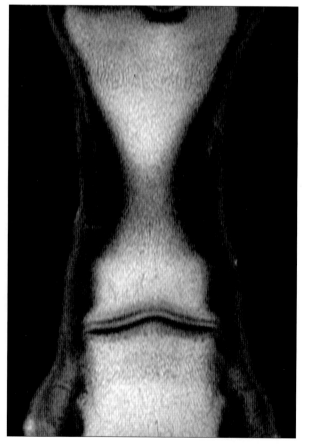

F9: Frontal Section of the Pastern

1 Metacarpal condyle
  1a Sagittal ridge
2 Proximal phalanx (P1)
  2a Proximal sagittal groove
  2b Medial glenoid cavity
  2c Lateral glenoid cavity
  2d Medial condyle
  2e Lateral condyle
  2f Distal sagittal groove
3 Middle phalanx
  3a Medial glenoid cavity
  3b Lateral glenoid cavity
4 Metacarpophalangeal (MP) joint
5 Collateral ligament of the MP joint
6 Collateral recess of the MP joint
7 Proximal interphalangeal (PIP) joint
8 Collateral ligament of the PIP joint
9 Abaxial palmar ligament of the PIP joint
10 Extensor branch of the third interosseus muscle
11 Dorsal ramus (artery) of P1
12 Dorsal ramus (vein) of P1
13 Coronal vein
14 Ungular cartilage
15 Skin

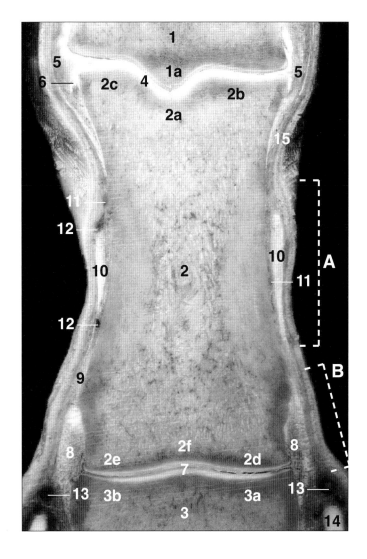

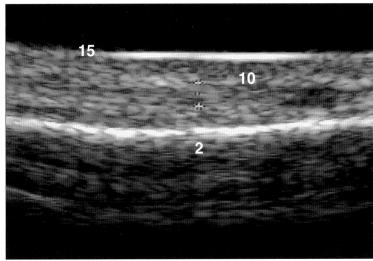

A Frontal ultrasound scan of the equine pastern, medial approach (see dotted area in illustration above, right).

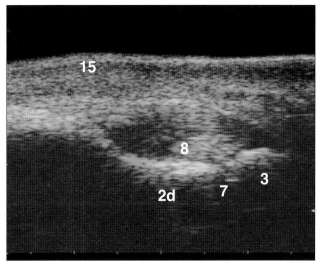

B Frontal ultrasound scan of the equine pastern, medial approach (see dotted area in illustration above).

F10: Frontal Section of the Pastern

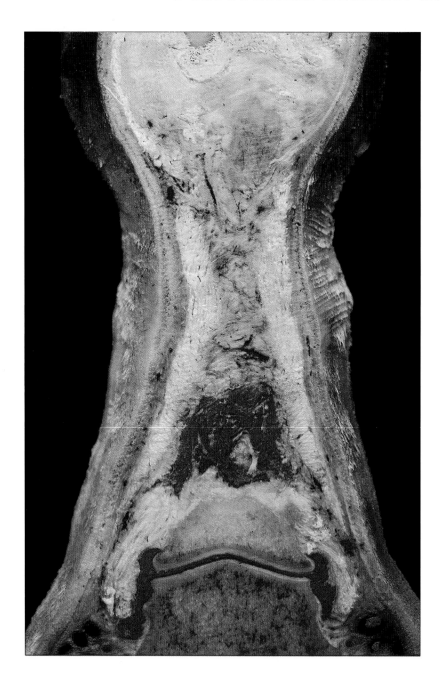

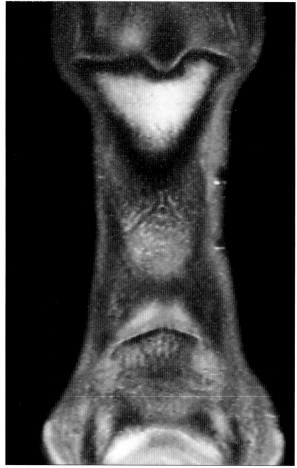

Frontal MRI scan of the pastern after injection of latex into the arteries and veins.

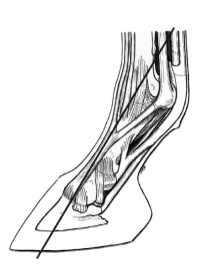

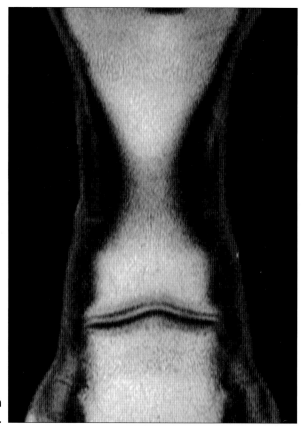

Frontal MRI scan of the pastern.

F10: Frontal Section of the Pastern

1 Metacarpal condyle (sagittal ridge)
2 Proximal phalanx
  2a Dorsal cortex
  2b Medial condyle
  2c Lateral condyle
  2d Distal sagittal groove
3 Middle phalanx (P2)
  3a Extensor process
4 Metacarpophalangeal (MP) joint
  4a Dorsal articular capsule
  4b Dorsal recess
  4c Distodorsal recess
  4d Distodorsal synovial fold
  4e Dorsal metacarpophalangeal fascia
5 Proximal interphalangeal (PIP) joint
  5a Collateral sesamoidean ligament
  5b Dorsal recess
  5c Distodorsocollateral recess
  5d Synovial membrane
6 Dorsal digital extensor tendon
7 Extensor branch of the third interosseus muscle
8 Dorsal ramus (artery) of P1
9 Dorsal ramus (artery) of P2
10 Dorsal ramus (vein) of P2
11 Coronal vein
12 Skin

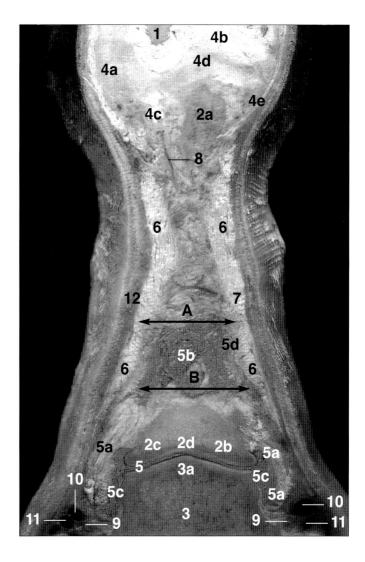

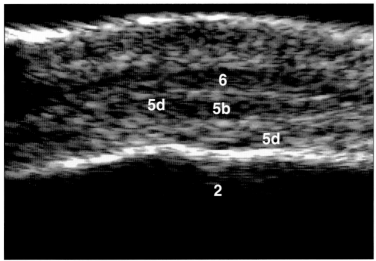

A Transverse ultrasound scan of the pastern, dorsal approach (see dotted area in illustration above, right).

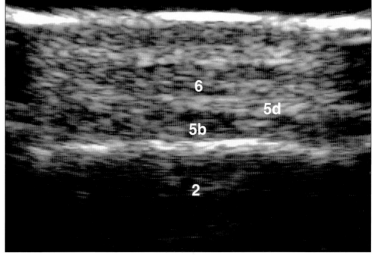

B Transverse ultrasound scan of the pastern, dorsal approach (see dotted area in illustration above).

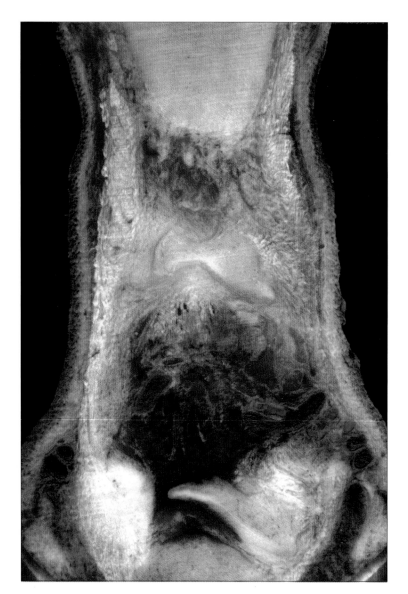

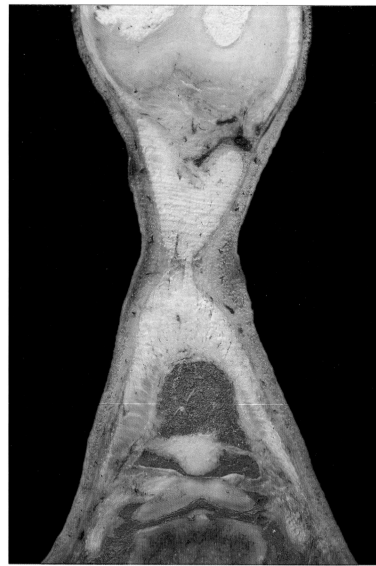

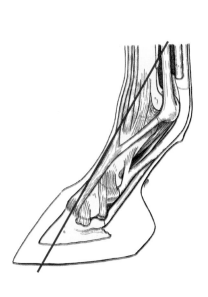

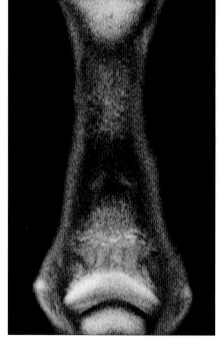

Frontal MRI scan
of the pastern.

1 Proximal phalanx (P1)
 1a Medial distal condyle
 1b Lateral distal condyle
2 Middle phalanx (P2)
 2a Extensor process
 2b Medial distal condyle
 2c Dorsal articular margin
3 Distal phalanx
 3a Extensor process
4 Metacarpophalangeal joint
 4a Dorsal articular capsule
 4b Dorsal recess
 4c Distodorsal recess
 4d Lateral digital extensor tendon
 4e Dorsal metacarpophalangeal fascia
5 Proximal interphalangeal joint
 5a Collateral sesamoidean ligament
 5b Dorsal recess
 5c Distodorsocollateral recess
6 Distal interphalangeal joint
 6a Collateral ligament
 6b Dorsal recess
7 Dorsal digital extensor tendon
8 Extensor branch of the third interosseus muscle
9 Dorsal rami (artery and vein) of P1
10 Dorsal rami (artery and vein) of P2
11 Coronal artery
12 Coronal vein
13 Coronal cushion
14 Corium coronae
15 Corium parietis
16 Hoof wall
17 Skin

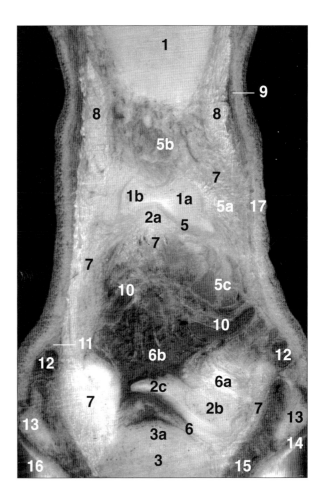

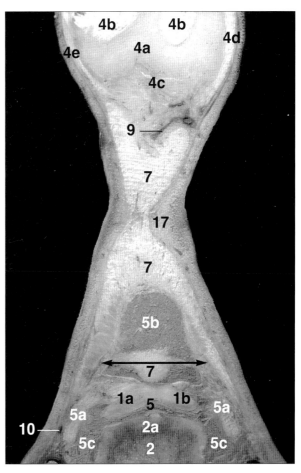

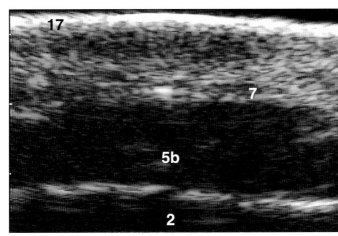

Transverse ultrasound scan of the pastern, dorsal approach (see arrows in illustration at right).

The Equine Fetlock

Dissections of the Equine Fetlock

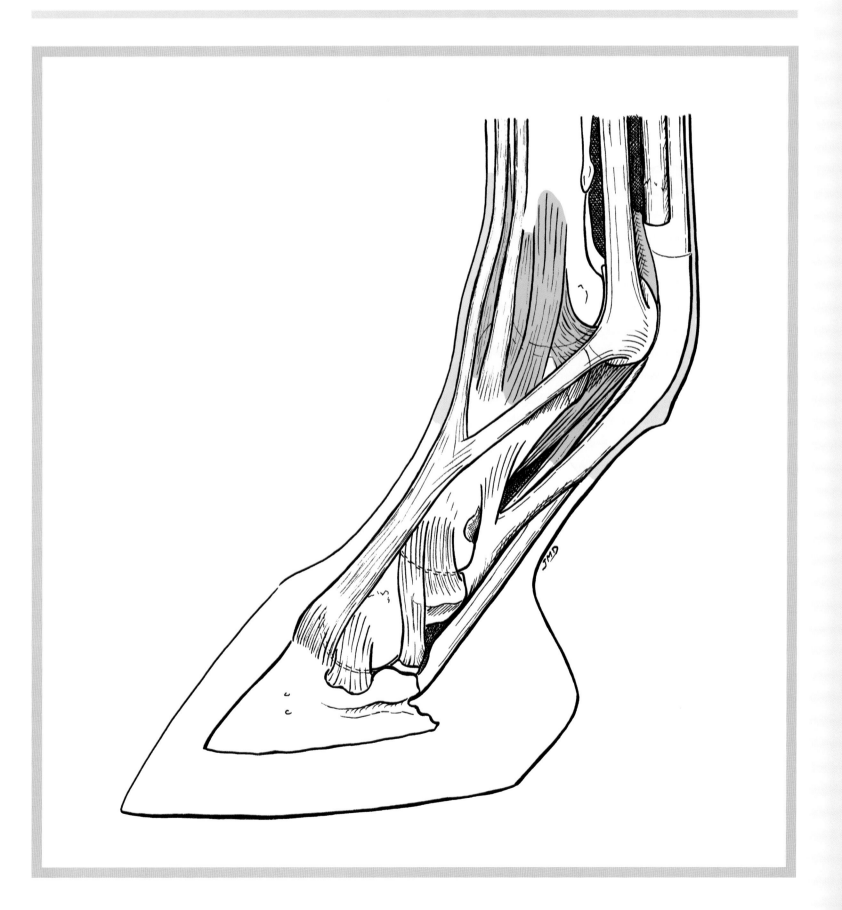

Dissection 1: Fetlock Area – Medial Aspect
(Superficial Elements)

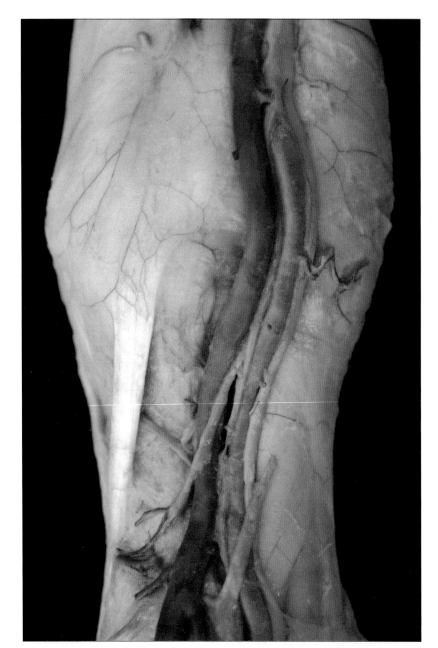

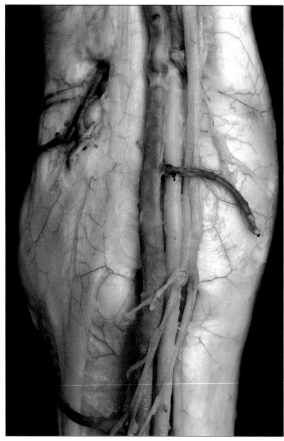

Digital and metacarpal vessels and nerves of the fetlock, medial aspect.

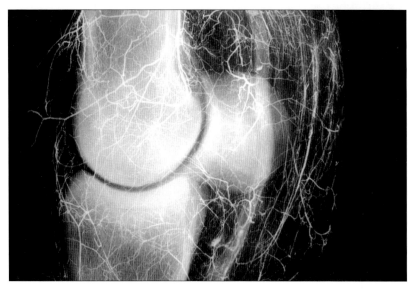

Contrast radiographic study of the arteries (arteriography) of the fetlock, lateromedial projection.

Dissection 1: Fetlock Area – Medial Aspect
(Superficial Elements)

1 Third metacarpal bone
2 Proximal phalanx (P1)
3 Medial proximal sesamoid bone
4 Dorsal capsule of the metacarpophalangeal joint
5 Metacarpophalangeal fascia
6 Dorsal digital extensor tendon
7 Third interosseus muscle
  7a Medial branch
  7b Medial extensor branch
8 Superficial digital flexor tendon (medial branch)
9 Deep digital flexor tendon (covered by the digital sheath wall)
10 Palmar annular ligament
11 Proximal digital annular ligament
12 Digital sheath wall
13 Vascular network of the metacarpophalangeal joint
14 Medial proper palmar digital artery
  14a Ergot ramus
  14b Dorsal ramus of P1
15 Medial common palmar digital vein
16 Medial proper palmar digital vein
  16a Dorsal ramus of P1
17 Medial common palmar digital nerve
18 Medial proper palmar digital nerve
  18a Dorsal ramus
  18b Intermediate ramus
19 Ergot ligament

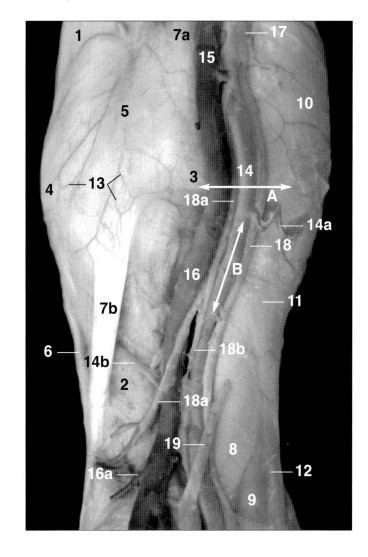

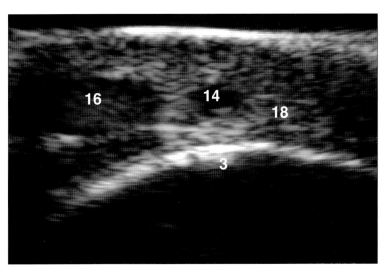

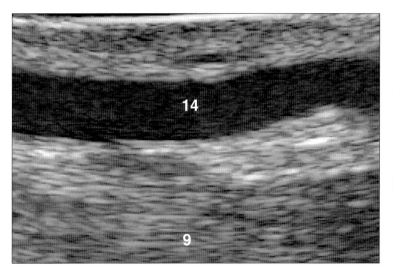

A Transverse ultrasound dscan of the vessels and nerves of the fetlock, palmaromedial approach (see arrow in illustration above, right).

B Longitudinal ultrasound scan of the proper palmar digital artery (see arrow in illustration above).

Dissection 2: Fetlock Area – Medial Aspect

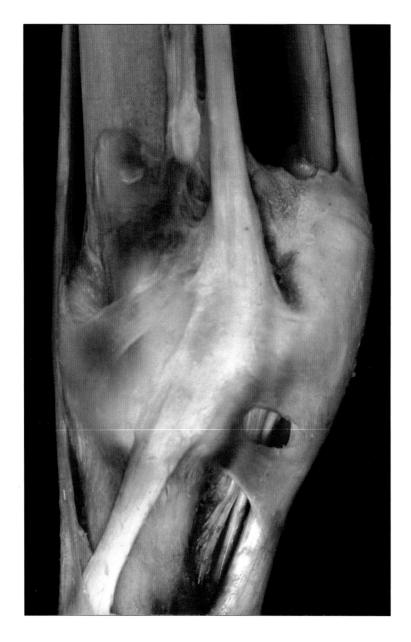

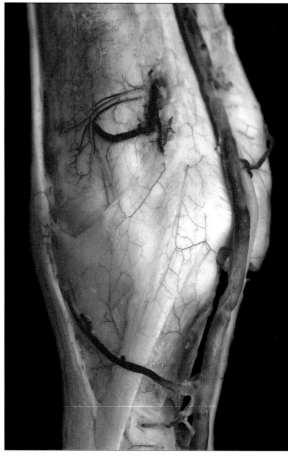

Dissected specimen after injection of coloured latex into the vessels.

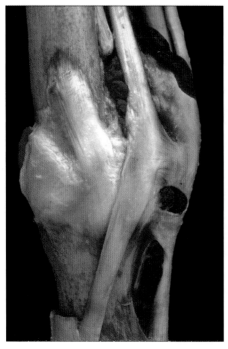

Dissected specimen after latex injection into the synovial cavities, medial aspect.

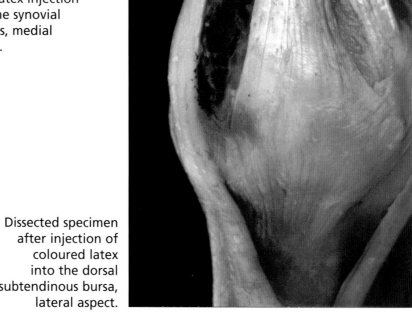

Dissected specimen after injection of coloured latex into the dorsal subtendinous bursa, lateral aspect.

1 Third metacarpal bone
2 Second metacarpal bone
3 Proximal phalanx
4 Dorsal metacarpophalangeal fascia
5 Dorsal capsule of the metacarpophalangeal joint
6 Medial collateral ligament (superficial part)
7 Palmar (intersesamoidean) ligament
8 Straight sesamoidean ligament
9 Medial oblique sesamoidean ligament
10 Abaxial palmar ligament of the proximal interphalangeal joint
11 Dorsal digital extensor tendon
12 Third interosseus muscle
    12a Medial branch
    12b Medial extensor branch
13 Superficial digital flexor tendon
    13a Manica flexoria
    13b Medial branch
14 Deep digital flexor tendon
15 Palmar annular ligament
16 Proximal digital annular ligament
    16a Proximal attachment
17 Digital sheath cavity
    17a Collateral recess

Ultrasound scans A and B below:
a Medial proper palmar digital artery
b Medial proper palmar digital vein (collapsed)
c Medial proper palmar digital nerve
d Medial proximal sesamoid bone

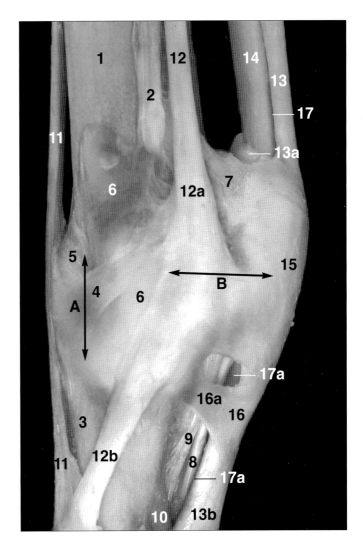

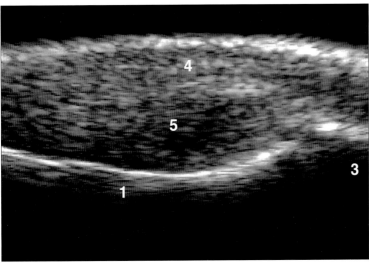

A Longitudinal ultrasound scan of the fetlock, dorsomedial approach (see arrow in illustration above, right).

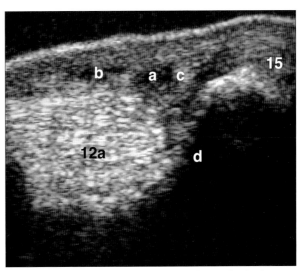

B Transverse ultrasound scan of the fetlock, medial approach (see arrow in illustration above).

Dissection 3: Fetlock Area
(Flexor Tendons)

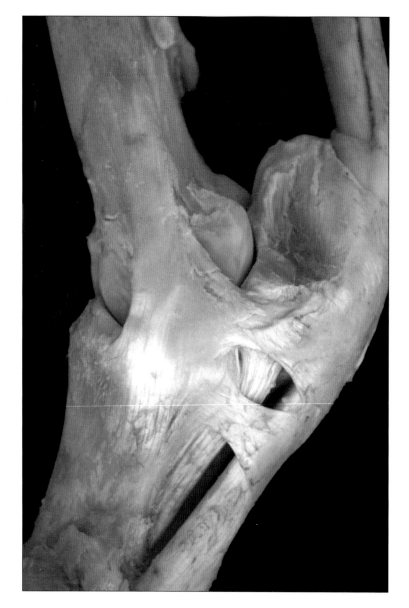

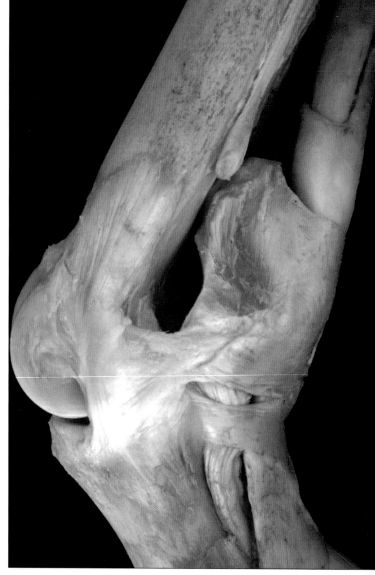

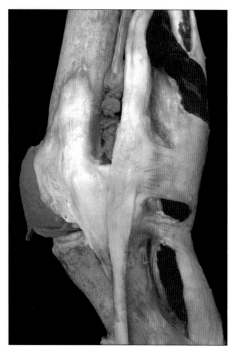

Flexor tendons and suspensory apparatus on the flexed fetlock after injection of coloured latex into the synovial cavities.

1 Third metacarpal bone
  1a Metacarpal condyle
2 Second metacarpal bone
3 Fourth metacarpal bone
4 Proximal phalanx
  4a Palmar eminence
5 Proximal sesamoid bone
  5a Interosseus face
  5b Articular surface
6 Collateral ligament of the metacarpophalangeal joint
  6a Superficial part
  6b Deep part

(Flexor Tendons)

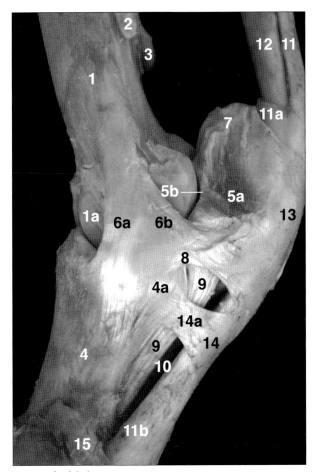

Extended joint.

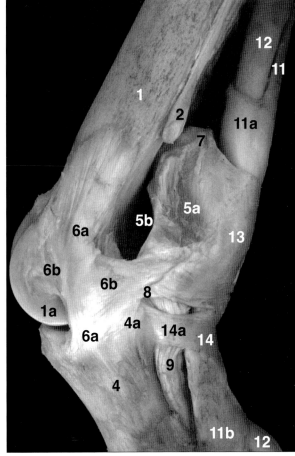

Flexed joint.

7 Palmar (intersesamoidean) ligament
8 Collateral sesamoidean ligament
9 Oblique sesamoidean ligament
10 Straight sesamoidean ligament
11 Superficial digital flexor tendon
    11a Manica flexoria
    11b Distal branch
12 Deep digital flexor tendon
13 Palmar annular ligament
14 Proximal digital annular ligament
    14a Proximal attachment
15 Distal digital annular ligament
    (proximal attachment)

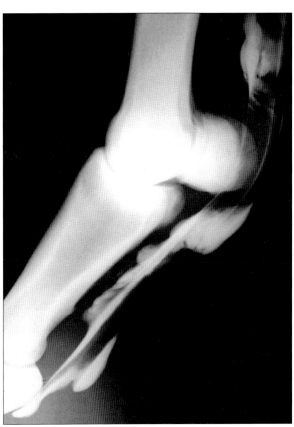

Single contrast radiographic study (tenography) of the digital sheath, lateromedial view.

Dissection 4: Metacarpophalangeal Joint – Medial Aspect
(Deep Elements)

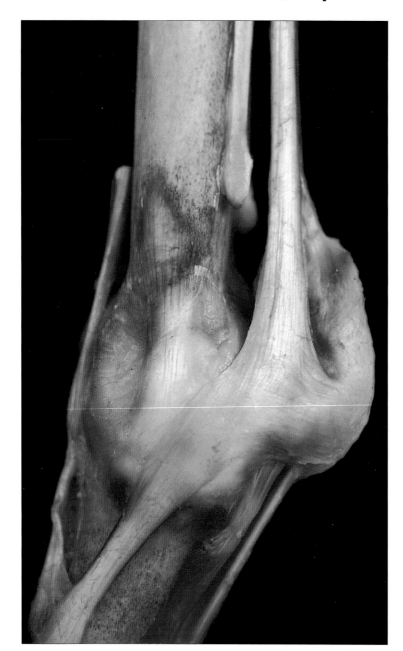

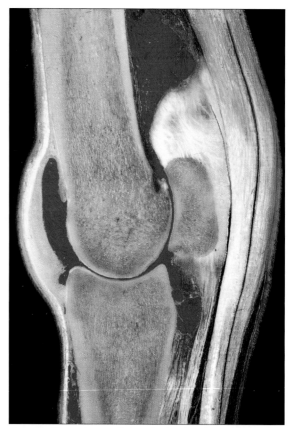

Sagittal section of the fetlock after injection of coloured latex into the synovial cavities.

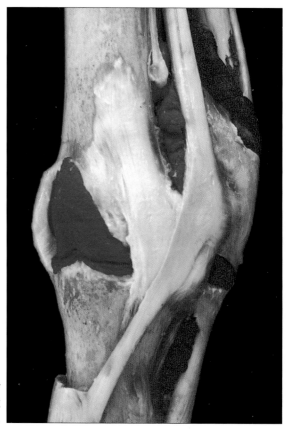

Dissected specimen after injection of coloured latex into the synovial cavities.

Dissection 4: Metacarpophalangeal Joint – Medial Aspect
(Deep Elements)

1 Third metacarpal bone
   1a Metacarpal condyle
2 Second metacarpal bone
3 Fourth metacarpal bone
4 Proximal phalanx
   4a Palmar eminence
5 Medial proximal sesamoid bone
6 Dorsal capsule of the metacarpophalangeal joint
7 Medial collateral ligament (superficial part)
8 Palmar (intersesamoidean) ligament
9 Straight sesamoidean ligament
10 Medial oblique sesamoidean ligament
11 Dorsal digital extensor tendon
12 Third interosseus muscle
   12a Medial branch
   12b Medial extensor branch
13 Proximal attachment of the proximal digital annular ligament

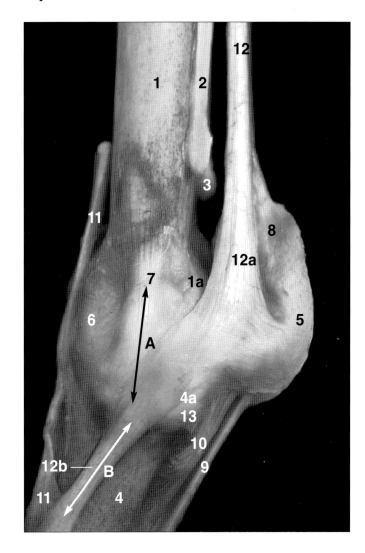

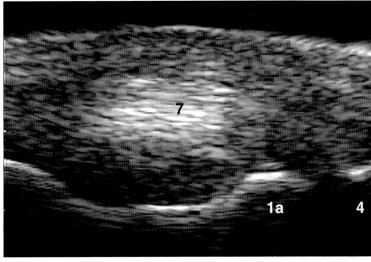

A Longitudinal ultrasound scan of the medial collateral ligament (see arrow in illustration above, right).

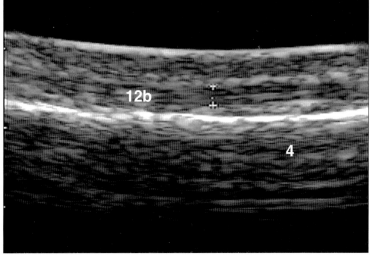

B Longitudinal ultrasound scan of the extensor branch of the third interosseus muscle (see arrow in illustration above).

Dissection 5: Metacarpophalangeal Joint
(Extended Joint – Collateral and Sesamoidean Ligaments)

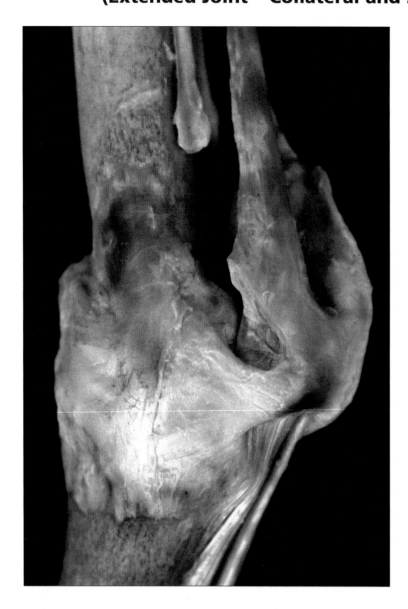

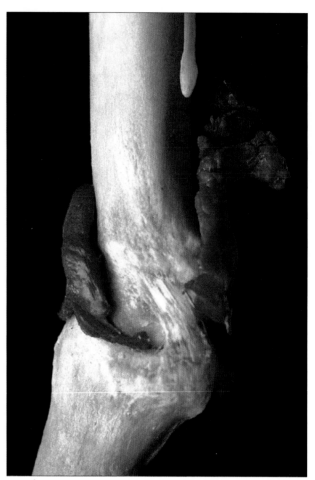

Casting preparation of the metacarpophalangeal joint synovial cavity.

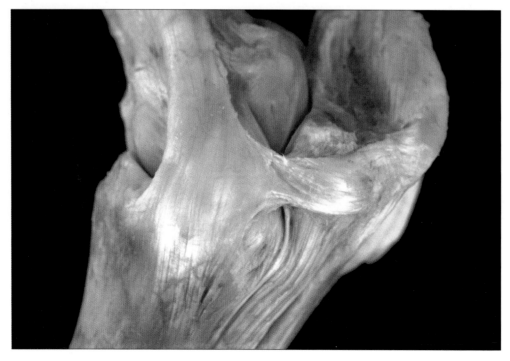

Dissection 5: Metacarpophalangeal Joint
(Extended Joint – Collateral and Sesamoidean Ligaments)

1 Third metacarpal bone
 1a Metacarpal condyle
2 Second metacarpal bone
3 Fourth metacarpal bone
4 Proximal phalanx
 4a Medial palmar eminence
5 Medial proximal sesamoid bone
 5a Interosseus face
 5b Articular surface
6 Dorsal capsule of the metacarpophalangeal joint
7 Medial collateral ligament
 7a Superficial part
 7b Deep part
8 Medial collateral sesamoidean ligament
9 Palmar (intersesamoidean) ligament
10 Straight sesamoidean ligament
11 Medial oblique sesamoidean ligament
12 Third interosseus muscle
 12a Medial branch
 12b Medial extensor branch
  (sectioned and removed)

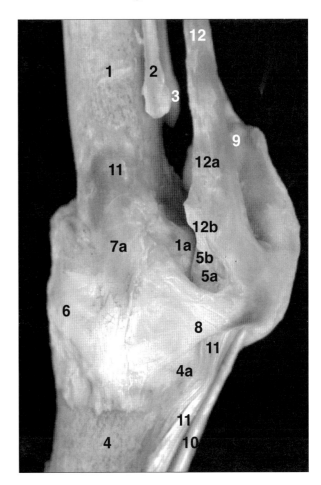
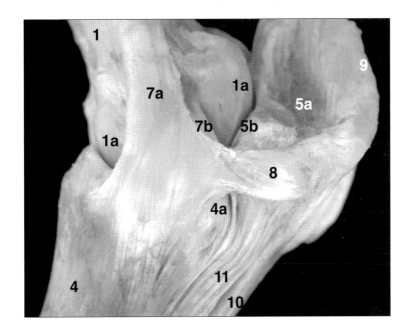
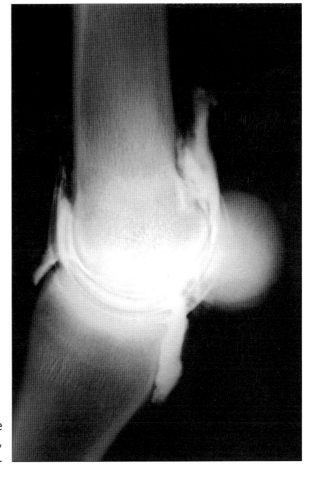

Contrast arthrography of the metacarpophalangeal joint, lateromedial projection.

Dissection 6: Metacarpophalangeal Joint
(Flexed Joint – Collateral and Sesamoidean Ligaments)

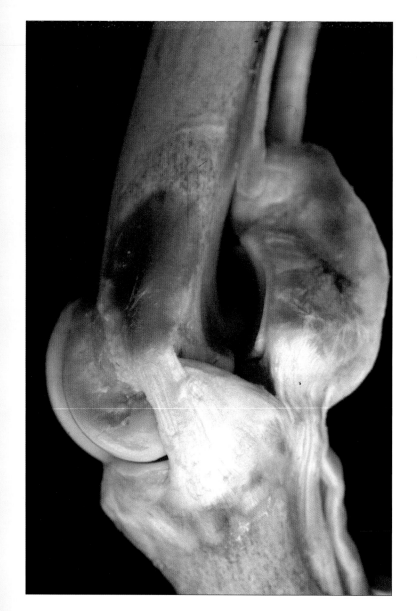

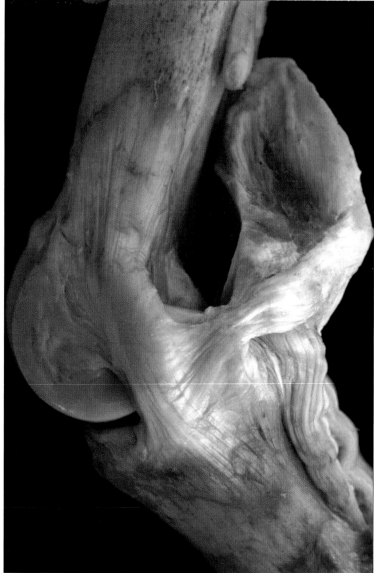

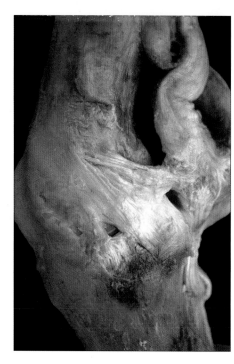

Deep part of the lateral
collateral ligament.

Dissection 6: Metacarpophalangeal Joint
(Flexed Joint – Collateral and Sesamoidean Ligaments)

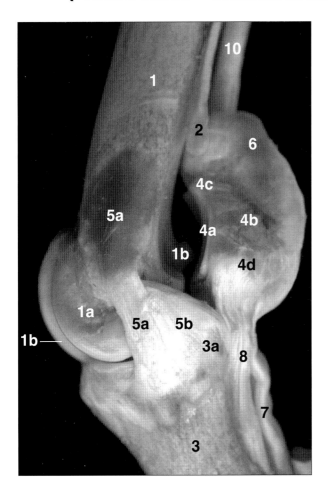

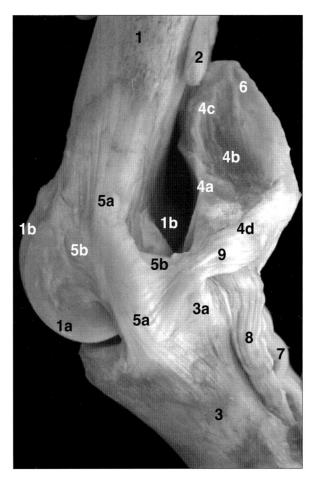

1 Third metacarpal bone
  1a Metacarpal condyle
  1b Sagittal ridge
2 Fourth metacarpal bone
3 Proximal phalanx
  3a Lateral palmar eminence
4 Lateral proximal sesamoid bone
  4a Articular surface
  4b Interosseus face
  4c Apex
  4d Base
5 Lateral collateral ligament
  5a Superficial part
  5b Deep part
6 Palmar (intersesamoidean) ligament
7 Straight sesamoidean ligament
8 Oblique sesamoidean ligament
9 Lateral collateral sesamoidean ligament
10 Third interosseus muscle medial branch

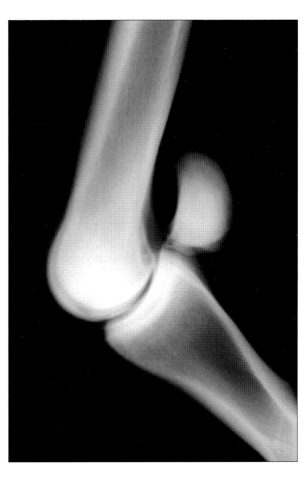

Lateromedial radiographic view
of the flexed fetlock.

Dissection 7: Metacarpophalangeal Joint
(Collateral Ligament)

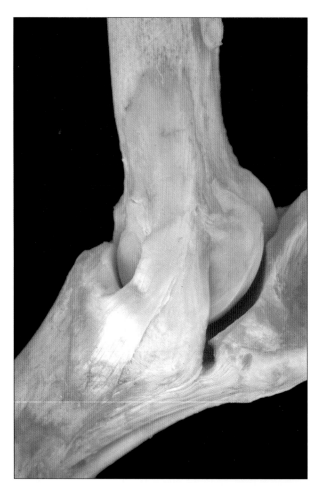

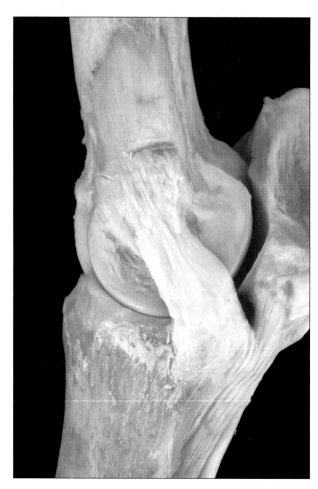

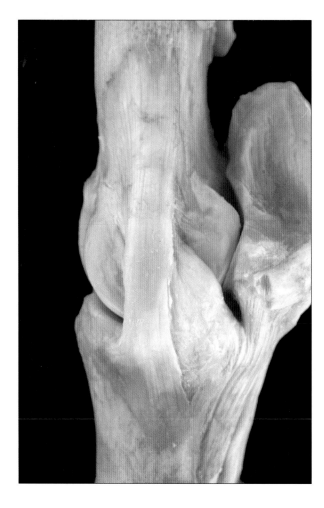

(Collateral Ligament)

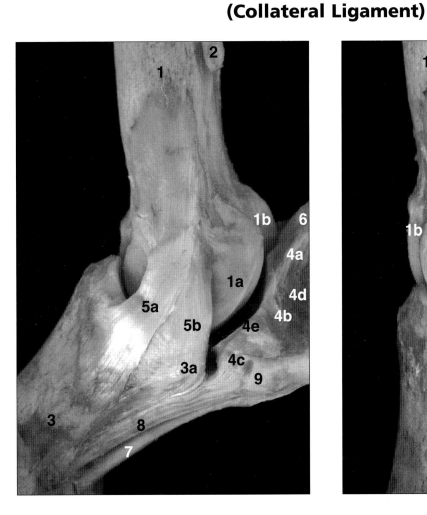

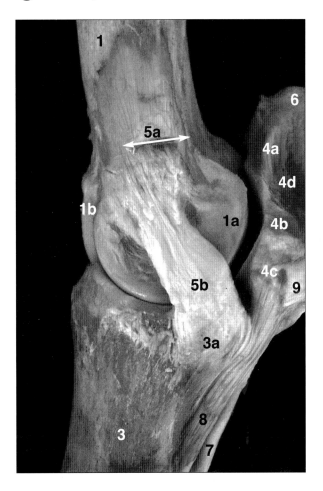

1 Third metacarpal bone
  1a Metacarpal condyle
  1b Sagittal ridge
2 Fourth metacarpal bone
3 Proximal phalanx
  3a Lateral palmar eminence
4 Lateral proximal sesamoid bone
  4a Apex
  4b Body
  4c Base
  4d Interosseus face
  4e Articular surface
5 Lateral collateral ligament
  5a Superficial part (↔ section)
  5b Deep part
6 Palmar (intersesamoidean)
  ligament
7 Straight sesamoidean ligament
8 Lateral oblique sesamoidean
  ligament
9 Collateral sesamoidean ligament
  (sectioned)

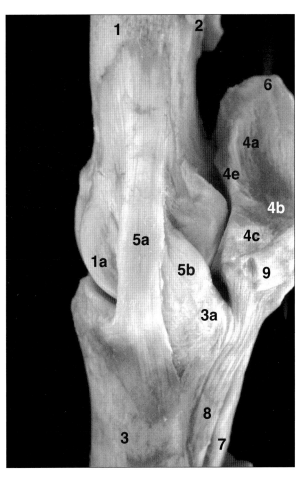

Dissection 8: Fetlock Area – Palmarolateral Aspect

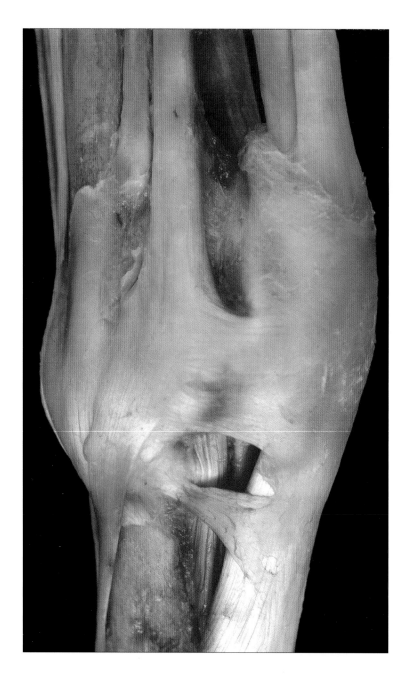

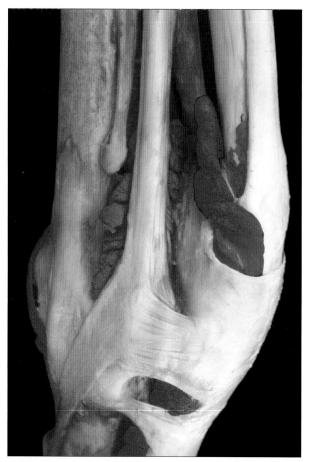

Dissected fetlock with injection of coloured latex into the synovial cavities.

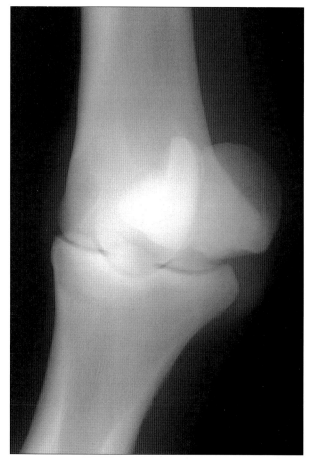

Dorsomedial-palmarolateral oblique radiographic view of the metacarpophalangeal joint.

Dissection 8: Fetlock Area – Palmarolateral Aspect

1 Third metacarpal bone
2 Fourth metacarpal bone
3 Proximal phalanx
4 Dorsal capsule of the metacarpophalangeal joint
5 Lateral collateral ligament (superficial part)
6 Collateral sesamoidean ligament
7 Palmar (intersesamoidean) ligament
8 Straight sesamoidean ligament
9 Oblique sesamoidean ligament
10 Lateral digital extensor tendon
11 Dorsal digital extensor tendon
12 Third interosseus muscle
    12a Lateral branch
    12b Medial branch
    12c Lateral extensor branch
13 Superficial digital flexor tendon
    13a Manica flexoria
    13b Lateral branch
14 Deep digital flexor tendon
15 Palmar annular ligament
16 Proximal digital annular ligament
    16a Proximal attachment

Ultrasound scans A and B below:
a Lateral proper palmar digital artery
b Lateral proper palmar digital vein
c Lateral proper palmar digital nerve

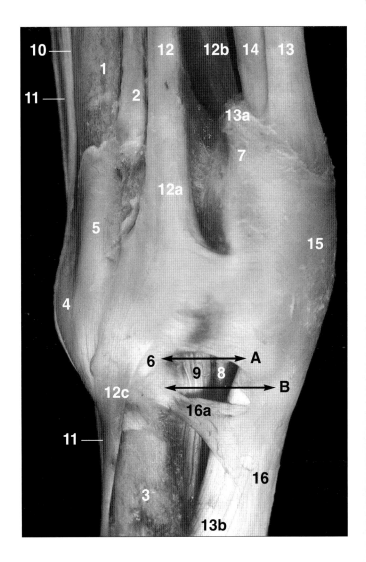

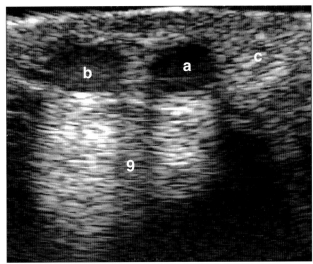

A Transverse ultrasound scan of the lateral oblique sesamoidean ligament, palmarolateral approach (see arrow in illustration above, right).

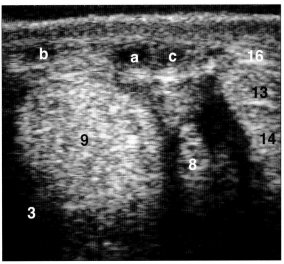

B Transverse ultrasound scan of the proximal pastern, palmarolateral approach (see arrow in illustration above).

Dissection 9: Metacarpophalangeal Joint – Palmarolateral Aspect

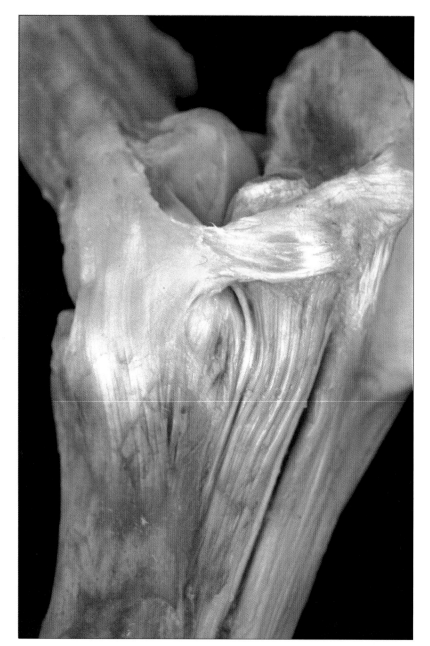

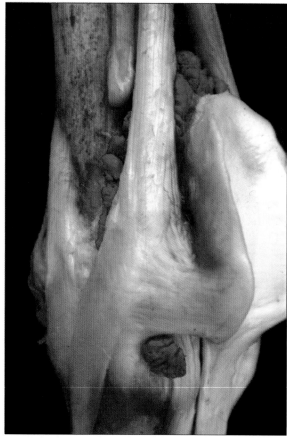

Injection of coloured latex into the synovial cavity demonstrating the palmar recesses of the joint.

1 Third metacarpal bone
  1a Metacarpal condyle
  1b Sagittal ridge
2 Second metacarpal bone
3 Proximal phalanx
  3a Palmar eminence
4 Lateral proximal sesamoid bone
  4a Apex
  4b Base
  4c Interosseus face
5 Lateral collateral ligament
  5a Superficial part
  5b Deep part

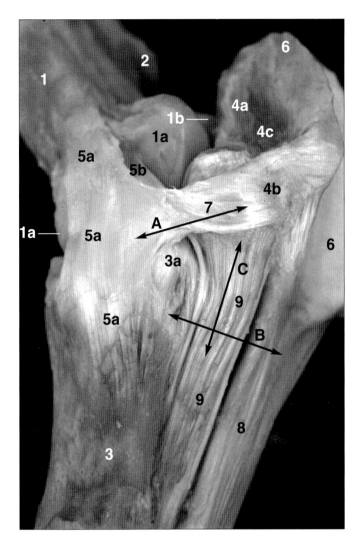

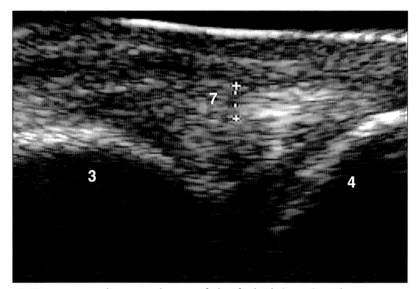

A Transverse ultrasound scan of the fetlock imaging the collateral sesamoidean ligament, palmarolateral approach (see arrow in illustration at left).

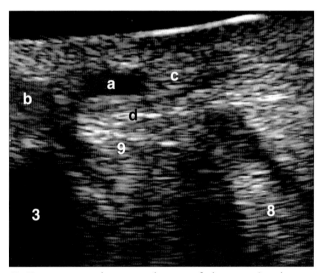

B Transverse ultrasound scan of the proximal pastern, palmarolateral approach (see arrow in illustration above, left).

6 Palmar (intersesamoidean) ligament
7 Collateral sesamoidean ligament
8 Straight sesamoidean ligament
9 Oblique sesamoidean ligament

Ultrasound scans A, B and C:
a Lateral proper palmar digital artery
b Lateral proper palmar digital vein
c Lateral proper palmar digital nerve
d Proximal digital annular ligament (proximal attachment)

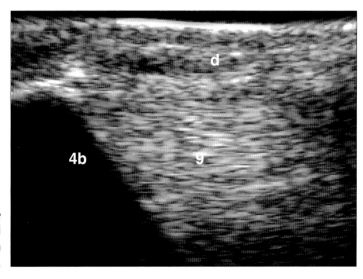

C Longitudinal ultrasound scan of the oblique sesamoidean ligament (proximal attachment), palmarolateral approach (see arrow in illustration above, left).

Dissection 10: Metacarpophalangeal Joint – Palmar Aspect

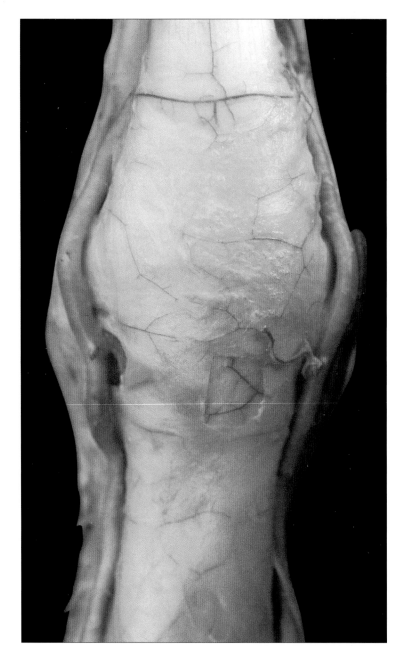

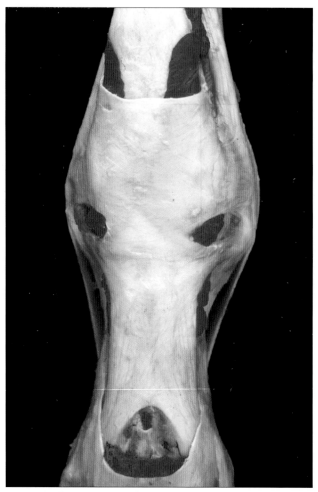

Dissected specimen after injection of coloured latex into the digital sheath cavity.

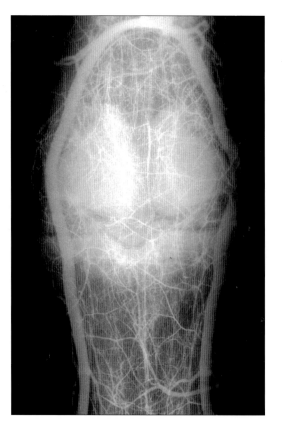

Contrast radiographic study of the arteries (arteriography) of the fetlock, dorsopalmar view.

1 Third interosseus muscle
  1a Lateral branch
  1b Lateral extensor branch
2 Superficial digital flexor tendon (SDFT)
  2a Lateral branch
  2b Medial branch (covered by the
    proximal digital annular ligament)
3 Deep digital flexor tendon (covered by the
  digital sheath wall)
4 Palmar annular ligament
5 Proximal digital annular ligament
  5a Window dissected at the junction
    between the palmar annular ligament
    and the proximal digital annular ligament
6 Digital sheath wall
7 Lateral proper palmar digital artery
8 Medial proper palmar digital artery
  8a Ergot ramus
9 Distal metacarpal arterial anastomosis of the SDFT
10 Proximal digital arterial anastomosis of the SDFT
11 Medial proper palmar digital vein
12 Ergot ligament

Ultrasound scans A and B:
a Proximal sesamoid bone
b Medial proper palmar digital nerve

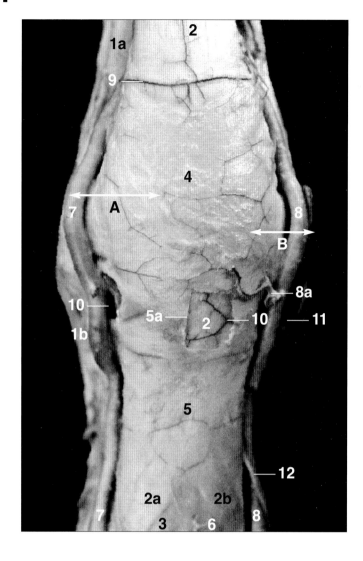

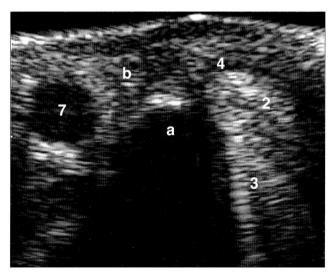

A Transverse ultrasound scan of the fetlock, palmarolateral approach (see arrow in illustration above, right).

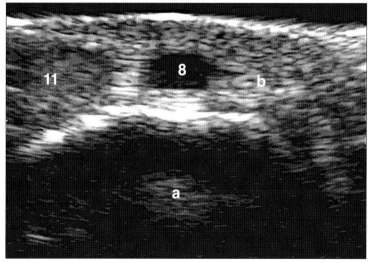

B Transverse ultrasound scan of the proper palmar digital vessels, palmarolateral approach (see arrow in illustration above).

Dissection 11: Fetlock Area – Palmar Aspect

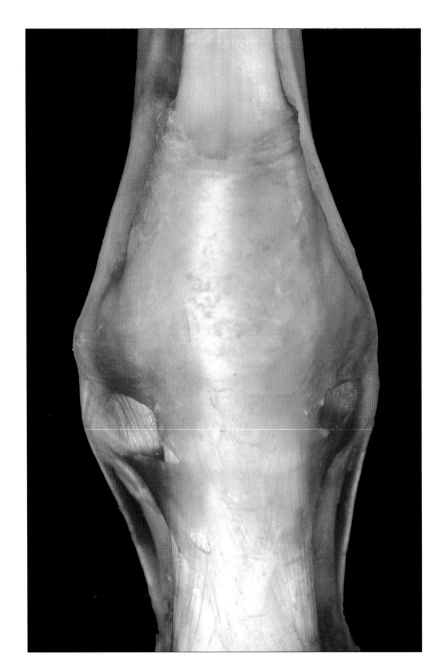

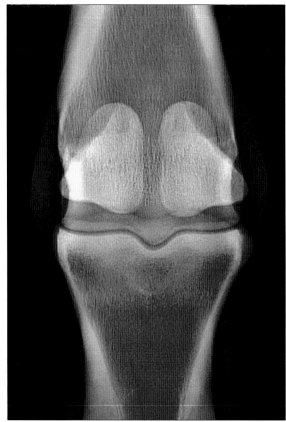

Dorsopalmar radiographic projection of the metacarpophalangeal joint.

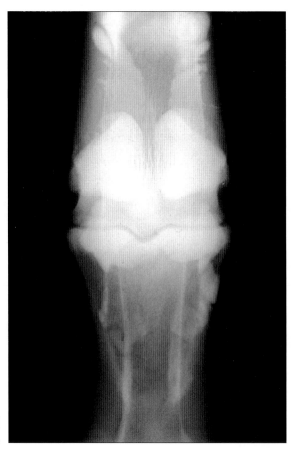

Contrast radiographic study of the digital sheath (tenography), dorsopalmar view.

1 Third metacarpal bone
2 Proximal phalanx
3 Superficial digital flexor tendon
   3a Distal branch
4 Palmar annular ligament
5 Proximal digital annular ligament
   5a Proximal attachment
6 Third interosseus muscle
   6a Distal branch
   6b Extensor branch
7 Collateral sesamoidean ligament
8 Oblique sesamoidean ligament
9 Digital sheath wall

Ultrasound scans A and B:
a Proximal sesamoid bone
b Palmar (intersesamoidean) ligament
c Deep digital flexor tendon

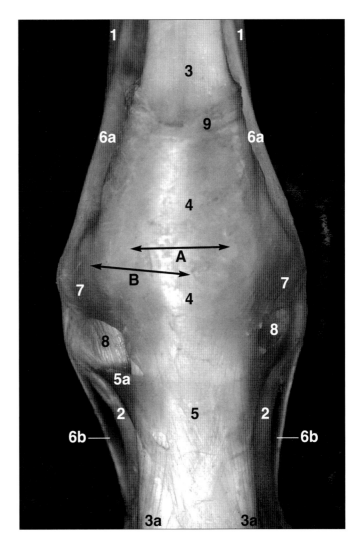

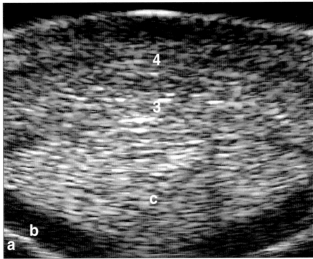

A Transverse ultrasound scan of the fetlock, palmar approach (see arrow in illustration above, right).

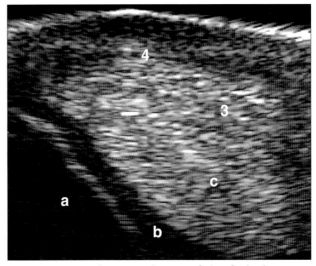

B Transverse ultrasound scan of the fetlock, palmarolateral approach (see arrow in illustration above).

Dissection 12: Fetlock Area – Palmar Aspect
(Palmar Ligament Reflected)

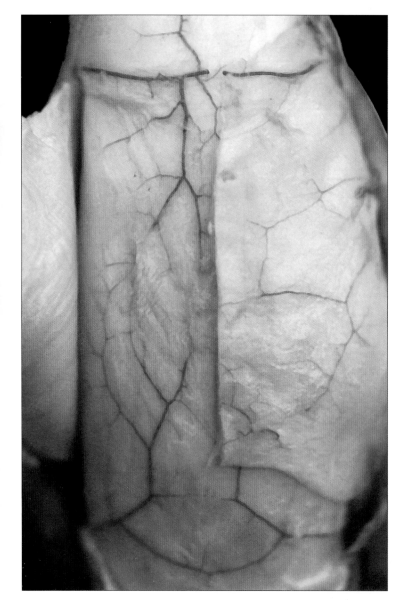

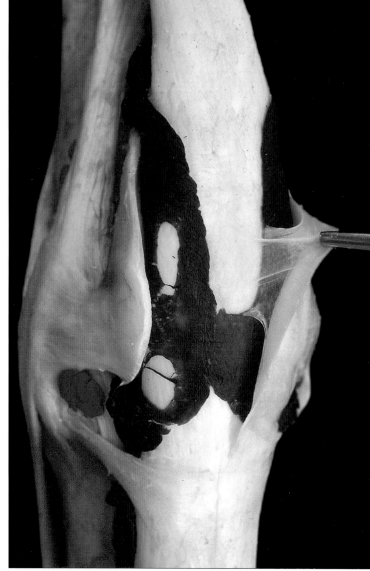

Dissected specimen after injection of coloured latex into the digital sheath cavity.

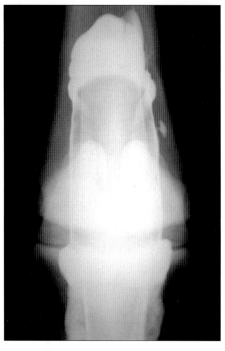

Contrast radiographic study of the digital sheath (tenography), dorsopalmar view.

1 Superficial digital flexor tendon (SDFT)
2 Palmar annular ligament
  2a Medial part
  2b Lateral part (reclined)
3 Proximal digital annular ligament
  3a Proximal attachment
4 Digital sheath cavity
  4a Cavity
  4b Synovial membrane
5 Third interosseus muscle
  5a Distal branch
  5b Extensor branch
6 Medial palmar proper digital artery
7 Lateral palmar proper digital artery
8 Distal metacarpal arterial anastomosis of the SDFT
9 Proximal digital arterial anastomosis of the SDFT
10 Ergot ramus

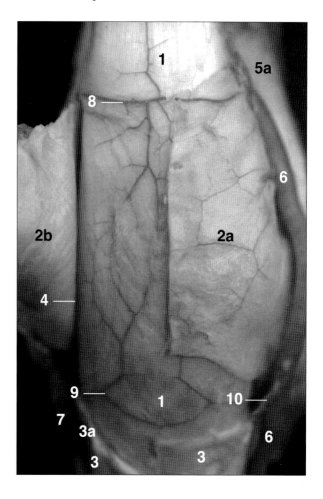

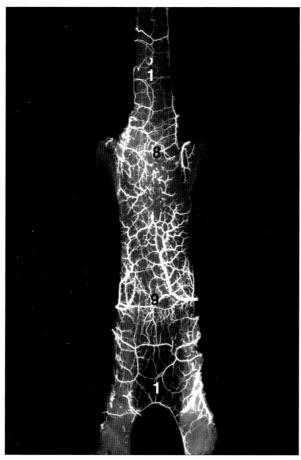

Contrast radiographic study of the arteries (arteriography) of the isolated superficial digital flexor tendon.

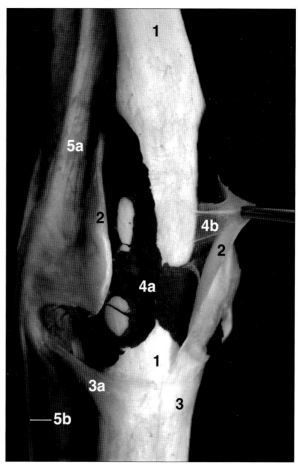

Dissection 13: Fetlock Area – Metacarpophalangeal Joint
Palmar Aspect (Suspensory Apparatus)

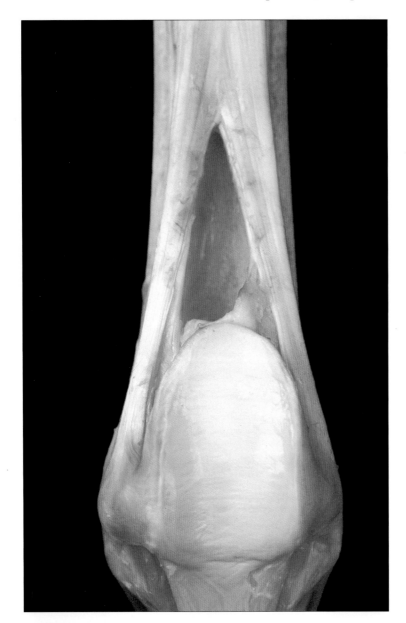

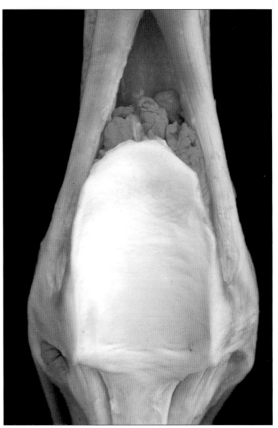

Dissected specimen after injection of coloured latex into the metacarpo-phalangeal joint cavity.

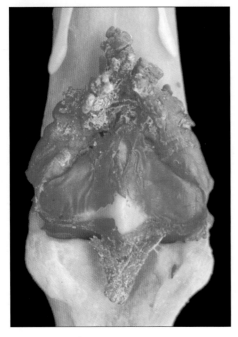

Casting preparation of the palmar recesses of the metacarpo-phalangeal joint, palmar aspect.

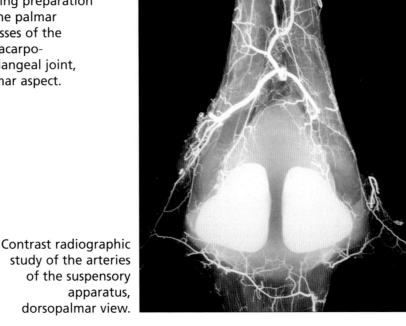

Contrast radiographic study of the arteries of the suspensory apparatus, dorsopalmar view.

1 Third metacarpal bone
2 Second metacarpal bone
3 Fourth metacarpal bone
4 Proximal phalanx (palmar eminence)
5 Medial proximal sesamoid bone
6 Lateral proximal sesamoid bone
7 Palmar (intersesamoidean) ligament
8 Straight sesamoidean ligament
9 Medial oblique sesamoidean ligament
10 Lateral oblique sesamoidean ligament
11 Third interosseus muscle
    11a Medial branch
    11b Lateral branch
    11c Medial extensor branch
12 Fibrous union between the third interosseus
    muscle and the palmar ligament

Ultrasound scans A and B:
a Superficial digital flexor tendon
b Deep digital flexor tendon

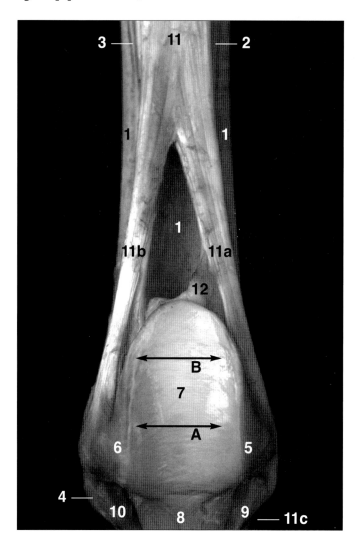

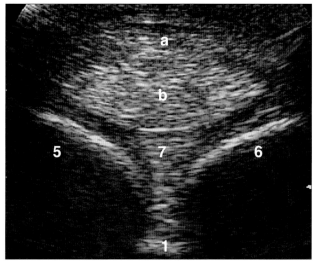

A Transverse ultrasound scan of the fetlock, palmar approach (see arrow in illustration above, right).

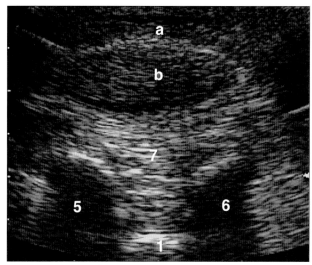

B Transverse ultrasound scan of the fetlock, palmar approach (see arrow in illustration above).

Dissection 14: Metacarpophalangeal Joint – Palmar Aspect
(Oblique and Cruciate Sesamoidean Ligaments)

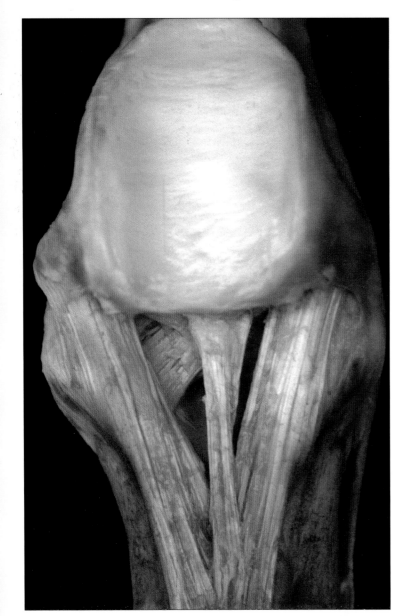

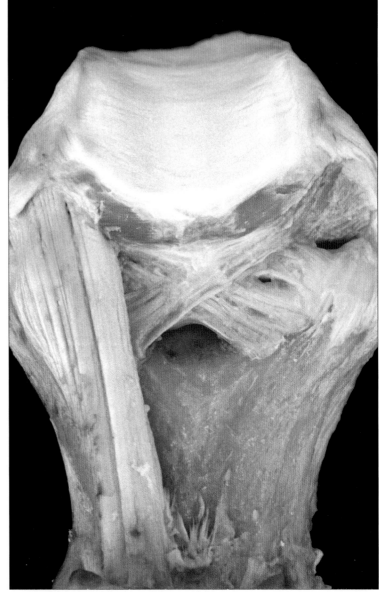

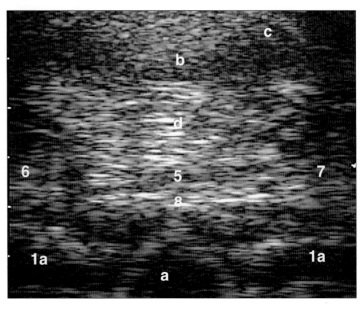

A Transverse ultrasound scan of the distal fetlock, palmar approach (see arrow on illustration opposite).

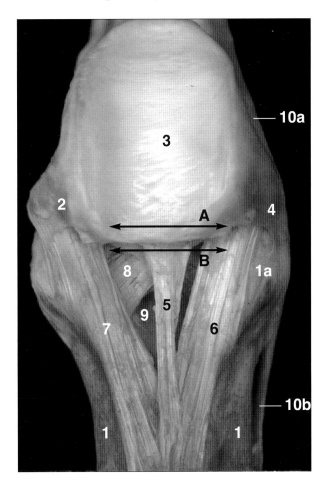

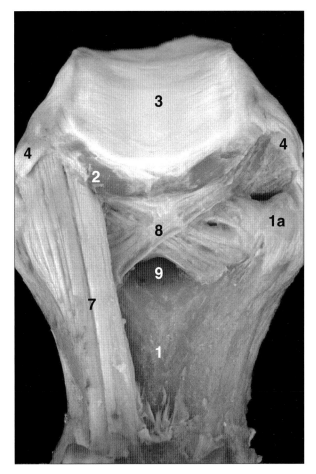

1 Proximal phalanx
   1a Palmar eminence
2 Lateral proximal sesamoid bone
3 Palmar (intersesamoidean) ligament
4 Collateral sesamoidean ligament
5 Sagittal bundle of the oblique
   sesamoidean ligament
6 Medial oblique sesamoidean ligament
7 Lateral oblique sesamoidean ligament
8 Cruciate sesamoidean ligament
9 Distopalmar recess of the
   metacarpophalangeal joint
10 Third interosseus muscle
   10a Medial branch
   10b Medial extensor branch

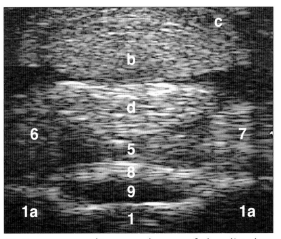

B Transverse ultrasound scan of the distal
fetlock, palmar approach (see arrow in
illustration above, left).

Ultrasound scans A (left) and B (right):
a Sagittal ridge of the third metacarpal bone
b Deep digital flexor tendon
c Superficial digital flexor tendon
d Straight sesamoidean ligament

Dissection 15: Metacarpophalangeal Joint
(Deep Palmar Structures)

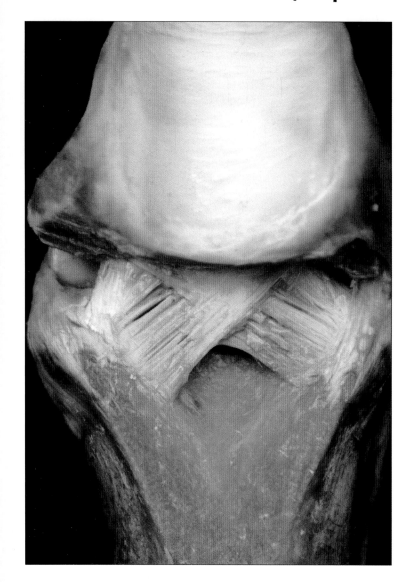

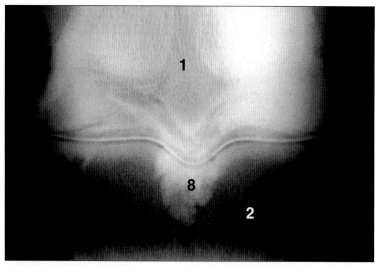

Contrast radiographic study of the metacarpophalangeal joint cavity (arthrography), dorsopalmar view.

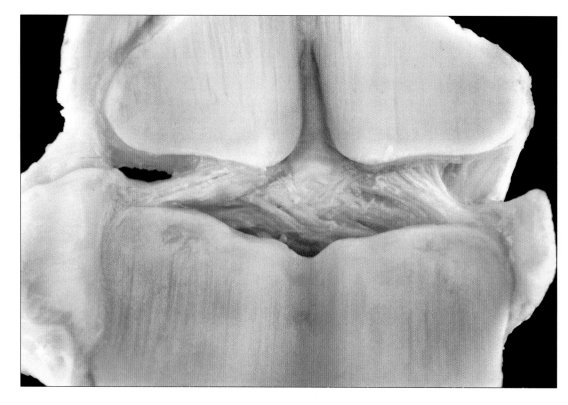

Dissection 15: Metacarpophalangeal Joint
(Deep Palmar Structures)

1 Metacarpal condyle
2 Proximal phalanx (PI)
   2a Palmar eminence
   2b Insertion surface of the oblique sesamoidean ligament (trigone of PI)
3 Medial proximal sesamoid bone
4 Lateral proximal sesamoid bone
5 Palmar (intersesamoidean) ligament
6 Cruciate sesamoidean ligament
7 Short sesamoidean ligament
8 Distopalmar recess of the metacarpophalangeal joint
9 Oblique sesamoidean ligament
10 Collateral sesamoidean ligament
11 Collateral ligament of the metacarpophalangeal joint
12 Distal branch of the third interosseus muscle

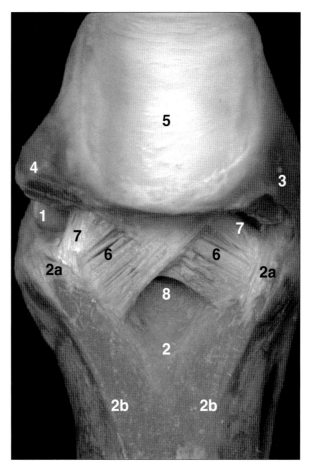

Palmar aspect.

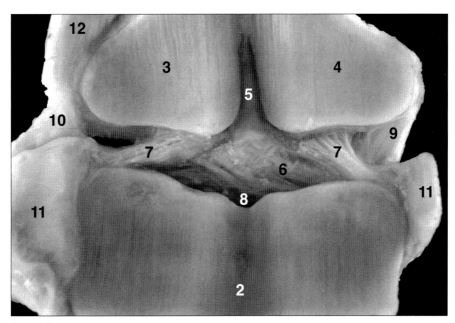

Dorsal aspect.

Dissection 16: Fetlock Area – Dorsal Aspect
(Superficial Structures)

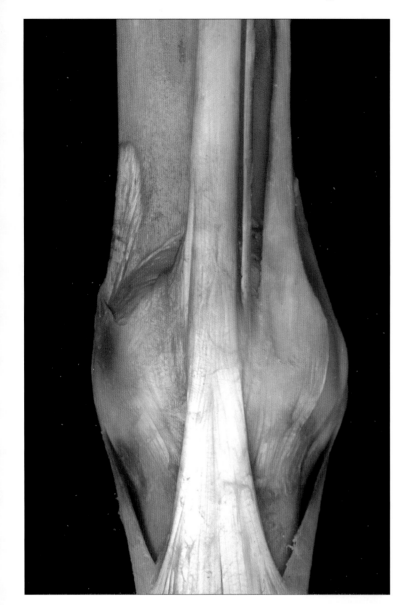

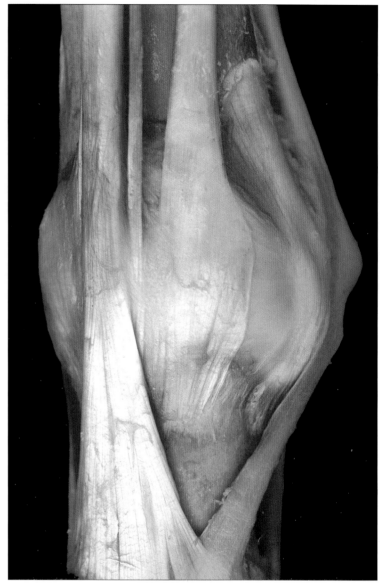

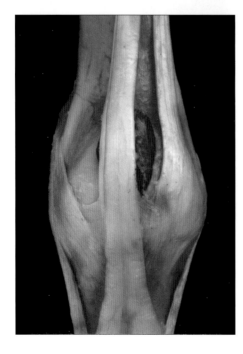

Dissected specimen after injection of coloured latex into the subtendinous extensor bursa.

Dissection 16: Fetlock Area – Dorsal Aspect
(Superficial Structures)

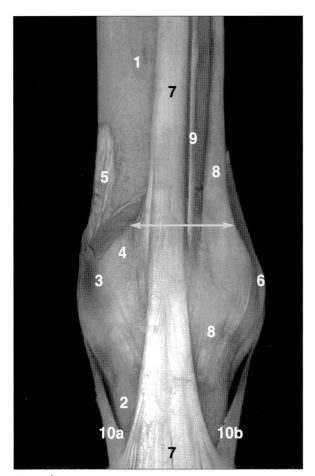

Dorsal aspect.

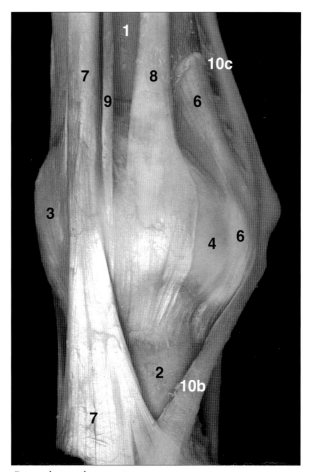

Dorsolateral aspect.

1 Third metacarpal bone
2 Proximal phalanx
3 Dorsal metacarpophalangeal fascia
4 Dorsal articular capsule
5 Medial collateral ligament (superficial part)
6 Lateral collateral ligament (superficial part)
7 Dorsal digital extensor tendon
8 Lateral digital extensor tendon
9 Accessory digital extensor tendon
10 Third interosseus muscle
    10a Medial extensor branch
    10b Lateral extensor branch
    10c Lateral branch

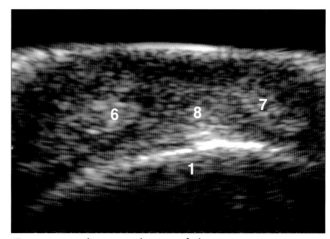

Transverse ultrasound scan of the extensor tendons, dorsal approach (see arrow above).

Dissection 17: Fetlock Area – Metacarpophalangeal Joint
(Dorsal Aspect – Deep Structures)

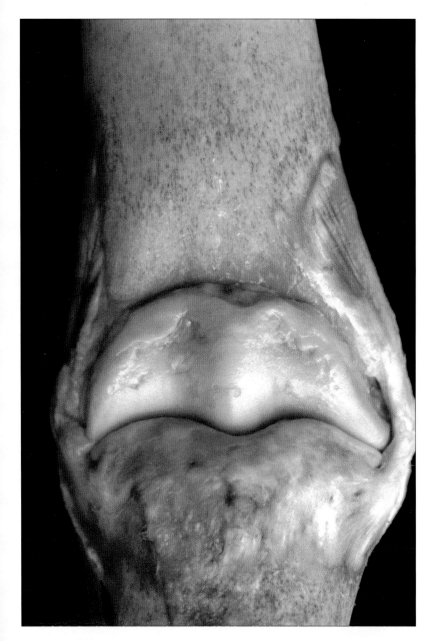

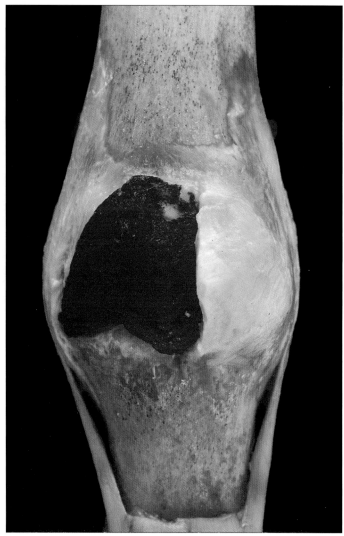

Dissected specimen with injection of coloured latex into the metacarpophalangeal cavity.

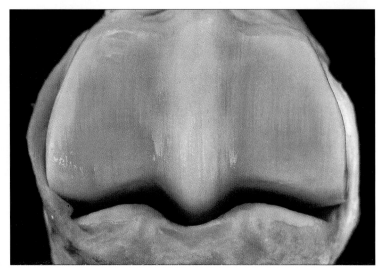

Metacarpophalangeal joint in flexion, dorsal aspect.

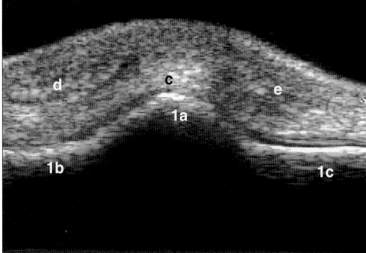

A Transverse ultrasound scan of the flexed fetlock, dorsal approach (see arrow on illustration opposite).

Dissection 17: Fetlock Area – Metacarpophalangeal Joint
(Dorsal Aspect – Deep Structures)

1 Third metacarpal bone
    1a Metacarpal condyle sagittal ridge
    1b Metacarpal condyle medial part
    1c Metacarpal condyle lateral part
    1d Metacarpal condyle dorsal margin
2 Proximal phalanx
3 Metacarpophalangeal joint
4 Medial collateral ligament (superficial part)
5 Lateral collateral ligament (superficial part)

Ultrasound scans A and B:
a Subchondral bone
b Articular cartilage
c Dorsal articular capsule
d Dorsal digital extensor tendon
e Lateral digital extensor tendon
f Skin

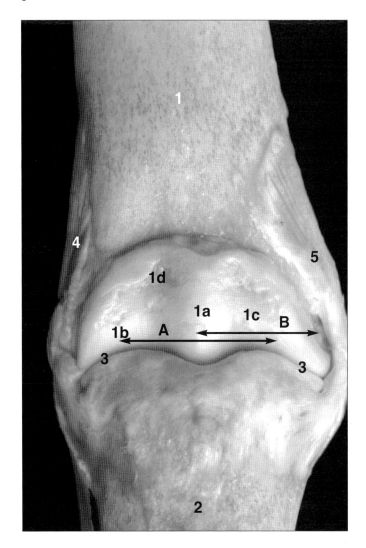

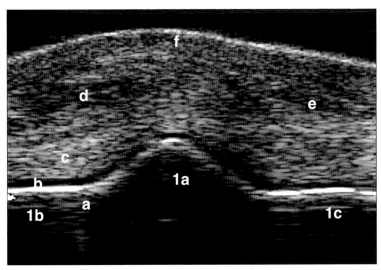

A Transverse ultrasound scan of the fetlock, dorsal approach (see arrow in illustration above, right).

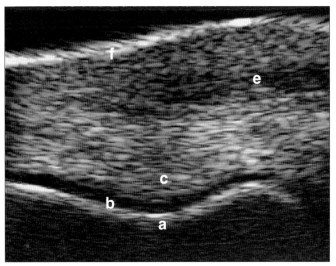

B Transverse ultrasound scan of the fetlock, dorsolateral approach (see arrow in illustration above).

Sagittal and Parasagittal Sections of the Equine Fetlock

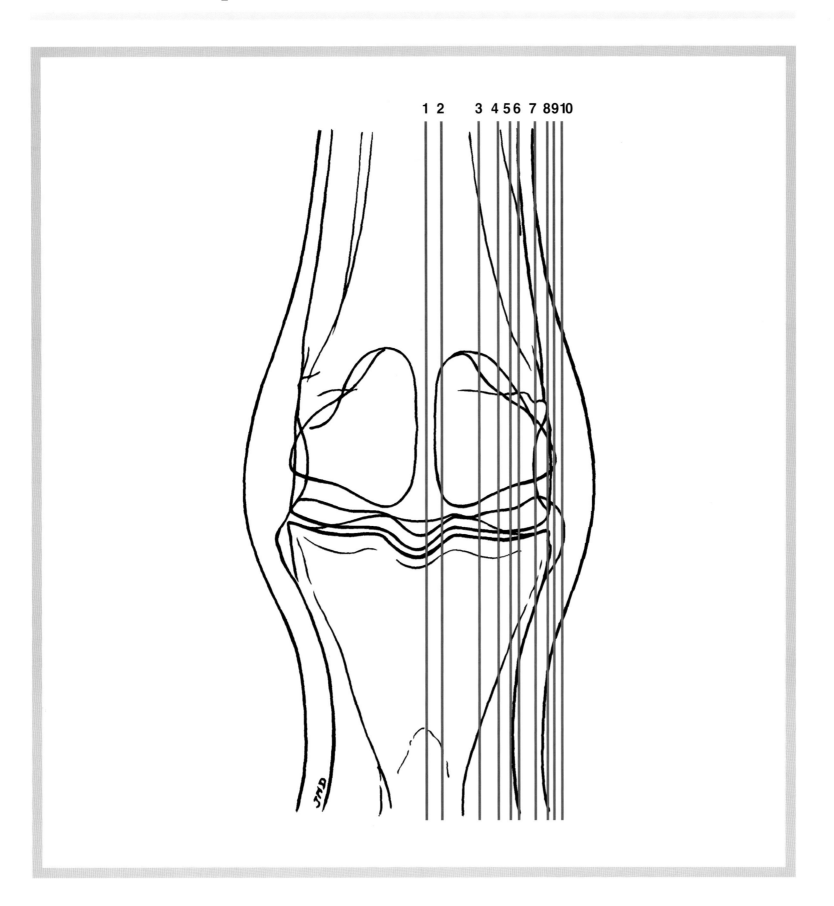

S1a: Sagittal Section of the Digit

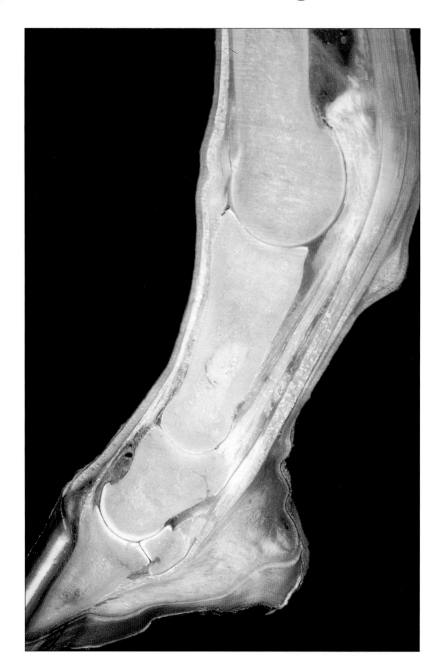

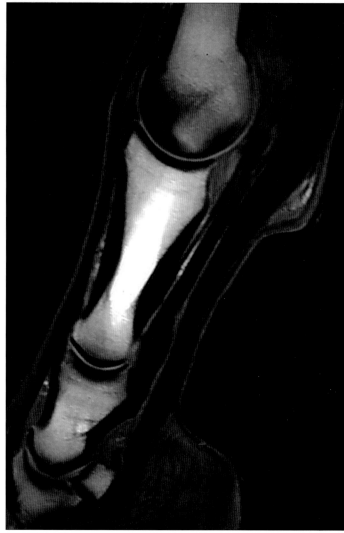

Sagittal MRI scan of the digit after injection of latex into the arteries and fat material into the veins.

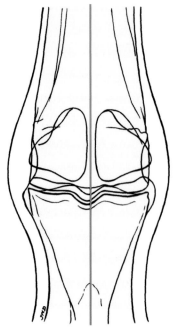

1 Third metacarpal bone
   1a Metacarpal condyle (sagittal ridge)
2 Proximal phalanx
   2a Proximal sagittal groove
   2b Distal sagittal groove
3 Middle phalanx
   3a Flexor tuberosity
4 Distal phalanx
5 Distal sesamoid bone
6 Dorsal capsule of the metacarpophalangeal joint
7 Synovial cavity of the metacarpophalangeal joint
     7a Dorsal recess
     7b Proximopalmar recess
     7c Distopalmar recess
8 Palmar (intersesamoidean) ligament
9 Synovial cavity of the proximal interphalangeal joint
     9a Dorsal recess
     9b Sagittal palmar recess
10 Middle scutum
11 Synovial cavity of the distal interphalangeal joint
     11a Dorsal recess
     11b Proximopalmar recess
12 Collateral sesamoidean ligament
13 Straight sesamoidean ligament
14 Oblique sesamoidean ligament
15 Cruciate sesamoidean ligaments
16 Dorsal digital extensor tendon
17 Superficial digital flexor tendon
     17a Manica flexoria
18 Deep digital flexor tendon
19 Palmar annular ligament
20 Digital sheath cavity
21 Skin
22 Ergot
23 Digital cushion
24 Hoof wall
25 Sole
26 Frog

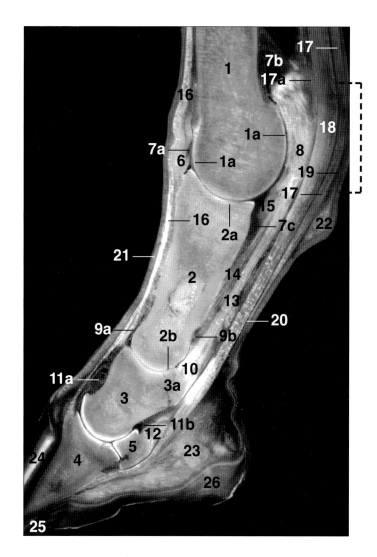

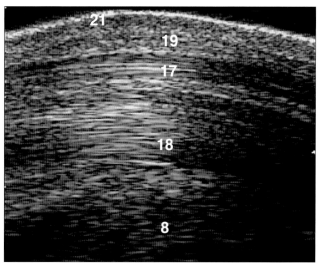

Sagittal ultrasound scan of the fetlock, palmar approach (see dotted area in illustration above).

S1b: Sagittal Section of the Metacarpophalangeal Joint

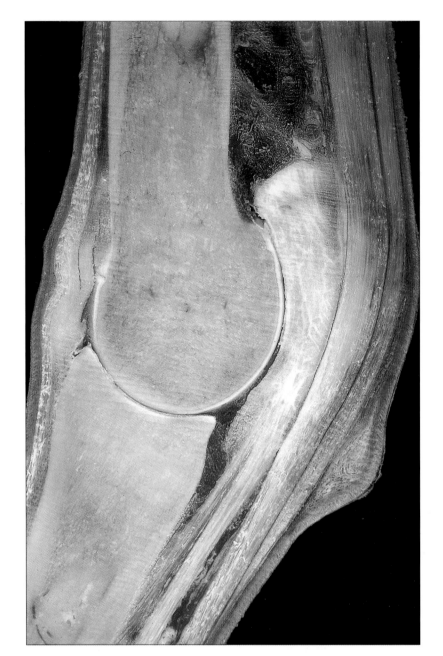

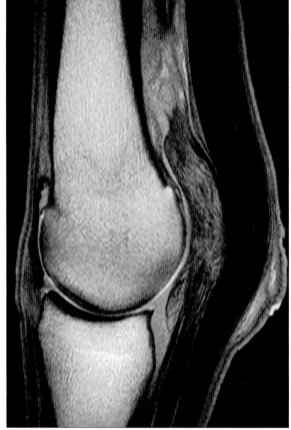

Sagittal MRI scan of the fetlock.

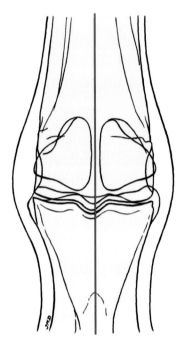

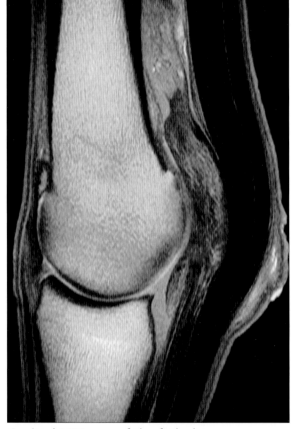

Sagittal MRI scan of the fetlock.

1 Third metacarpal bone
2 Metacarpal condyle
    2a Sagittal ridge
    2b Dorsal margin
    2c Palmar margin
3 Proximal phalanx
    3a Proximal sagittal groove
    3b Proximodorsal articular margin
    3c Proximopalmar articular margin
4 Dorsal capsule of the metacarpophalangeal joint
5 Synovial membrane
    5a Proximodorsal synovial fold
    5b Distodorsal synovial fold
6 Synovial cavity
    6a Dorsal recess
    6b Distodorsal recess
    6c Proximopalmar recess
    6d Synovial villi
    6e Distopalmar recess
7 Palmar (intersesamoidean) ligament
8 Proximal scutum (palmar surface)
9 Straight sesamoidean ligament
10 Oblique sesamoidean ligament
11 Cruciate sesamoidean ligaments
12 Dorsal digital extensor tendon
13 Subtendinous bursa
14 Superficial digital flexor tendon
    14a Manica flexoria
15 Deep digital flexor tendon
    15a Metacarpophalangeal fibrocartilaginous
        part
16 Palmar annular ligament
17 Digital sheath
    17a Synovial membrane
    17b Synovial cavity
18 Common palmar digital artery
19 Common palmar digital vein
20 Palmar metacarpal artery
21 Ergot
22 Skin

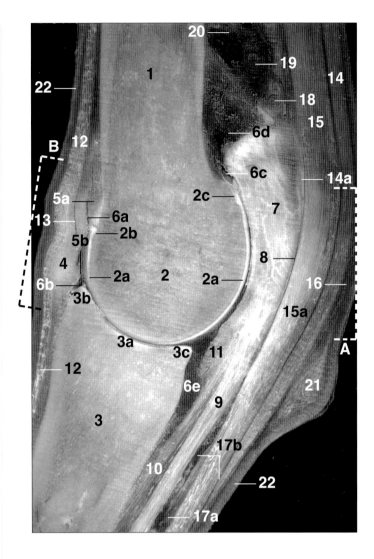

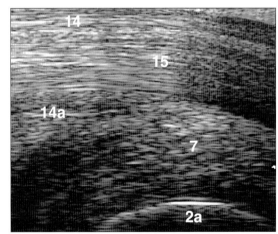

A Sagittal ultrasound scan of the fetlock, palmar approach (see dotted area in illustration above).

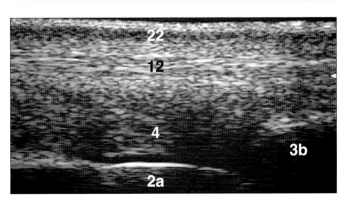

B Sagittal ultrasound scan of the fetlock, dorsal approach (see dotted area in illustration at top of page).

S2: Parasagittal Section of the Metacarpophalangeal Joint

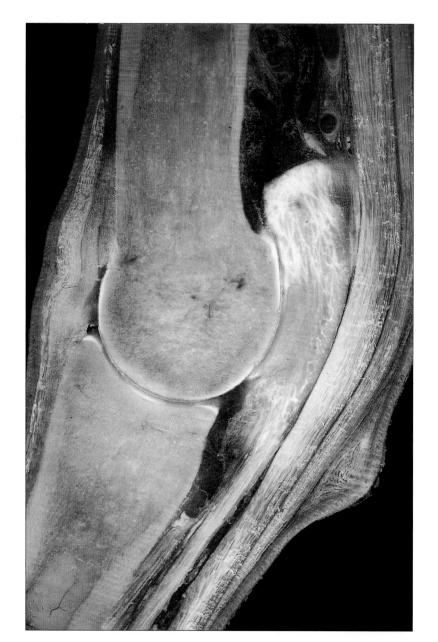

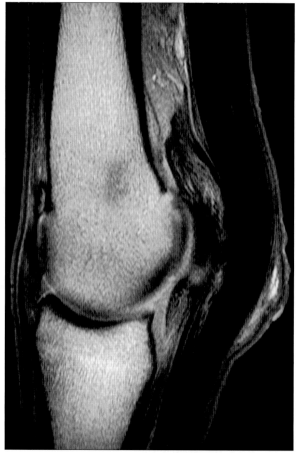

Parasagittal MRI scan of the fetlock.

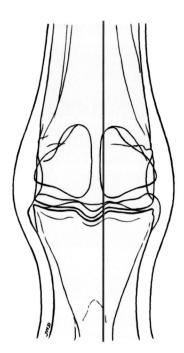

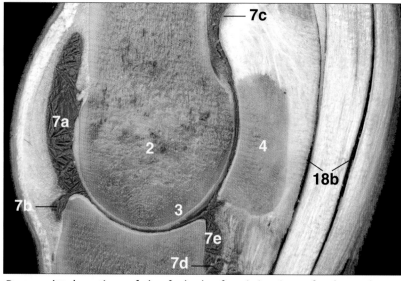

Parasagittal section of the fetlock after injection of coloured latex into the synovial cavities.

1 Third metacarpal bone
2 Metacarpal condyle
   2a Base of the sagittal ridge
   2b Dorsal margin
   2c Palmar margin
3 Proximal phalanx
   3a Border of the proximal sagittal groove
   3b Proximodorsal articular margin
   3c Proximopalmar articular margin
4 Proximal sesamoid bone (axial border)
5 Dorsal capsule of the metacarpophalangeal joint
6 Synovial membrane
   6a Proximodorsal synovial fold
   6b Distodorsal synovial fold
7 Synovial cavity
   7a Dorsal recess
   7b Distodorsal recess
   7c Proximopalmar recess
   7d Synovial villi
   7e Distopalmar recess
8 Palmar (intersesamoidean) ligament
9 Proximal scutum (palmar surface)
10 Straight sesamoidean ligament
11 Oblique sesamoidean ligament
12 Cruciate sesamoidean ligaments
13 Dorsal digital extensor tendon
14 Subtendinous bursa
15 Superficial digital flexor tendon
   15a Manica flexoria
16 Deep digital flexor tendon
   16a Metacarpophalangeal fibrocartilaginous part
17 Palmar annular ligament
18 Digital sheath
   18a Synovial membrane
   18b Synovial cavity
19 Medial common palmar digital artery
20 Lateral proper palmar digital artery
21 Palmar metacarpal artery
22 Medial common palmar digital vein
23 Ergot
24 Skin

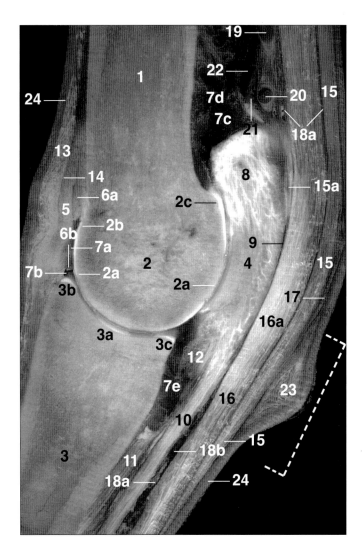

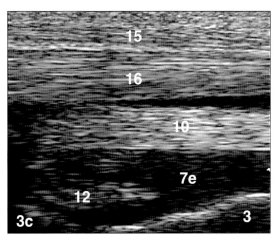

Parasagittal ultrasound scan of the fetlock, palmar approach (see dotted area in illustration above).

S3a: Parasagittal Section of the Metacarpophalangeal Joint

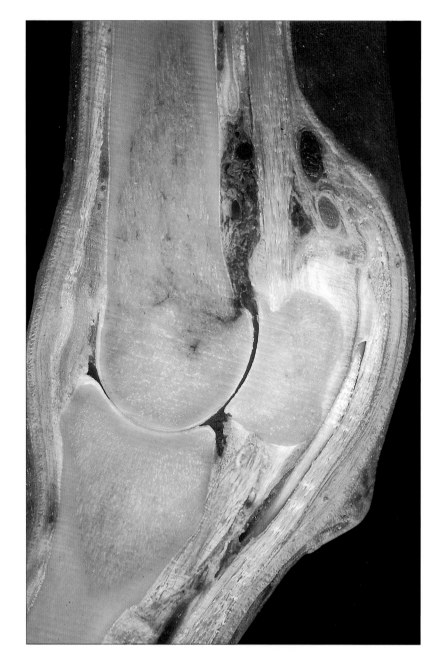

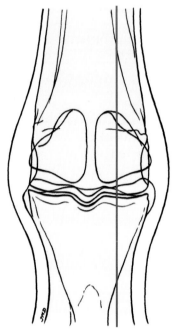

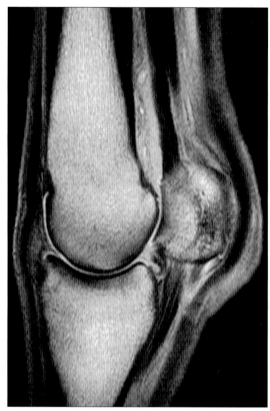

Parasagittal MRI scan of the fetlock.

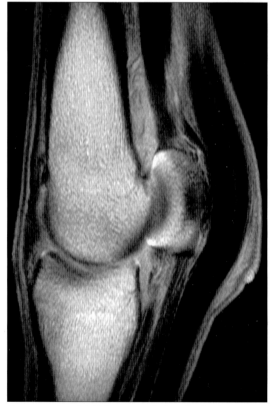

Parasagittal MRI scan of the fetlock.

1 Third metacarpal bone
 1a Metacarpal condyle (lateral part)
2 Fourth metacarpal bone
3 Proximal phalanx
 3a Lateral glenoidal cavity
 3b Dorsal margin
 3c Palmar margin
4 Lateral proximal sesamoid bone
 4a Base
 4b Apex
 4c Articular surface
 4d Flexor surface
5 Dorsal capsule of the metacarpophalangeal joint
6 Synovial membrane
 6a Proximodorsal synovial fold
 6b Distodorsal synovial fold
7 Synovial cavity
 7a Dorsal recess
 7b Proximopalmar recess
 7c Synovial villi
 7d Distopalmar recess
8 Palmar (intersesamoidean) ligament
9 Proximal scutum (palmar surface)
10 Straight sesamoidean ligament
11 Oblique sesamoidean ligament
12 Cruciate sesamoidean ligaments
13 Third interosseus muscle (lateral branch)
14 Lateral digital extensor tendon
15 Superficial digital flexor tendon
 15a Manica flexoria
16 Deep digital flexor tendon
17 Palmar annular ligament
18 Digital sheath
 18a Synovial membrane
 18b Synovial cavity
19 Lateral proper palmar digital artery
20 Lateral proper palmar digital vein
21 Palmar metacarpal artery and vein
22 Ergot
23 Skin

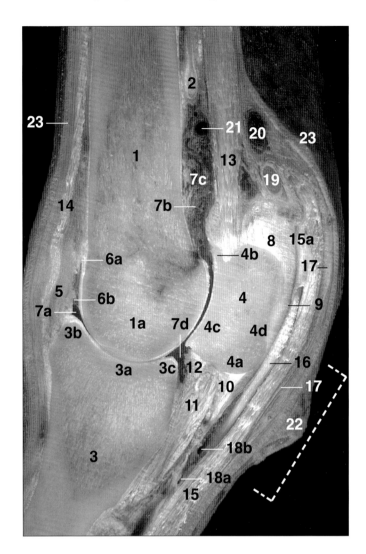

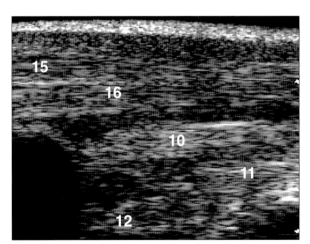

Parasagittal ultrasound scan of the distal fetlock, palmar approach (see dotted area in illustration above).

S3b: Parasagittal Section of the Metacarpophalangeal Joint

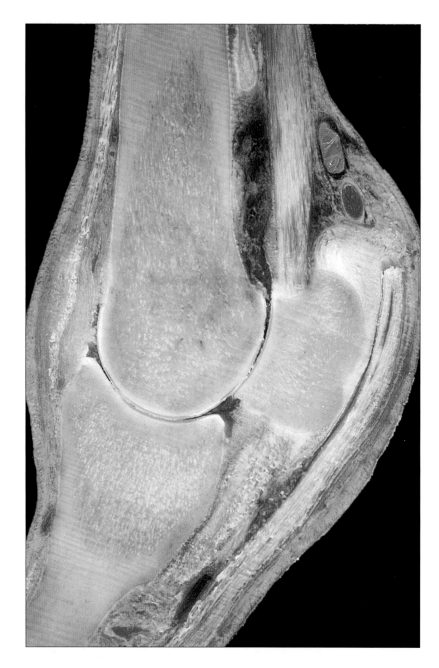

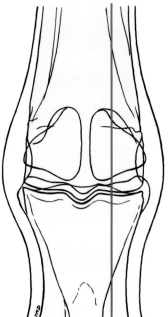

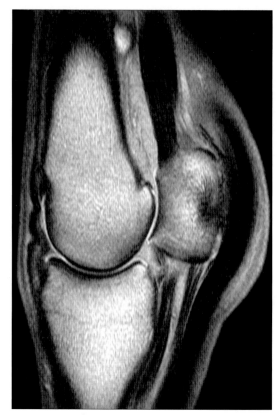

Parasagittal MRI scan of the fetlock.

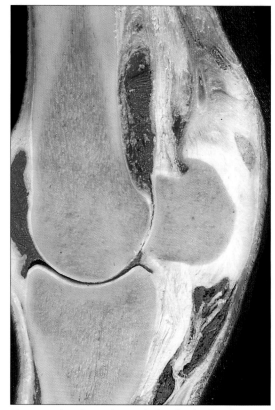

Parasagittal section of the fetlock after injection of coloured latex into the synovial cavities and vessels.

1 Third metacarpal bone
   1a Metacarpal condyle (lateral part)
2 Fourth metacarpal bone
3 Proximal phalanx
   3a Lateral glenoidal cavity
   3b Proximodorsal articular margin
   3c Proximopalmar articular margin
4 Lateral proximal sesamoid bone
   4a Base
   4b Articular surface
   4c Flexor surface
   4d Interosseus face
5 Dorsal capsule of the metacarpophalangeal joint
6 Synovial membrane
   6a Proximodorsal synovial fold
   6b Distodorsal synovial fold
7 Synovial cavity
   7a Dorsal recess
   7b Proximopalmar recess
   7c Synovial villi
   7d Distopalmar recess
8 Palmar (intersesamoidean) ligament
9 Proximal scutum (palmar surface)
10 Straight sesamoidean ligament
11 Oblique sesamoidean ligament
12 Cruciate sesamoidean ligaments
13 Third interosseus muscle (lateral branch)
14 Lateral digital extensor tendon
15 Superficial digital flexor tendon
16 Palmar annular ligament
17 Digital sheath
   17a Synovial membrane
   17b Synovial cavity
18 Lateral proper palmar digital artery
19 Lateral proper palmar digital vein
20 Palmar metacarpal artery and vein
21 Skin

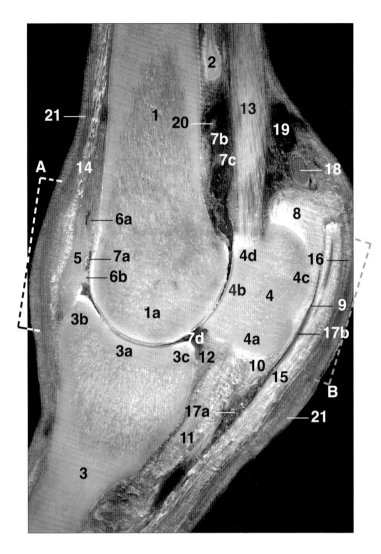

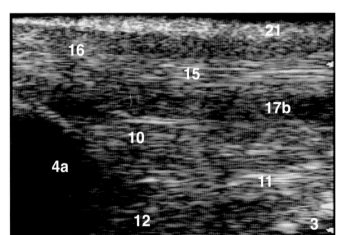

B Parasagittal ultrasound scan of the fetlock, palmar approach (see dotted area in illustration above).

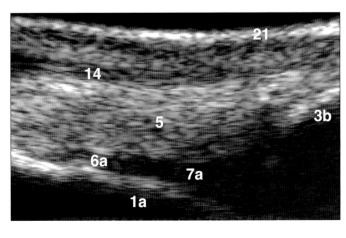

A Parasagittal ultrasound scan of the fetlock, dorsal approach (see dotted area in illustration above, right).

S4: Parasagittal Section of the Metacarpophalangeal Joint

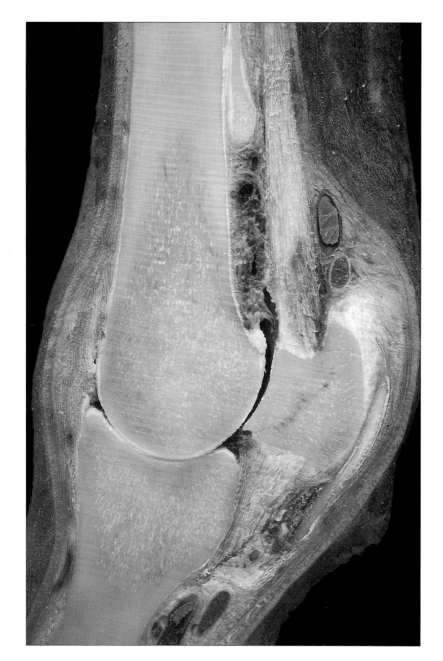

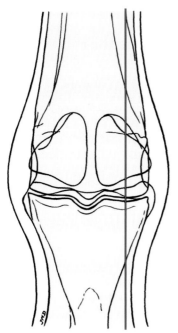

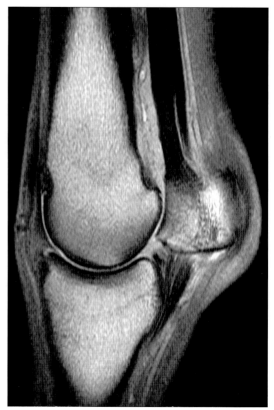

Parasagittal MRI scan of the fetlock.

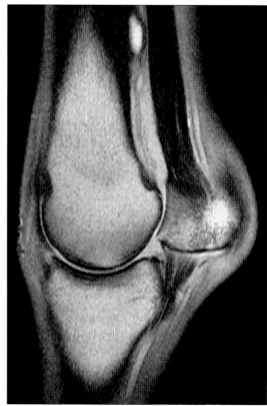

Parasagittal MRI scan of the fetlock.

1 Third metacarpal bone
   1a Metacarpal condyle (medial part)
2 Second metacarpal bone
3 Proximal phalanx
   3a Medial glenoidal cavity
   3b Dorsal margin
   3c Palmar margin
   3d Medial palmar eminence
4 Medial proximal sesamoid bone
   4a Base
   4b Articular surface
   4c Interosseus face
   4d Palmar border
   4e Flexor surface
5 Dorsal capsule of the metacarpophalangeal joint
6 Synovial membrane
   6a Proximodorsal synovial fold
7 Synovial cavity
   7a Dorsal recess
   7b Proximopalmar recess
   7c Synovial villi
   7d Distopalmar recess
8 Palmar (intersesamoidean) ligament
9 Proximal scutum
10 Oblique sesamoidean ligament
11 Short sesamoidean ligament
12 Third interosseus muscle
   12a Medial branch
   12b Medial extensor branch
13 Superficial digital flexor tendon
14 Palmar annular ligament
15 Digital sheath (collateral recess)
16 Medial proper palmar digital artery
17 Medial proper palmar digital vein
18 Medial proper palmar digital nerve
19 Palmar metacarpal vein and artery
20 Ergot
21 Skin

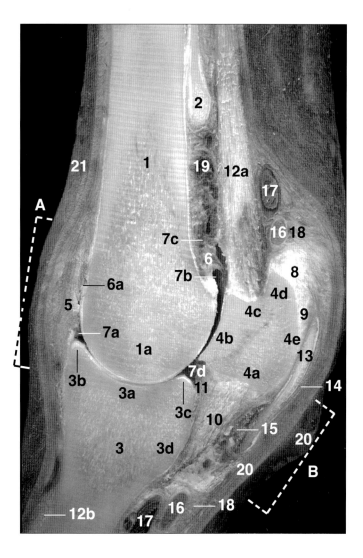

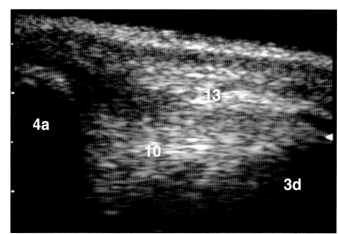

B Parasagittal ultrasound scan of the distal fetlock, palmar approach (see dotted area in illustration above).

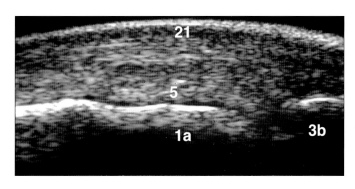

A Parasagittal ultrasound scan of the distal fetlock, palmar approach (see dotted area in illustration above, right).

S5: Parasagittal Section of the Metacarpophalangeal Joint

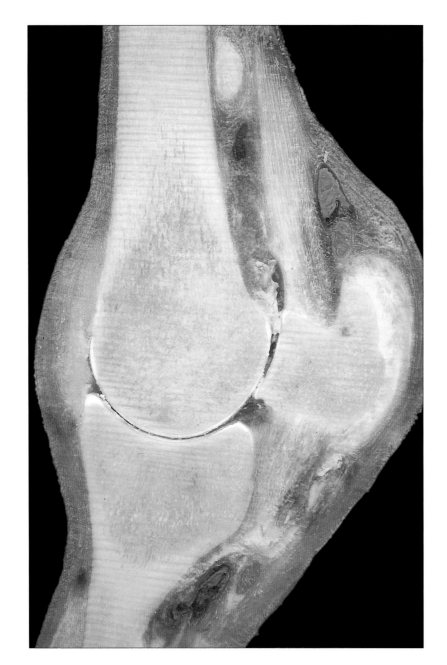

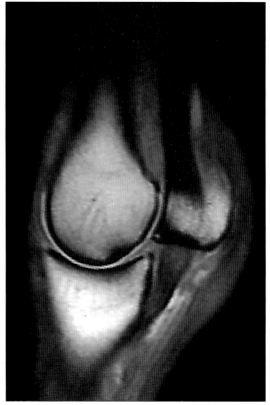

Parasagittal MRI scan of the fetlock after injection of latex into the arteries and fat material into the veins.

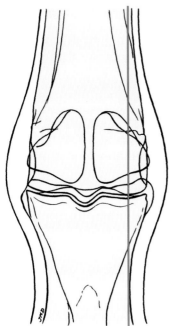

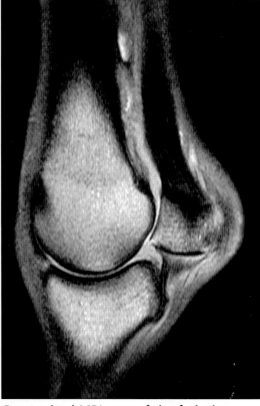

Parasagittal MRI scan of the fetlock.

1 Third metacarpal bone
   1a Metacarpal condyle (medial part)
2 Second metacarpal bone
3 Proximal phalanx (P1)
   3a Medial glenoidal cavity
   3b Proximodorsal articular margin
   3c Proximopalmar articular margin
   3d Palmar eminence
4 Medial proximal sesamoid bone
   4a Base
   4b Articular surface
   4c Interosseus face
   4d Palmar border
   4e Flexor surface
5 Dorsal capsule of the metacarpophalangeal joint
6 Synovial membrane
7 Synovial cavity
   7a Dorsal recess
   7b Proximopalmar recess
   7c Synovial villi
   7d Distopalmar recess
8 Palmar (intersesamoidean) ligament
9 Oblique sesamoidean ligament
10 Short sesamoidean ligament
11 Third interosseus muscle
   11a Medial branch
   11b Medial extensor branch
12 Palmar annular ligament
13 Digital sheath (collateral recess)
14 Medial proper palmar digital artery
   14a Palmar ramus of P1
   14b Ramus of the proximal sesamoid bone
15 Medial proper palmar digital vein
   15a Palmar ramus of P1
   15b Dorsal ramus of P1
16 Medial palmar metacarpal artery and vein
17 Medial proper palmar digital nerve
18 Skin

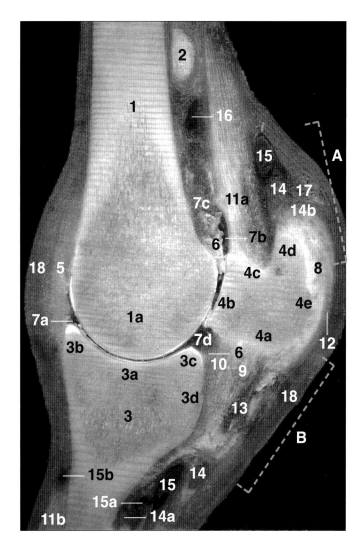

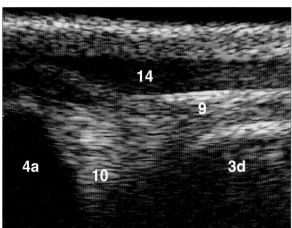

B Parasagittal ultrasound scan of the fetlock, palmar approach (see dotted area in illustration above).

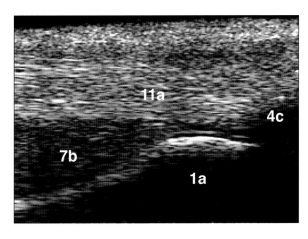

A Parasagittal ultrasound scan of the fetlock, palmar approach (see dotted area in illustration above, right).

S6: Parasagittal Section of the Metacarpophalangeal Joint

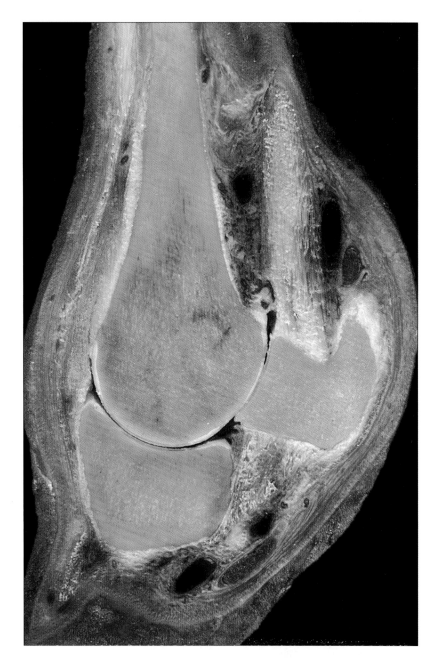

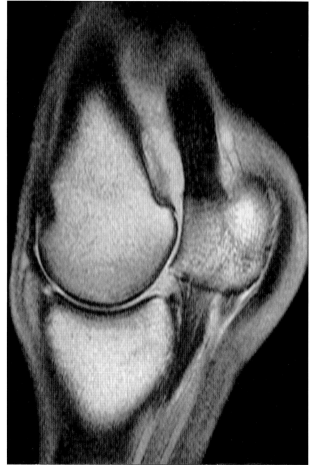

Parasagittal MRI scan of the fetlock.

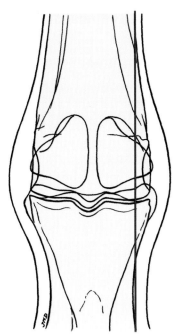

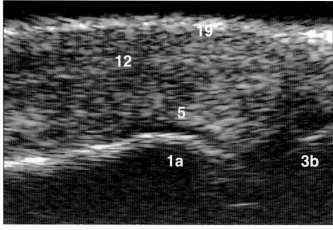

A Parasagittal ultrasound scan of the fetlock, dorsal approach (see dotted area in illustration on facing page).

1 Third metacarpal bone
    1a Metacarpal condyle (lateral part)
2 Fourth metacarpal bone
3 Proximal phalanx
    3a Lateral glenoidal cavity
    3b Proximodorsal articular margin
    3c Proximopalmar articular margin
    3d Lateral palmar eminence
4 Lateral proximal sesamoid bone
    4a Base
    4b Articular surface
    4c Interosseus face
    4d Palmar border
5 Dorsal capsule of the metacarpophalangeal
    joint
6 Lateral collateral ligament
7 Synovial cavity
    7a Dorsal recess
    7b Proximopalmar recess
    7c Synovial villi
    7d Distopalmar recess
8 Palmar (intersesamoidean) ligament
9 Oblique sesamoidean ligament
10 Short sesamoidean ligament
11 Third interosseus muscle
    11a Lateral branch
    11b Lateral extensor branch
12 Lateral digital extensor tendon
13 Lateral proper palmar digital artery
    13a Ramus for the proximal sesamoid
          bone
14 Lateral proper palmar digital vein
15 Lateral proper palmar digital nerve
16 Lateral palmar metacarpal artery
17 Lateral palmar metacarpal vein
18 Dorsal metacarpophalangeal fascia
19 Skin

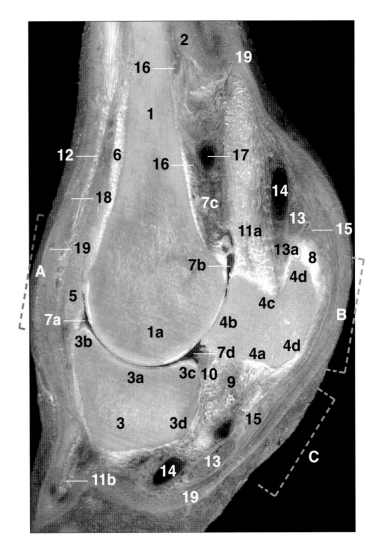

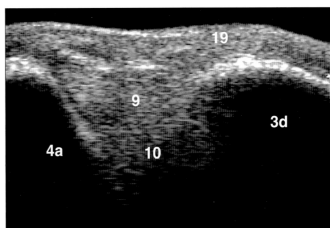

C Parasagittal ultrasound scan of the fetlock, palmar approach (see dotted area in illustration above).

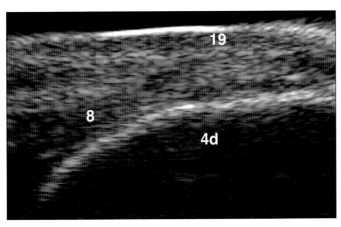

B Parasagittal ultrasound scan of the fetlock, palmar approach (see dotted area in illustration at top, right).

S7: Parasagittal Section of the Metacarpophalangeal Joint

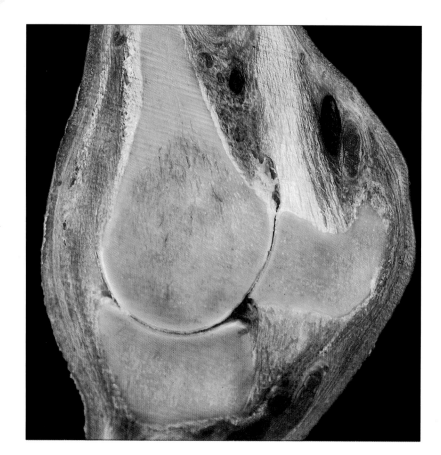

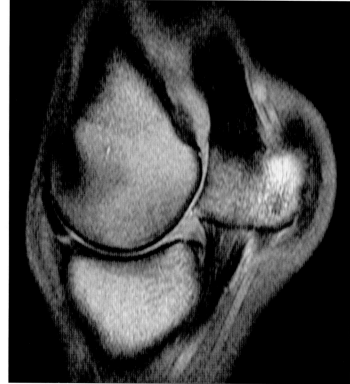

Parasagittal MRI scan of the fetlock.

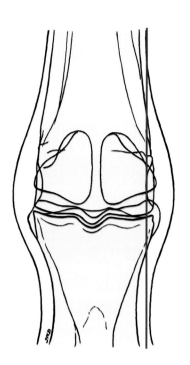

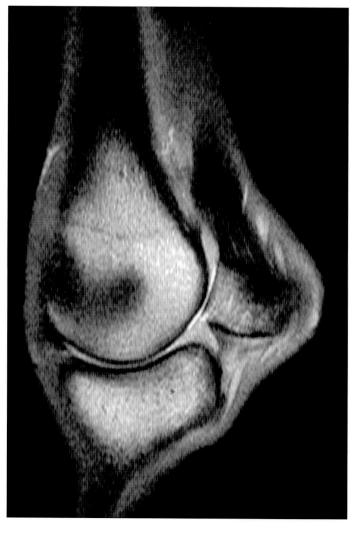

Parasagittal MRI
scan of the fetlock.

1 Third metacarpal bone
   1a Metacarpal condyle (lateral part)
2 Proximal phalanx
   2a Lateral glenoidal cavity
   2b Proximodorsal articular margin
   2c Proximopalmar articular margin
   2d Lateral palmar eminence
3 Lateral proximal sesamoid bone
   3a Base
   3b Articular surface
   3c Interosseus face
   3d Palmar border
4 Dorsal capsule of the metacarpophalangeal joint
5 Lateral collateral ligament
6 Synovial cavity
   6a Dorsal recess
   6b Proximopalmar recess
   6c Synovial villi
   6d Distopalmar recess
7 Palmar (intersesamoidean) ligament
8 Lateral oblique sesamoidean ligament
9 Third interosseus muscle
   9a Lateral branch
   9b Lateral extensor branch
10 Lateral digital extensor tendon
11 Lateral proper palmar digital artery
12 Lateral proper palmar digital vein
13 Lateral proper palmar digital nerve
14 Lateral palmar metacarpal artery
15 Lateral palmar metacarpal vein
16 Dorsal metacarpophalangeal fascia
17 Skin

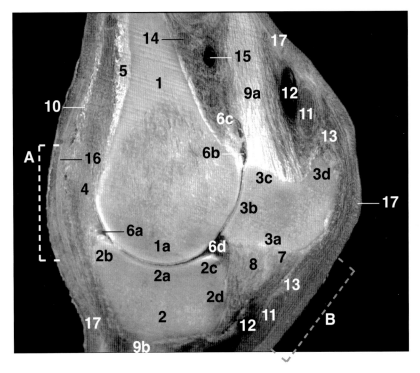

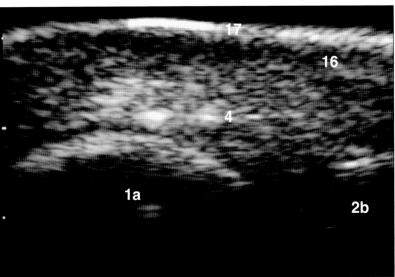

A Parasagittal ultrasound scan of the half-flexed fetlock, dorsal approach (see dotted area in illustration above).

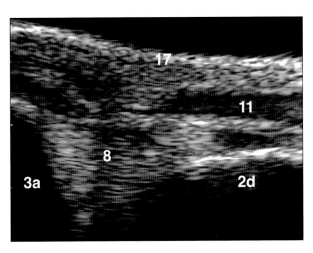

B Parasagittal ultrasound scan of the fetlock, palmar approach (see dotted area in illustration at top, right).

S8: Parasagittal Section of the Metacarpophalangeal Joint
(The Joint is Half-flexed)

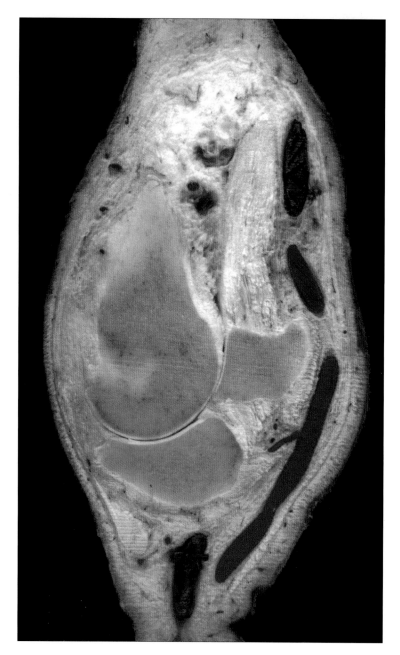

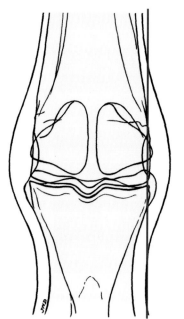

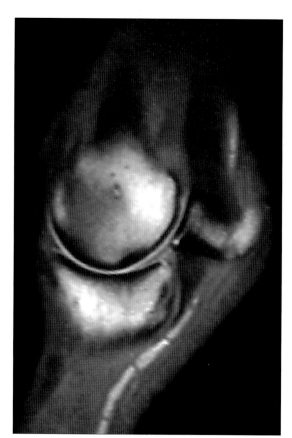

Parasagittal MRI scan of the fetlock after injection of latex into the arteries and fat material into the veins.

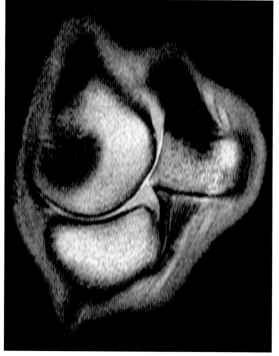

Parasagittal MRI scan of the fetlock.

1 Third metacarpal bone
   1a Metacarpal condyle (lateral part)
2 Proximal phalanx
   2a Lateral glenoidal cavity
   2b Lateral palmar eminence
3 Lateral proximal sesamoid bone
   3a Articular surface
   3b Interosseus face
   3c Palmar border
   3d Base
4 Dorsal capsule of the
   metacarpophalangeal joint
5 Synovial membrane (distodorsal
   synovial fold)
6 Synovial cavity
   6a Proximopalmar recess
   6b Synovial villi
7 Palmar (intersesamoidean) ligament
8 Lateral oblique sesamoidean ligament
9 Third interosseus muscle
   9a Lateral branch
   9b Lateral extensor branch
10 Lateral digital extensor tendon
11 Lateral proper palmar digital artery
   11a Articular branch
12 Lateral palmar common digital vein
13 Lateral palmar proper digital vein
14 Lateral palmar proper digital nerve
15 Lateral palmar metacarpal artery
16 Ergot ligament
17 Skin

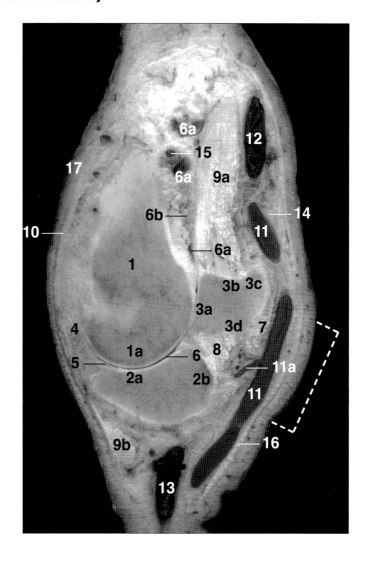

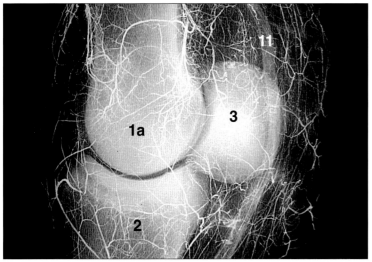

Contrast radiographic study of the arteries (arteriography) of the fetlock, lateromedial projection.

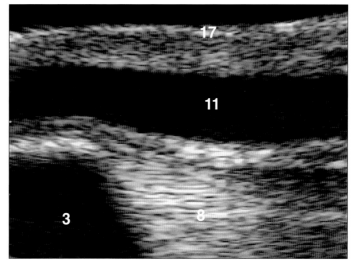

Parasagittal ultrasound scan of the fetlock, palmar approach (see dotted area in illustration above).

S9: Parasagittal Section of the Metacarpophalangeal Joint

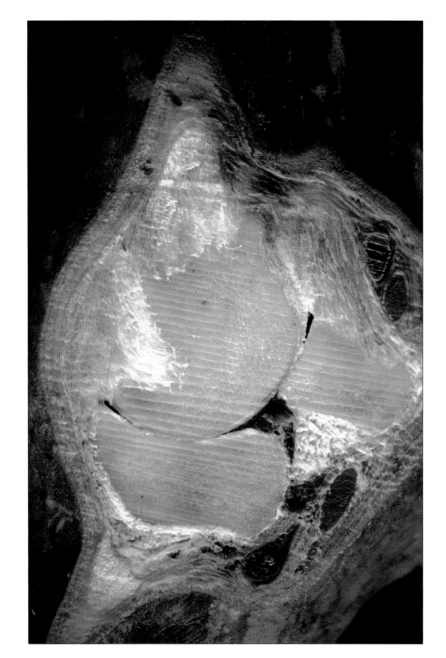

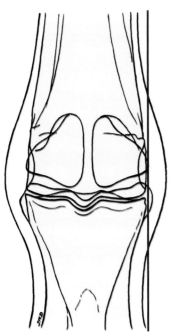

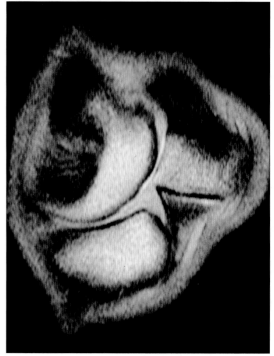

Parasagittal MRI scan of the fetlock.

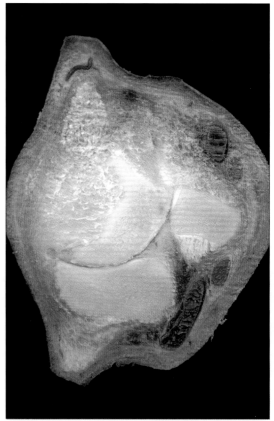

Parasagittal section of the fetlock after injection of coloured latex into the vessels.

1 Metacarpal condyle
   1a Collateral fossa
2 Proximal phalanx
   2a Glenoidal cavity
   2b Dorsal margin
   2c Palmar eminence
3 Proximal sesamoid bone
   3a Articular surface
   3b Interosseus face
4 Dorsal articular capsule
5 Synovial cavity
   5a Collateral recess
6 Collateral ligament of the
   metacarpophalangeal joint
   6a Deep part
   6b Superficial part
7 Oblique sesamoidean ligament
8 Third interosseus muscle
   8a Distal branch
   8b Extensor branch
9 Proper palmar digital artery
10 Proper palmar digital vein
11 Proper palmar digital nerve
12 Metacarpal artery
13 Dorsal metacarpophalangeal fascia
14 Skin
   14a Skin section

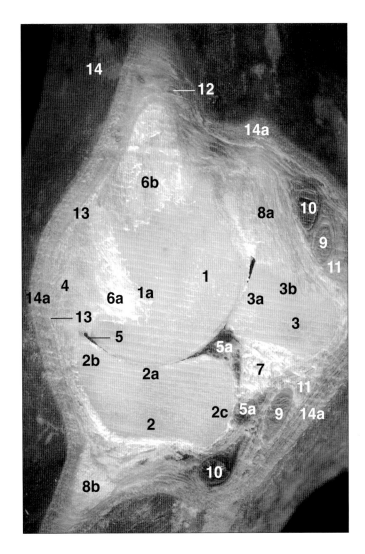

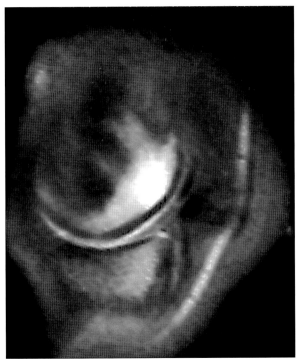

Parasagittal MRI scan of the fetlock after injection of latex into the arteries and fat material into the veins.

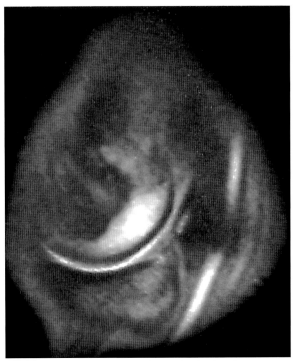

Parasagittal MRI scan of the fetlock after injection of latex into the arteries and fat material into the veins.

S10: Parasagittal Section of the Metacarpophalangeal Joint

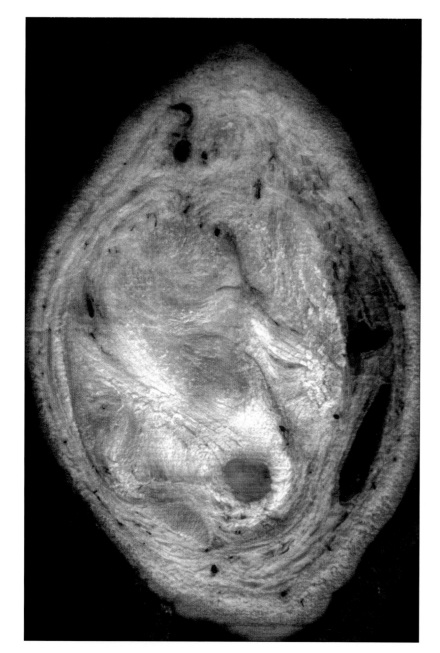

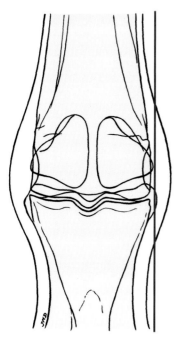

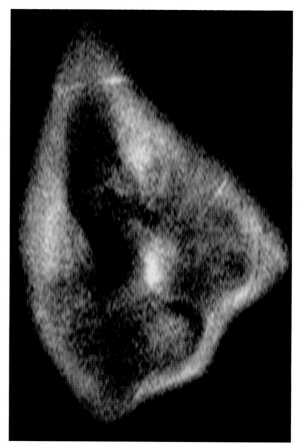

Parasagittal MRI scan of the fetlock.

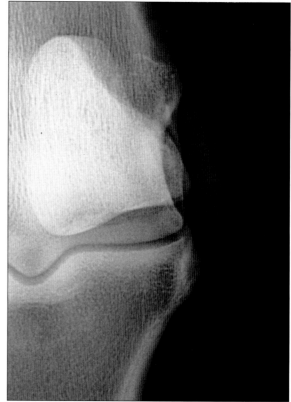

Dorsopalmar radiograph of the sectioned structures.

1 Proximal phalanx (palmar eminence)
2 Collateral ligament of the metacarpophalangeal joint (deep part)
3 Third interosseus muscle
   3a Distal branch
   3b Extensor branch
4 Proper palmar digital vein
5 Vascular network of the metacarpophalangeal joint
6 Dorsal metacarpophalangeal fascia
7 Skin
   7a Skin section

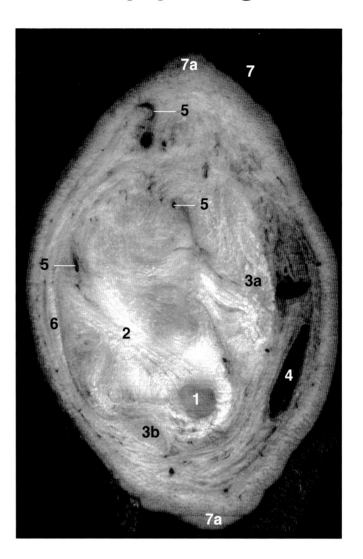

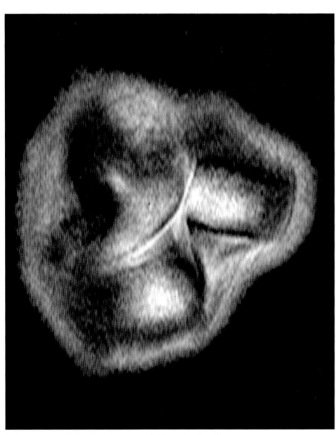

Parasagittal MRI scan of the fetlock.

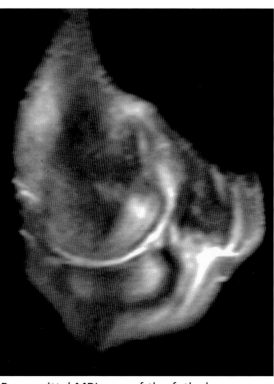

Parasagittal MRI scan of the fetlock.

Transverse Sections of the Equine Fetlock

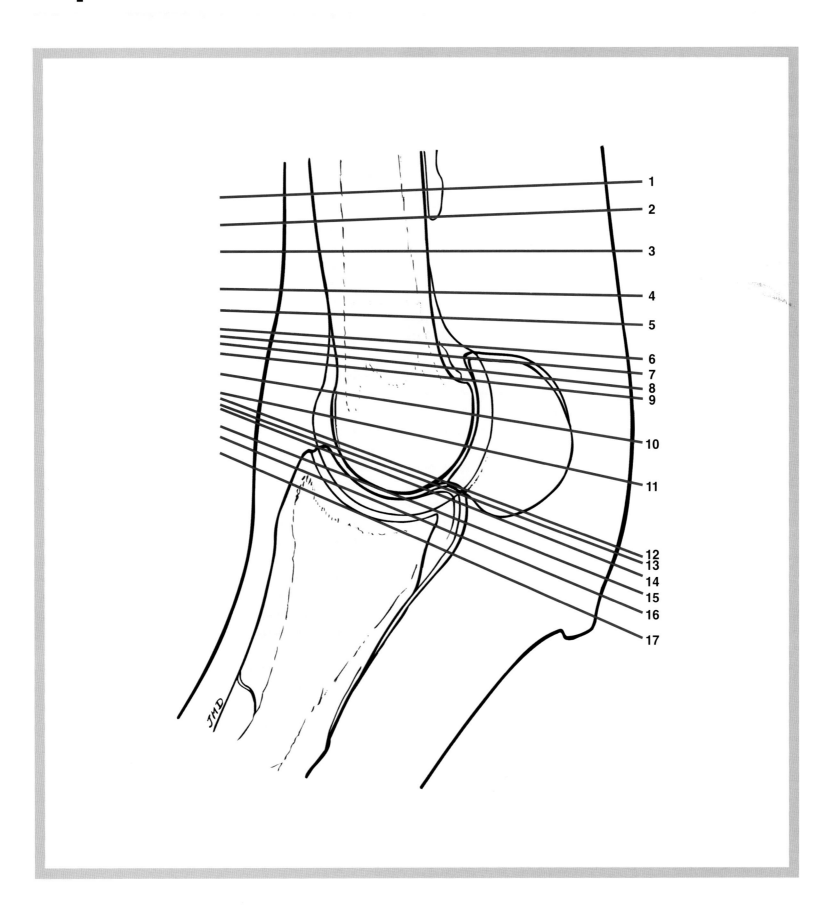

T1: Transverse Section of the Metacarpophalangeal Joint

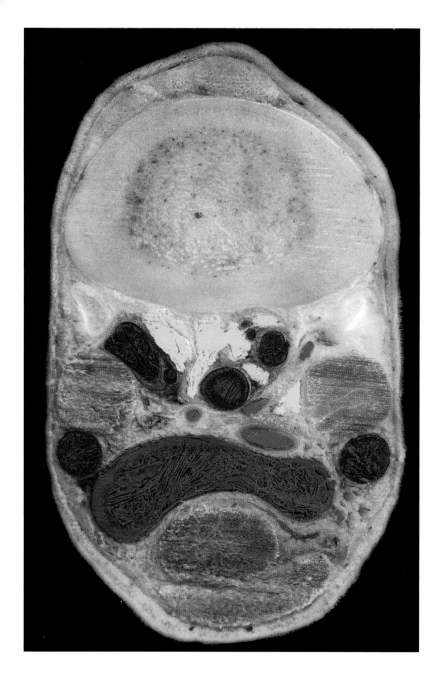

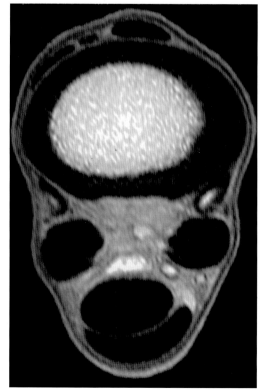

Transverse MRI scan of the fetlock.

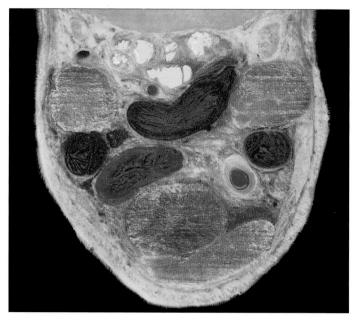

Transverse anatomical section of the fetlock area after injection of coloured latex into the synovial cavities and vessels.

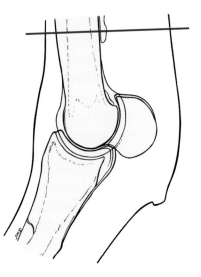

1 Third metacarpal bone
2 Second metacarpal bone
3 Fourth metacarpal bone
4 Proximopalmar recess of the metacarpophalangeal joint cavity
   4a Synovial plica
5 Dorsal digital extensor tendon
6 Lateral digital extensor tendon
7 Accessory digital extensor tendon
8 Superficial digital flexor tendon
9 Deep digital flexor tendon
10 Third interosseus muscle (branches)
11 Digital sheath (synovial cavity)
   11a Synovial membrane
   11b Dorsal proximal recess
12 Medial common palmar digital artery
13 Common palmar digital veins
14 Common palmar digital nerves
15 Palmar metacarpal arteries
16 Palmar metacarpal veins
17 Dorsal metacarpal fascia
18 Palmar metacarpal fascia
19 Skin

Ultrasound scans A and B:
a Proper palmar digital artery
b Proper palmar digital vein

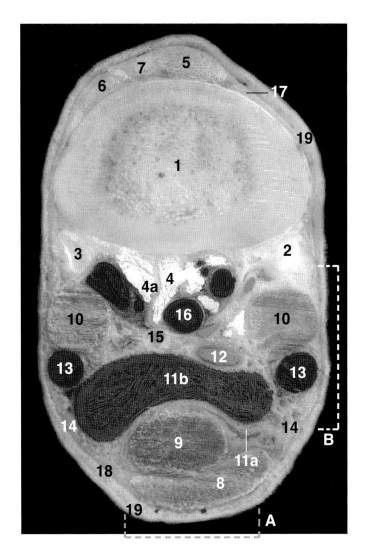

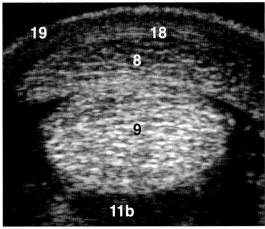

A Transverse ultrasound scan of the fetlock, palmar approach (see dotted area in illustration above, right).

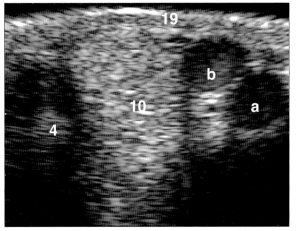

B Transverse ultrasound scan of the fetlock area, lateral approach (see dotted area in illustration above).

T2: Transverse Section of the Metacarpophalangeal Joint

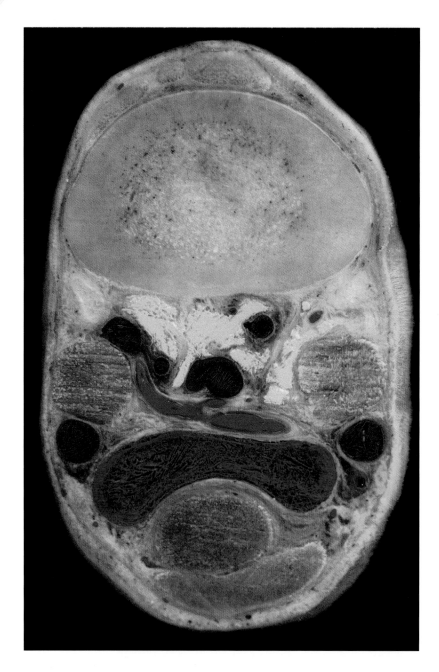

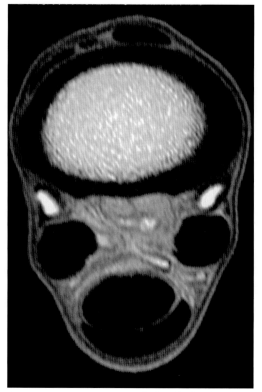

Transverse MRI scan of the fetlock.

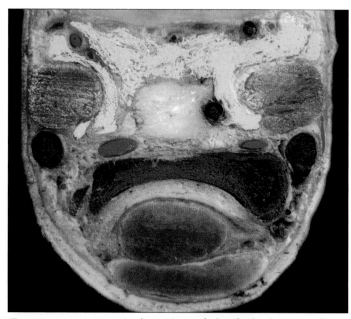

Transverse anatomical section of the fetlock area after injection of coloured latex into the synovial cavities and vessels.

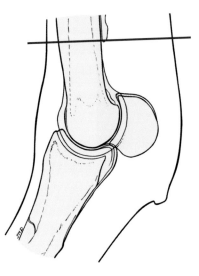

1 Third metacarpal bone
  1a Cancellous bone
  1b Cortical bone
  1c Periosteum
2 Fourth metacarpal bone
3 Proximopalmar recess of the metacarpophalangeal joint cavity
  3a Synovial plica
4 Dorsal digital extensor tendon
5 Lateral digital extensor tendon
6 Accessory digital extensor tendon
7 Superficial digital flexor tendon
8 Deep digital flexor tendon
9 Third interosseus muscle (branches)
10 Digital sheath (synovial cavity)
  10a Synovial membrane
  10b Dorsal proximal recess
11 Common palmar digital artery (bifurcation)
12 Common palmar digital vein
13 Common palmar digital nerve
14 Palmar metacarpal arteries
  14a Anastomosis with the digital arteries
15 Palmar metacarpal veins
16 Dorsal metacarpal fascia
17 Palmar metacarpal fascia
18 Skin

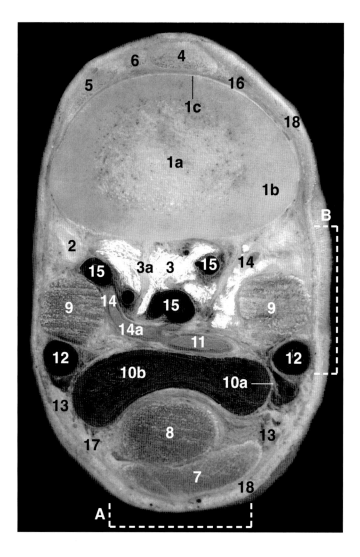

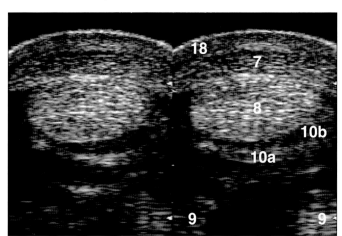

A Transverse ultrasound scan of the fetlock, palmar approach (see dotted area in illustration above, right).

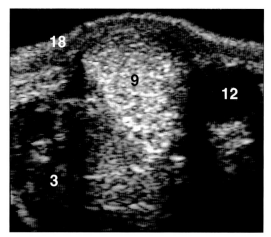

B Transverse ultrasound scan of the fetlock, medial approach (see dotted area in illustration above).

T3: Transverse Section of the Metacarpophalangeal Joint

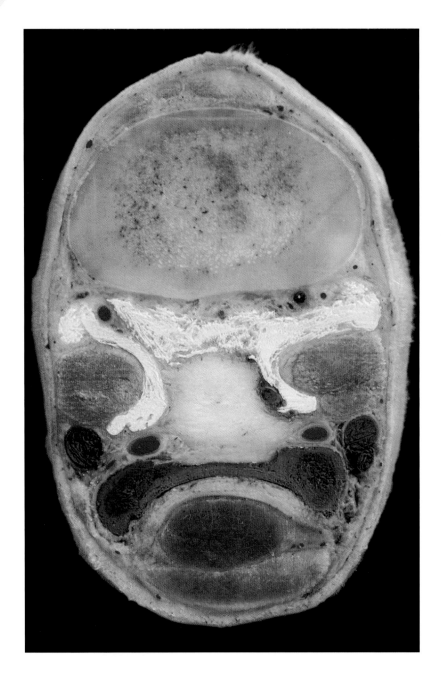

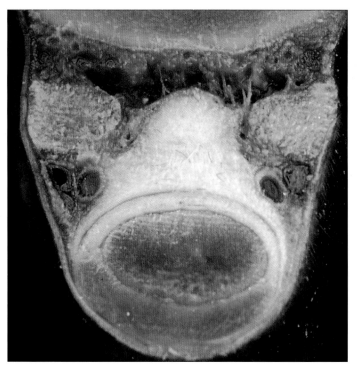

Transverse section of the fetlock after injection of coloured latex into the vessels.

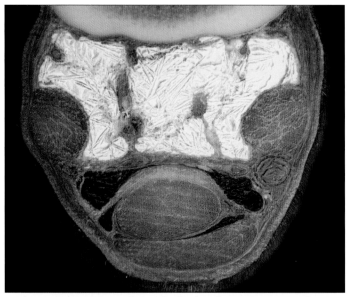

Transverse section of the fetlock after injection of coloured latex into the synovial cavities and vessels.

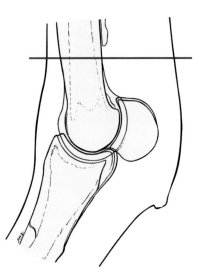

1 Third metacarpal bone
   1a Cancellous bone
   1b Cortical bone
   1c Periosteum
2 Dorsal capsule of the metacarpophalangeal (MP) joint
3 Synovial membrane
   3a Synovial plica
   3b Synovial villi
4 Proximopalmar recess of the MP joint cavity
5 Palmar (intersesamoidean) ligament
6 Proximal scutum (palmar surface)
7 Dorsal digital extensor tendon
8 Lateral digital extensor tendon
9 Accessory digital extensor tendon
10 Third interosseus muscle
   10a Lateral branch
   10b Medial branch
11 Superficial digital flexor tendon
   11a Manica flexoria
12 Deep digital flexor tendon
13 Digital sheath
   13a Synovial membrane
   13b Dorsal proximal recess
14 Lateral proper palmar digital artery
15 Medial proper palmar digital artery
16 Palmar metacarpal artery
17 Lateral proper palmar digital vein
18 Medial proper palmar digital vein
19 Palmar metacarpal vein
20 Vascular network of the MP joint
21 Lateral proper palmar digital nerve
22 Medial palmar proper digital nerve
23 Dorsal metacarpal fascia
24 Palmar metacarpal fascia
25 Skin

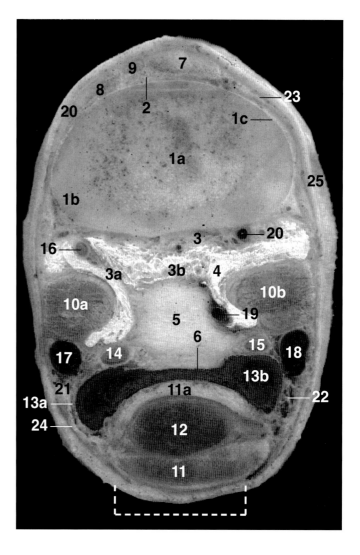

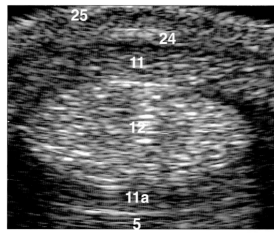

Transverse ultrasound scan of the fetlock area, palmar approach (see dotted area in illustration above, right).

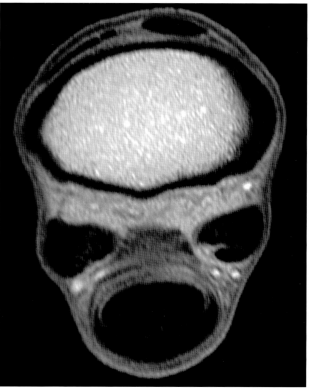

Transverse MRI scan of the fetlock.

T4: Transverse Section of the Metacarpophalangeal Joint

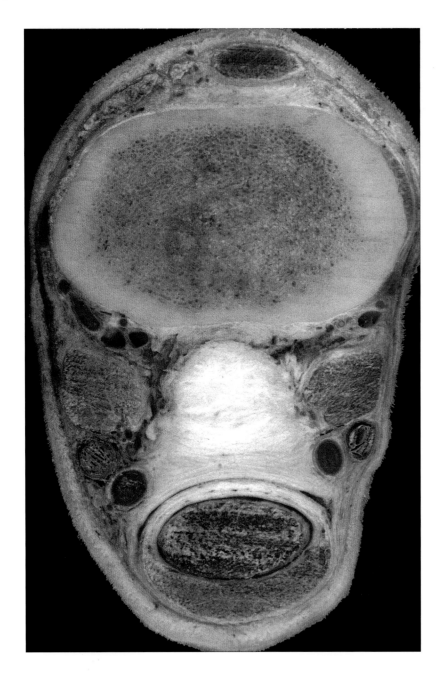

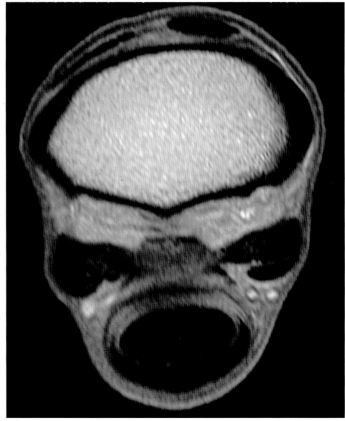

Transverse MRI scan of the fetlock.

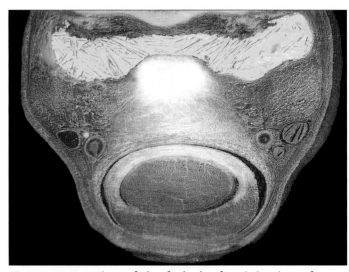

Transverse section of the fetlock after injection of coloured latex into the synovial cavities and vessels.

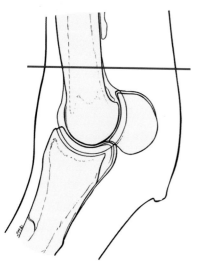

T4: Transverse Section of the Metacarpophalangeal Joint

1 Third metacarpal bone
   1a Cancellous bone
   1b Cortical bone
2 Dorsal capsule of the metacarpophalangeal (MP) joint
3 Synovial membrane
   3a Synovial villi
4 Proximopalmar recess of the MP joint cavity
5 Palmar (intersesamoidean) ligament
6 Proximal scutum (palmar surface)
7 Lateral collateral ligament (superficial part)
8 Medial collateral ligament (superficial part)
9 Dorsal digital extensor tendon
10 Lateral digital extensor tendon
11 Accessory digital extensor tendon
12 Third interosseus muscle
   12a Lateral branch
   12b Medial branch
13 Superficial digital flexor tendon
   13a Manica flexoria
14 Deep digital flexor tendon
15 Palmar annular ligament
16 Digital sheath (synovial cavity)
17 Lateral proper palmar digital artery
18 Medial proper palmar digital artery
19 Lateral proper palmar digital vein
20 Medial proper palmar digital vein
21 Vascular network of the MP joint
22 Lateral proper palmar digital nerve
23 Medial proper palmar digital nerve
24 Dorsal metacarpophalangeal fascia
25 Skin

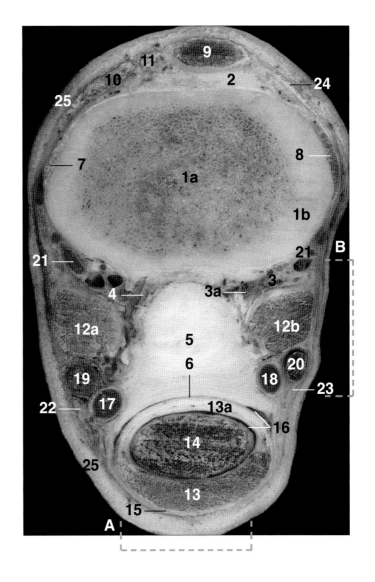

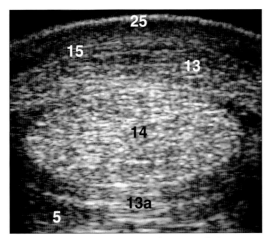

A Transverse ultrasound scan of the fetlock area, palmar approach (see dotted area in illustration above, right).

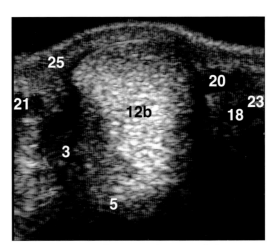

B Transverse ultrasound scan of the fetlock area, medial approach (see dotted area in illustration above).

T5: Transverse Section of the Metacarpophalangeal Joint

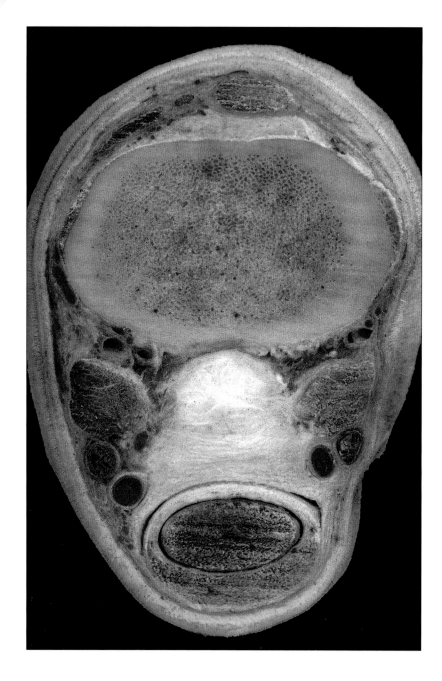

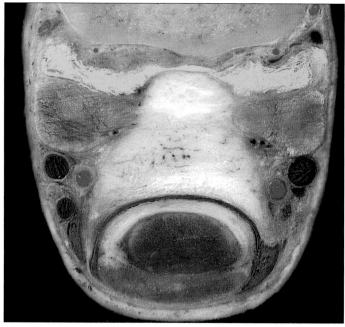

Transverse section of the fetlock after injection of latex into the synovial cavities and vessels.

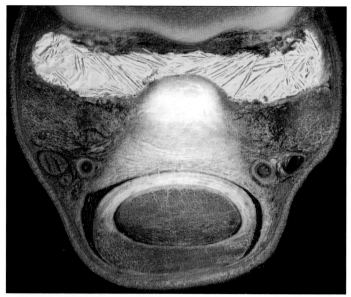

Transverse section of the fetlock after injection of coloured latex into the synovial cavities and vessels.

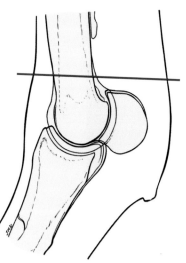

1 Third metacarpal bone
   1a Cancellous bone
   1b Cortical bone
2 Dorsal capsule of the metacarpophalangeal (MP) joint
3 Synovial membrane
   3a Synovial villi
4 Proximopalmar recess of the MP joint cavity
5 Palmar (intersesamoidean) ligament
6 Proximal scutum (palmar surface)
7 Lateral collateral ligament (superficial part)
8 Medial collateral ligament (superficial part)
9 Dorsal digital extensor tendon
10 Lateral digital extensor tendon
11 Accessory digital extensor tendon
12 Subtendinous bursa
13 Third interosseus muscle
   13a Lateral branch
   13b Medial branch
14 Superficial digital flexor tendon
   14a Manica flexoria
15 Deep digital flexor tendon
16 Palmar annular ligament
17 Digital sheath (synovial cavity)
18 Lateral proper palmar digital artery
19 Medial proper palmar digital artery
20 Lateral proper palmar digital vein
21 Medial proper palmar digital vein
22 Vascular network of the MP joint
23 Lateral proper palmar digital nerve
24 Medial proper palmar digital nerve
25 Dorsal metacarpophalangeal fascia
26 Skin

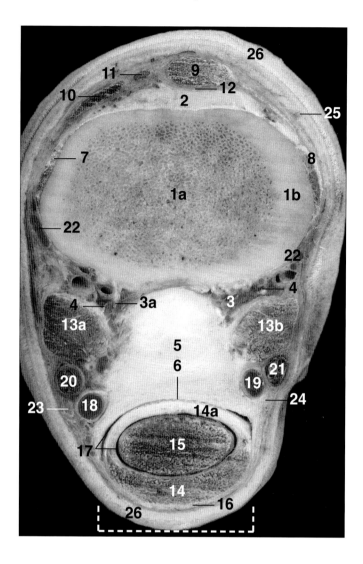

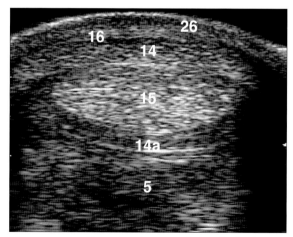

Transverse ultrasound scan of the fetlock area, palmar approach (see dotted area in illustration above, right).

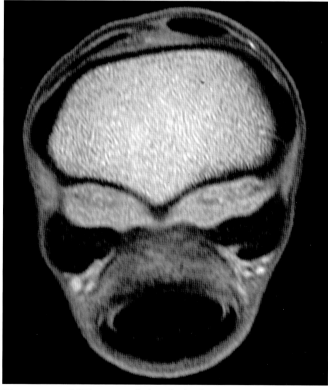

Transverse MRI scan of the fetlock.

T6: Transverse Section of the Metacarpophalangeal Joint

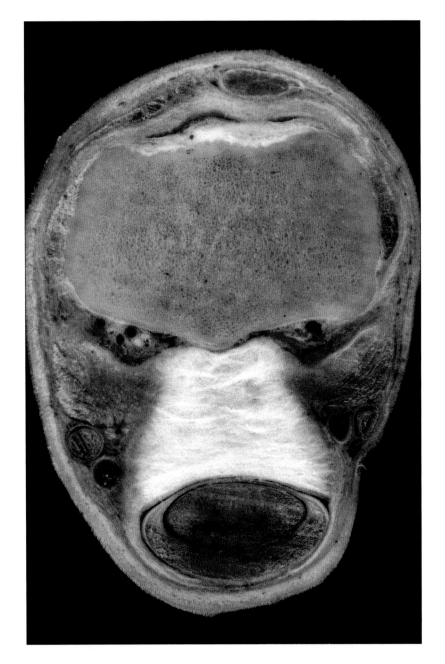

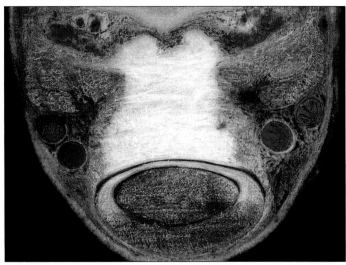

Transverse section of the fetlock after injection of latex into the synovial cavities and vessels.

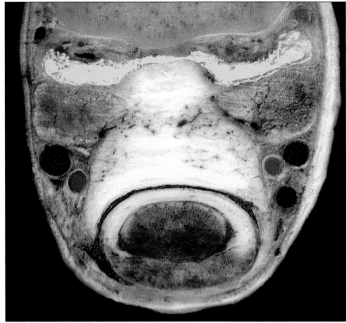

Transverse section of the fetlock after injection of coloured latex into the synovial cavities and vessels.

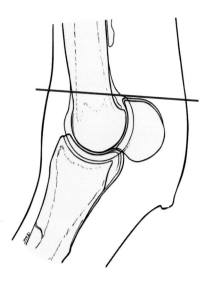

1 Third metacarpal bone
2 Sagittal ridge of the metacarpal condyle
3 Dorsal capsule of the metacarpophalangeal (MP) joint
4 Synovial membrane
    4a Proximodorsal synovial fold
    4b Synovial villi
5 Synovial cavity of the MP joint
    5a Dorsal recess
    5b Proximopalmar recess
6 Palmar (intersesamoidean) ligament
7 Proximal scutum (palmar surface)
8 Lateral collateral ligament (superficial part)
9 Medial collateral ligament (superficial part)
10 Dorsal digital extensor tendon
11 Lateral digital extensor tendon
12 Accessory digital extensor tendon
13 Subtendinous bursa
14 Third interosseus muscle
    14a Lateral branch
    14b Medial branch
15 Superficial digital flexor tendon
    15a Manica flexoria
16 Deep digital flexor tendon
17 Palmar annular ligament
18 Digital sheath
    18a Synovial membrane
    18b Synovial cavity
    18c Loose connective mesotendon
19 Lateral proper palmar digital artery
20 Medial proper palmar digital artery
21 Lateral proper palmar digital vein
22 Medial proper palmar digital vein
23 Vascular network of the MP joint
24 Lateral proper palmar digital nerve
25 Medial proper palmar digital nerve
26 Dorsal metacarpophalangeal fascia
27 Skin

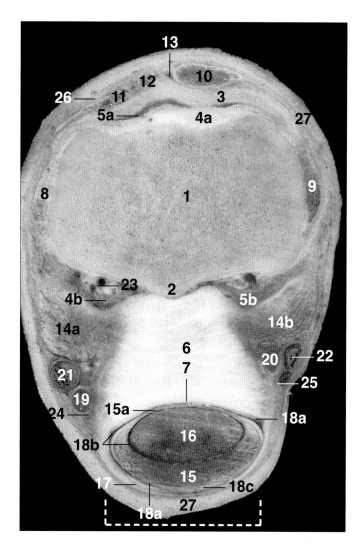

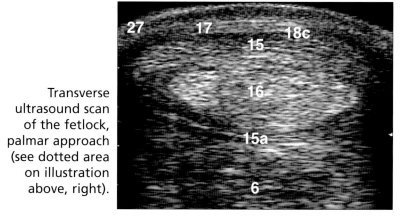

Transverse ultrasound scan of the fetlock, palmar approach (see dotted area on illustration above, right).

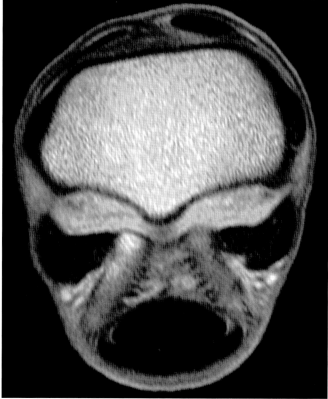

Transverse MRI scan of the fetlock.

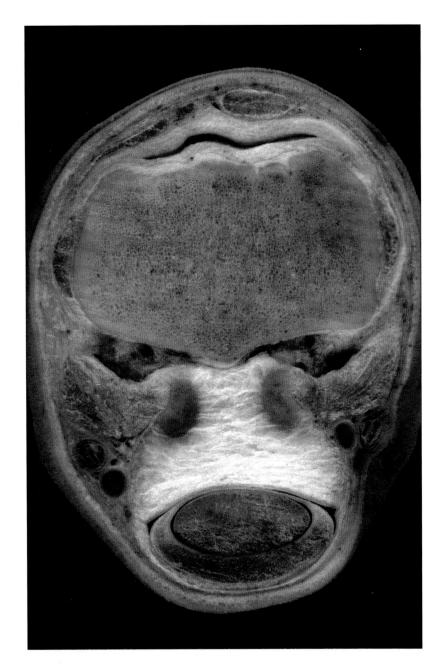

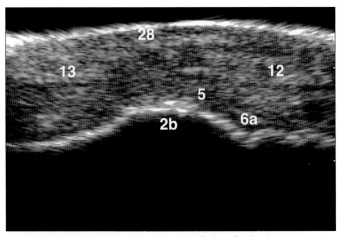

A Transverse ultrasound scan of the fetlock, dorsal approach (see dotted area in illustration on facing page).

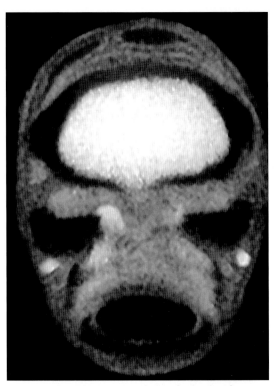

Transverse MRI scan of the fetlock after injection of latex into the arteries and fat material into the veins.

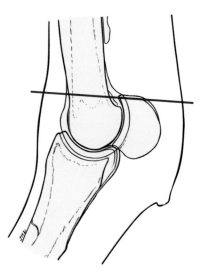

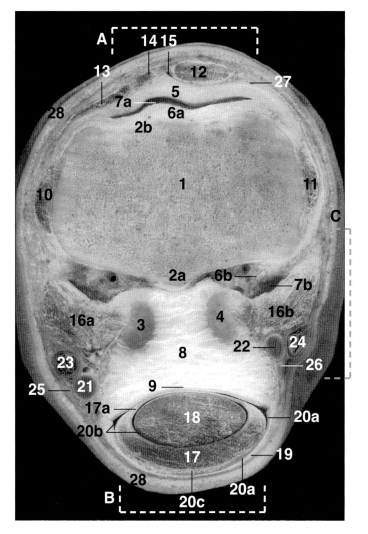

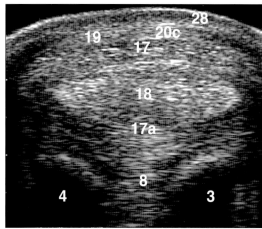

B Transverse ultrasound scan of the fetlock, palmar approach (see dotted area in illustration left).

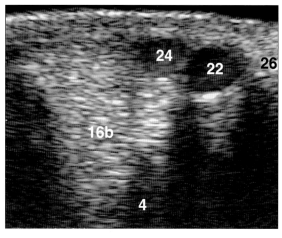

C Transverse ultrasound scan of the fetlock, medial approach (see dotted area in illustration left).

1 Third metacarpal bone
2 Metacarpal condyle
   2a Sagittal ridge
   2b Dorsal margin
3 Lateral proximal sesamoid bone (apex)
4 Medial proximal sesamoid bone (apex)
5 Dorsal capsule of the metacarpophalangeal (MP) joint
6 Synovial membrane of the MP joint
   6a Proximodorsal synovial fold
   6b Synovial villi
7 Synovial cavity of the MP joint
   7a Dorsal recess
   7b Proximopalmar recess
8 Palmar (intersesamoidean) ligament
9 Proximal scutum (palmar surface)
10 Lateral collateral ligament
11 Medial collateral ligament
12 Dorsal digital extensor tendon
13 Lateral digital extensor tendon
14 Accessory digital extensor tendon

15 Subtendinous bursa
16 Third interosseus muscle
   16a Lateral branch
   16b Medial branch
17 Superficial digital flexor tendon
   17a Manica flexoria
18 Deep digital flexor tendon
19 Palmar annular ligament
20 Digital sheath
   20a Synovial membrane
   20b Synovial cavity
   20c Loose connective mesotendon
21 Lateral proper palmar digital artery
22 Medial proper palmar digital artery
23 Lateral proper palmar digital vein
24 Medial proper palmar digital vein
25 Lateral proper palmar digital nerve
26 Medial proper palmar digital nerve
27 Dorsal metacarpophalangeal fascia
28 Skin

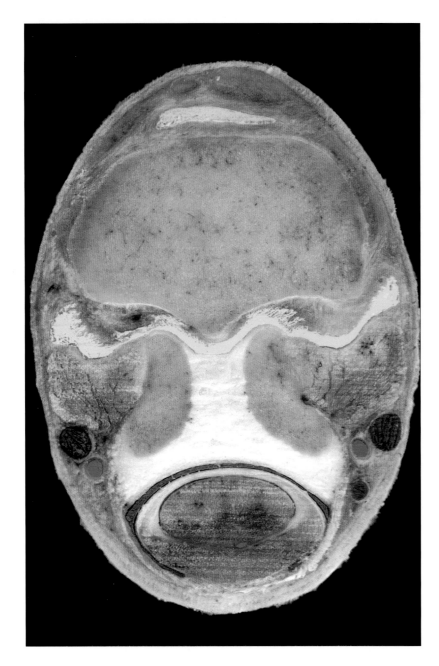

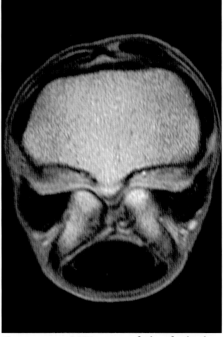

Transverse MRI scan of the fetlock.

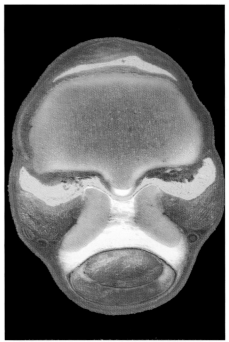

Transverse section of the fetlock after injection of coloured latex into the synovial cavities and vessels.

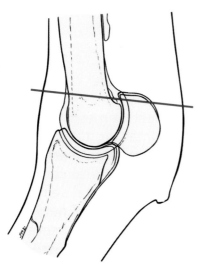

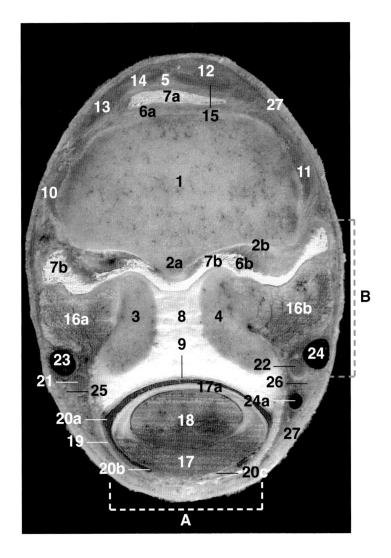

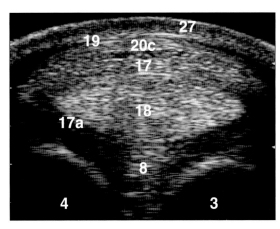

A Transverse ultrasound scan of the fetlock, palmar approach (see dotted area in illustration left).

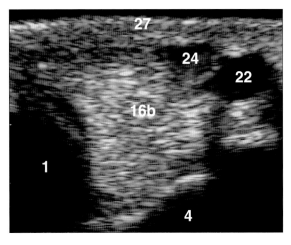

B Transverse ultrasound scan of the fetlock, medial approach (see dotted area in illustration left).

1 Third metacarpal bone
2 Metacarpal condyle
   2a Sagittal ridge
   2b Palmar margin
3 Lateral proximal sesamoid bone
4 Medial proximal sesamoid bone
5 Dorsal capsule of the metacarpophalangeal (MP) joint
6 Synovial membrane of the MP joint
   6a Proximodorsal synovial fold
   6b Synovial villi
7 Synovial cavity of the MP joint
   7a Dorsal recess
   7b Proximopalmar recess
8 Palmar (intersesamoidean) ligament
9 Proximal scutum (palmar surface)
10 Lateral collateral ligament (superficial part)
11 Medial collateral ligament (superficial part)
12 Dorsal digital extensor tendon
13 Lateral digital extensor tendon
14 Accessory digital extensor tendon

15 Subtendinous bursa
16 Third interosseus muscle
   16a Lateral branch
   16b Medial branch
17 Superficial digital flexor tendon
   17a Manica flexoria
18 Deep digital flexor tendon
19 Palmar annular ligament
20 Digital sheath
   20a Synovial cavity
   20b Synovial membrane
   20c Loose connective mesotendon
21 Lateral proper palmar digital artery
22 Medial proper palmar digital artery
23 Lateral proper palmar digital vein
24 Medial proper palmar digital vein
   24a Ergot ramus
25 Lateral proper palmar digital nerve
26 Medial proper palmar digital nerve
27 Skin

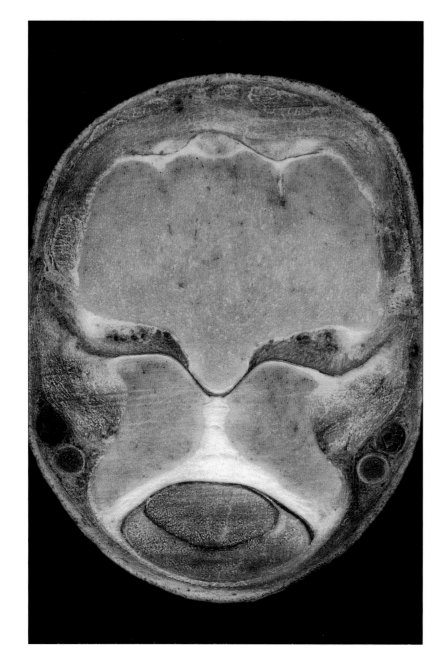

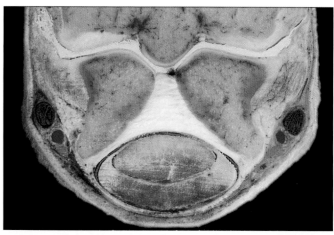

Transverse section of the fetlock after injection of coloured latex into the synovial cavities and vessels.

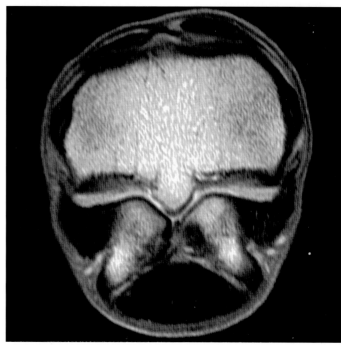

Transverse MRI scan of the fetlock.

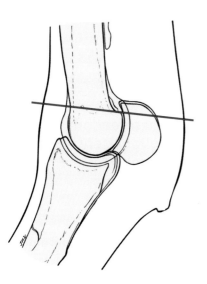

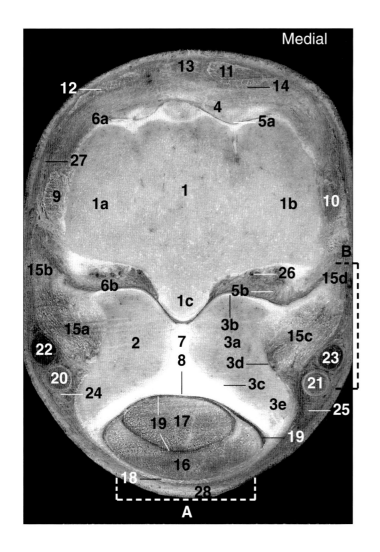

Medial

A

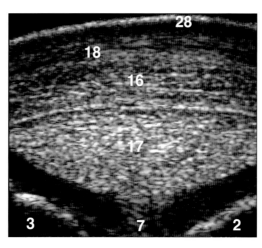

A Transverse ultrasound scan of the fetlock, palmar approach (see dotted area in illustration left).

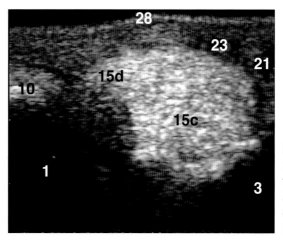

B Transverse ultrasound scan of the fetlock, medial approach (see dotted area in illustration left).

1 Metacarpal condyle
  1a Lateral part (lateral condyle)
  1b Medial part (medial condyle)
  1c Sagittal ridge
2 Lateral proximal sesamoid bone
3 Medial proximal sesamoid bone
  3a Body
  3b Articular surface
  3c Flexor surface
  3d Interosseus face
  3e Palmar border
4 Dorsal capsule of the MP joint
5 Synovial membrane
  5a Proximodorsal synovial fold
  5b Synovial villi
6 Synovial cavity
  6a Dorsal recess
  6b Proximopalmar recess
7 Palmar (intersesamoidean) ligament
8 Proximal scutum (palmar surface)
9 Lateral collateral ligament (superficial part)
10 Medial collateral ligament (superficial part)

11 Dorsal digital extensor tendon
12 Lateral digital extensor tendon
13 Accessory digital extensor tendon
14 Subtendinous bursa
15 Third interosseus muscle
  15a Lateral branch
  15b Lateral extensor branch
  15c Medial branch
  15d Medial extensor branch
16 Superficial digital flexor tendon
17 Deep digital flexor tendon
18 Palmar annular ligament
19 Digital sheath cavity
20 Lateral proper palmar digital artery
21 Medial proper palmar digital artery
22 Lateral proper palmar digital vein
23 Medial proper palmar digital vein
24 Lateral proper palmar digital nerve
25 Medial proper palmar digital nerve
26 Nutrient vessels for the metacarpal condyle
27 Dorsal metacarpophalangeal fascia
28 Skin

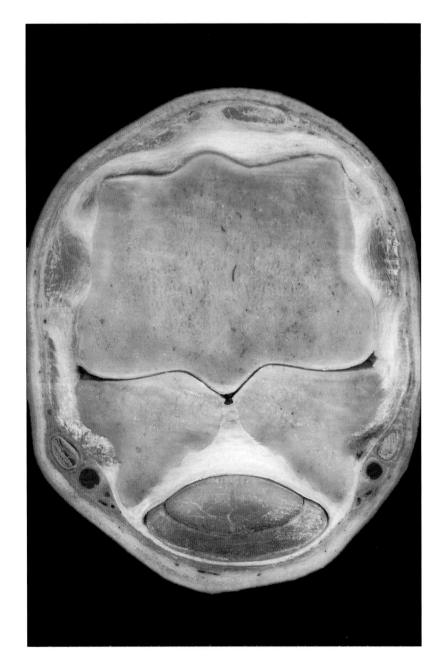

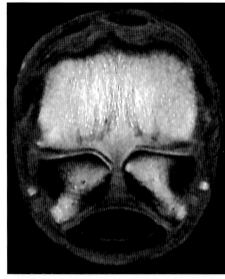

Transverse MRI scan of the fetlock after injection of latex into the arteries and fat material into the veins.

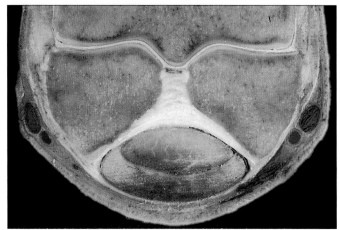

Transverse section of the fetlock after injection of coloured latex into the synovial cavities and vessels.

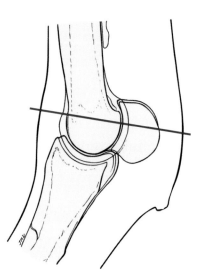

A Transverse ultrasound scan of the fetlock (zoom), palmar approach (see dotted area in illustration on facing page).

1 Metacarpal condyle
   1a Lateral part (lateral condyle)
   1b Medial part (medial condyle)
   1c Sagittal ridge
2 Lateral proximal sesamoid bone
3 Medial proximal sesamoid bone
   3a Body
   3b Articular surface
   3c Flexor surface
   3d Interosseus face
   3e Palmar border
4 Dorsal capsule of the metacarpophalangeal joint
5 Synovial membrane
6 Synovial cavity
   6a Dorsal recess
   6b Palmar recess
7 Palmar (intersesamoidean) ligament
8 Proximal scutum (palmar surface)
9 Lateral collateral ligament
10 Medial collateral ligament
   10a Superficial part
   10b Deep part
11 Lateral collateral sesamoidean ligament
12 Medial collateral sesamoidean ligament
13 Dorsal digital extensor tendon
14 Lateral digital extensor tendon
15 Accessory digital extensor tendon
16 Subtendinous bursa
17 Third interosseus muscle
   17a Lateral branch
   17b Lateral extensor branch
18 Superficial digital flexor tendon
19 Deep digital flexor tendon
20 Palmar annular ligament
21 Digital sheath cavity
22 Lateral proper palmar digital artery
23 Medial proper palmar digital artery
24 Lateral proper palmar digital vein
25 Medial proper palmar digital vein
26 Lateral proper palmar digital nerve
27 Medial proper palmar digital nerve
28 Metacarpophalangeal fascia
29 Skin

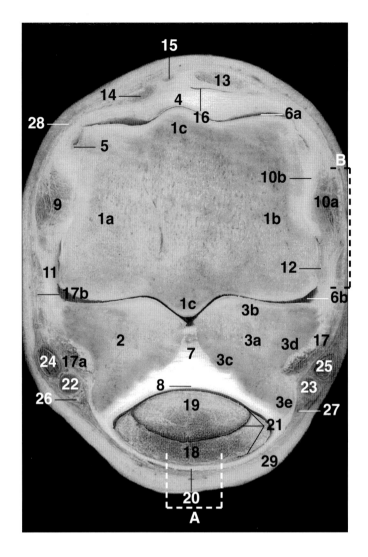

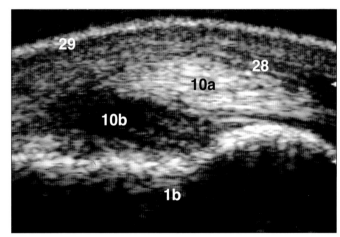

B Transverse ultrasound scan of the fetlock, medial approach (see dotted area in illustration above).

T11: Transverse Section of the Metacarpophalangeal Joint

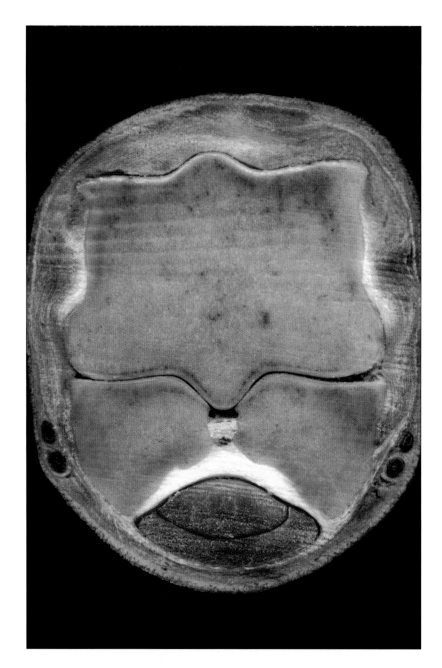

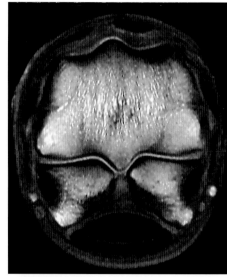

Transverse MRI scan of the fetlock after injection of latex into the arteries and fat material into the veins.

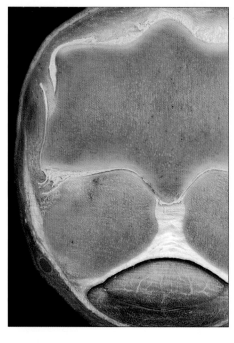

Transverse section of the fetlock after injection of coloured latex into the synovial cavities and vessels.

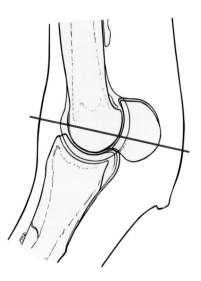

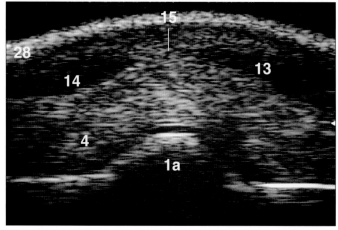

A Transverse ultrasound scan of the fetlock, dorsal approach (see dotted area in illustration on facing page).

1 Metacarpal condyle
  1a Sagittal ridge
  1b Collateral fossa
2 Lateral proximal sesamoid bone
3 Medial proximal sesamoid bone
  3a Body
  3b Articular surface
  3c Flexor surface
  3d Palmar border
4 Dorsal capsule of the metacarpophalangeal joint
5 Synovial membrane
6 Synovial cavity
  6a Dorsal recess
  6b Palmar recess
7 Palmar (intersesamoidean) ligament
8 Proximal scutum (palmar surface)
9 Lateral collateral ligament
10 Medial collateral ligament
  10a Superficial part
  10b Deep part
11 Lateral collateral sesamoidean ligament
12 Medial collateral sesamoidean
13 Dorsal digital extensor tendon
14 Lateral digital extensor tendon
15 Accessory digital extensor tendon
16 Third interosseus muscle
  16a Lateral extensor branch
  16b Medial extensor branch
17 Superficial digital flexor tendon
18 Deep digital flexor tendon
19 Palmar annular ligament
20 Digital sheath cavity
21 Lateral proper palmar digital artery
22 Medial proper palmar digital artery
23 Lateral proper palmar digital vein
24 Medial proper palmar digital vein
25 Lateral proper palmar digital nerve
26 Medial proper palmar digital nerve
27 Dorsal metacarpophalangeal fascia
28 Skin

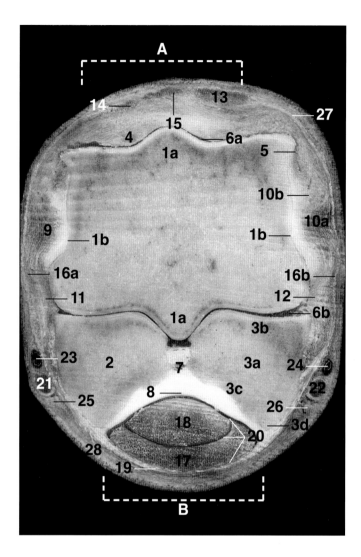

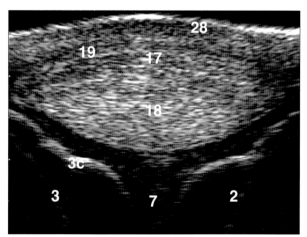

B Transverse ultrasound scan of the fetlock, palmar approach (see dotted area in illustration above).

T12: Transverse Section of the Metacarpophalangeal Joint

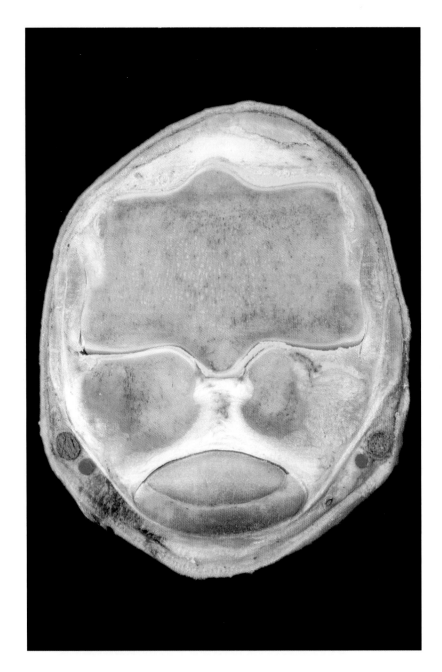

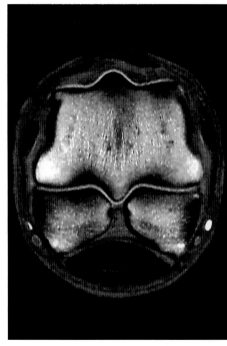

Transverse MRI scan of the fetlock after injection of latex into the arteries and fat material into the veins.

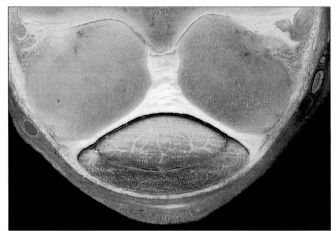

Transverse section of the fetlock after injection of coloured latex into the synovial cavities and vessels.

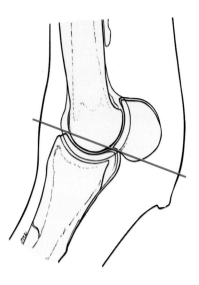

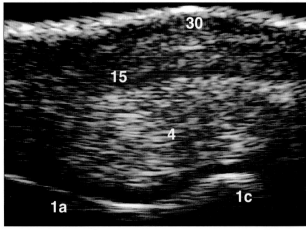

A Transverse ultrasound scan of the fetlock, dorsolateral approach (see dotted area in illustration on facing page).

1 Metacarpal condyle
  1a Lateral part (lateral condyle)
  1b Medial part (medial condyle)
  1c Sagittal ridge
  1d Collateral fossa
2 Lateral proximal sesamoid bone (base)
3 Medial proximal sesamoid bone (base)
4 Dorsal capsule of the metacarpophalangeal (MP) joint
5 Synovial cavity of the MP joint
  5a Dorsal recess
  5b Palmar recess
  5c Collateral recess
6 Palmar (intersesamoidean) ligament
7 Proximal scutum (palmar surface)
8 Lateral collateral ligament
  8a Superficial part
  8b Deep part
9 Medial collateral ligament
10 Lateral collateral sesamoidean ligament
11 Medial collateral sesamoidean ligament
12 Medial oblique sesamoidean ligament
13 Medial short sesamoidean ligament
14 Dorsal digital extensor tendon
15 Lateral digital extensor tendon
16 Accessory digital extensor tendon
17 Subtendinous bursa
18 Third interosseus muscle
  18a Lateral extensor branch
  18b Medial extensor branch
19 Superficial digital flexor tendon
20 Deep digital flexor tendon
21 Palmar annular ligament
22 Digital sheath cavity
23 Lateral proper palmar digital artery
24 Medial proper palmar digital artery
25 Lateral proper palmar digital vein
26 Medial proper palmar digital vein
27 Lateral proper palmar digital nerve
28 Medial proper palmar digital nerve
29 Ergot cushion
30 Skin

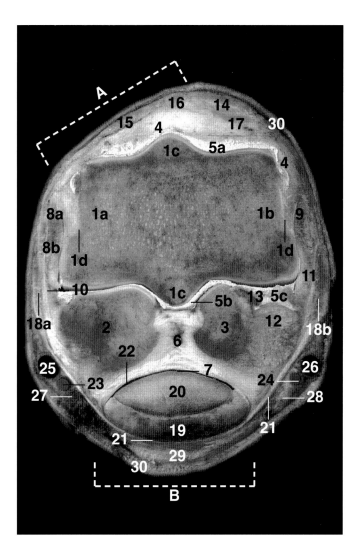

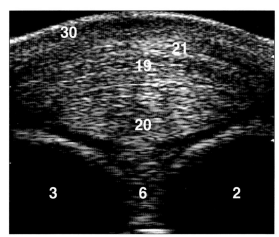

B Transverse ultrasound scan of the fetlock, palmar approach (see dotted area in illustration above).

T13: Transverse Section of the Metacarpophalangeal Joint

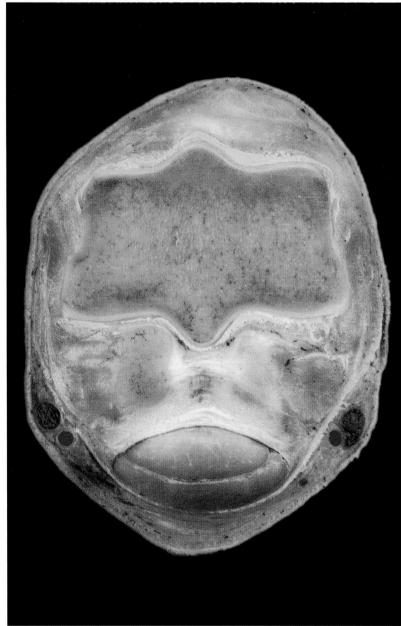

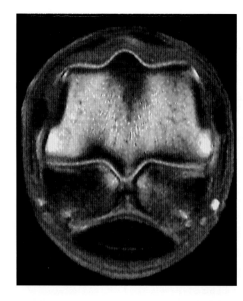

Transverse MRI scan of the fetlock after injection of latex into the arteries and fat material into the veins.

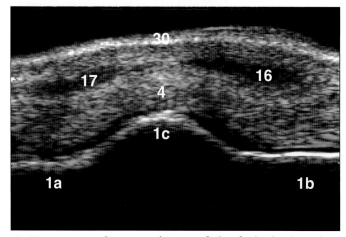

A Transverse ultrasound scan of the fetlock, dorsal approach (see dotted area in illustration on facing page).

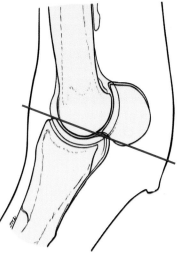

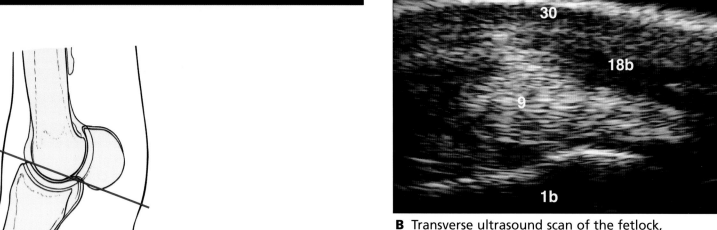

B Transverse ultrasound scan of the fetlock, dorsomedial approach (see dotted area in illustration on facing page).

1 Metacarpal condyle
  1a Lateral part (lateral condyle)
  1b Medial part (medial condyle)
  1c Sagittal ridge
  1d Collateral fossa
2 Lateral proximal sesamoid bone (base)
3 Medial proximal sesamoid bone (base)
4 Dorsal capsule of the metacarpophalangeal (MP) joint
5 Synovial cavity of the MP joint
  5a Dorsal recess
  5b Palmar recess
  5c Collateral recess
6 Palmar (intersesamoidean) ligament
7 Proximal scutum (palmar surface)
8 Lateral collateral ligament
  8a Superficial part
  8b Deep part
9 Medial collateral ligament
10 Lateral collateral sesamoidean ligament
11 Medial collateral sesamoidean ligament
12 Lateral oblique sesamoidean ligament
13 Medial oblique sesamoidean ligament
14 Lateral short sesamoidean ligament
15 Medial short sesamoidean ligament
16 Dorsal digital extensor tendon
17 Lateral digital extensor tendon
18 Third interosseus muscle
  18a Lateral extensor branch
  18b Medial extensor branch
19 Superficial digital flexor tendon
20 Deep digital flexor tendon
21 Palmar annular ligament
22 Digital sheath cavity
23 Lateral proper palmar digital artery
24 Medial proper palmar digital artery
25 Lateral proper palmar digital vein
26 Medial proper palmar digital vein
27 Lateral proper palmar digital nerve
28 Medial proper palmar digital nerve
29 Ergot cushion
30 Skin

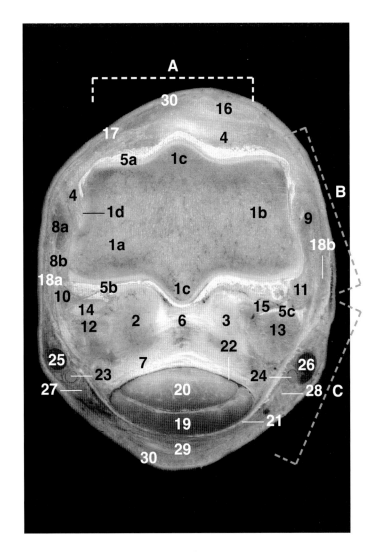

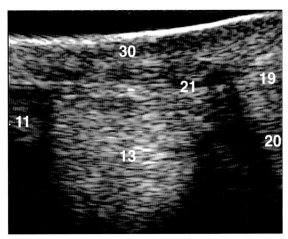

C Transverse ultrasound scan of the fetlock, palmaromedial approach (see dotted area in illustration above).

T14: Transverse Section of the Metacarpophalangeal Joint

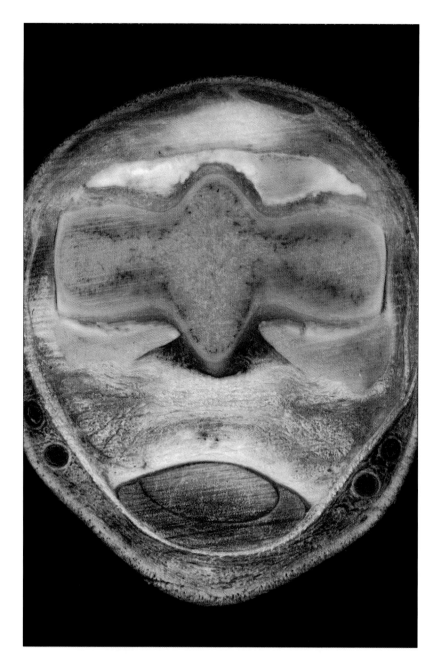

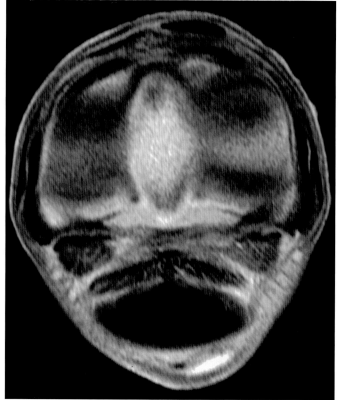

Transverse MRI scan of the fetlock.

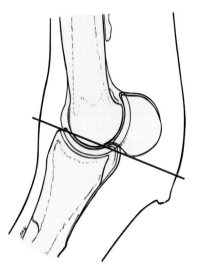

1 Metacarpal condyle
2 Proximal phalanx
    2a Sagittal groove
    2b Proximodorsal articular margin
    2c Proximopalmar articular margin
    2d Medial palmar eminence
3 Dorsal capsule of the metacarpophalangeal joint
4 Synovial cavity
    4a Distodorsal recess
    4b Distopalmar recess
5 Lateral collateral ligament
    5a Superficial part
    5b Deep part
6 Medial collateral ligament
7 Lateral collateral sesamoidean ligament
8 Medial collateral sesamoidean ligament
9 Straight sesamoidean ligament

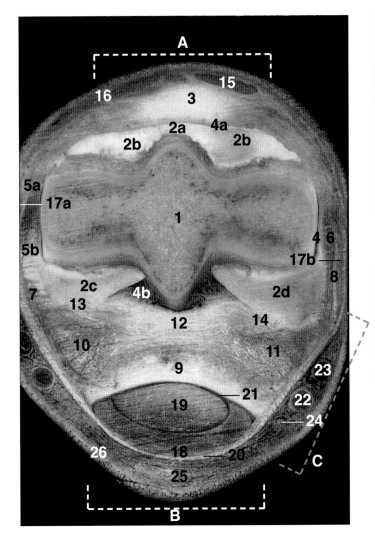

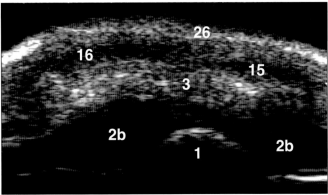

A Transverse ultrasound scan of the fetlock, dorsal approach (see dotted area in illustration at left).

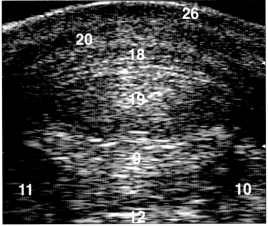

B Transverse ultrasound scan of the fetlock, palmar approach (see dotted area in illustration at left).

10 Lateral oblique sesamoidean ligament
11 Medial oblique sesamoidean ligament
12 Cruciate sesamoidean ligaments
13 Lateral short sesamoidean ligament
14 Medial short sesamoidean ligament
15 Dorsal digital extensor tendon
16 Lateral digital extensor tendon
17 Third interosseous muscle
    17a Lateral extensor branch
    17b Medial extensor branch
18 Superficial digital flexor tendon
19 Deep digital flexor tendon
20 Palmar annular ligament
21 Digital sheath cavity
22 Medial proper palmar digital artery
23 Medial proper palmar digital vein
24 Medial proper palmar digital nerve
25 Ergot cushion
26 Skin

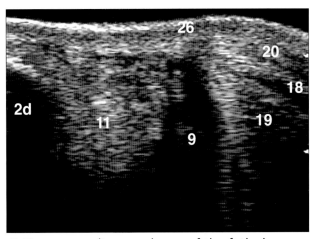

C Transverse ultrasound scan of the fetlock, palmaromedial approach (see dotted area in illustration above, left).

T15: Transverse Section of the Metacarpophalangeal Joint

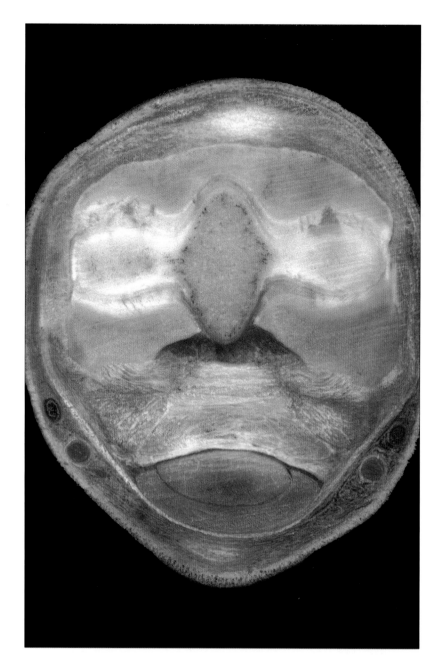

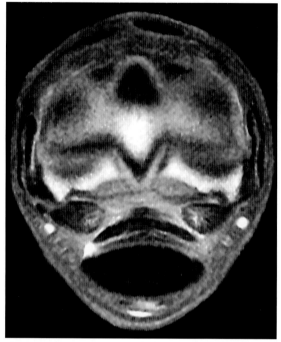

Transverse MRI scan of the fetlock after injection of latex into the arteries and fat material into the veins.

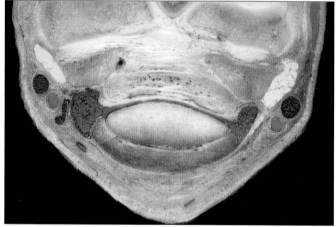

Transverse section of the fetlock after injection of coloured latex into the synovial cavities and vessels.

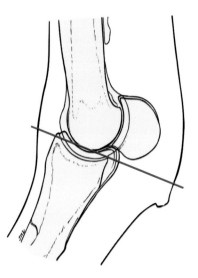

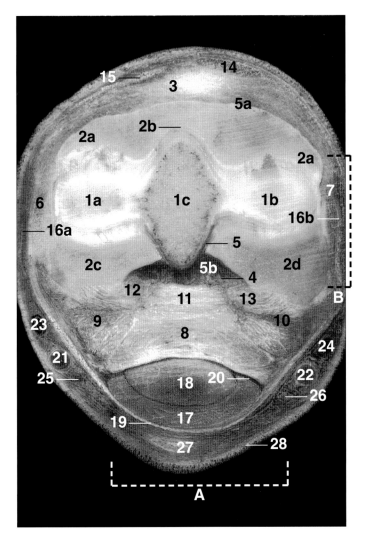

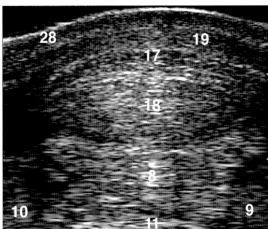

A Transverse ultrasound scan of the fetlock, palmar approach (see dotted area in illustration at left).

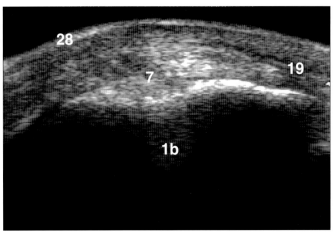

B Transverse ultrasound scan of the fetlock, medial approach (see dotted area in illustration at left).

1 Metacarpal condyle
  1a Lateral part (lateral condyle)
  1b Medial part (medial condyle)
  1c Sagittal ridge
2 Proximal phalanx
  2a Proximodorsal articular margin
  2b Sagittal groove
  2c Lateral palmar eminence
  2d Medial palmar eminence
3 Dorsal capsule of the metacarpophalangeal joint
4 Synovial membrane (synovial villi)
5 Synovial cavity
  5a Distodorsal recess
  5b Distopalmar recess
6 Lateral collateral ligament
7 Medial collateral ligament
8 Straight sesamoidean ligament
9 Lateral oblique sesamoidean ligament
10 Medial oblique sesamoidean ligament

11 Cruciate sesamoidean ligaments
12 Lateral short sesamoidean ligament
13 Medial short sesamoidean ligament
14 Dorsal digital extensor tendon
15 Lateral digital extensor tendon
16 Third interosseous muscle
  16a Lateral extensor branch
  16b Medial extensor branch
17 Superficial digital flexor tendon
18 Deep digital flexor tendon
19 Palmar annular ligament
20 Digital sheath cavity
21 Lateral proper palmar digital artery
22 Medial proper palmar digital artery
23 Lateral proper palmar digital vein
24 Medial proper palmar digital vein
25 Lateral proper palmar digital nerve
26 Medial proper palmar digital nerve
27 Ergot cushion
28 Skin

T16: Transverse Section of the Metacarpophalangeal Joint

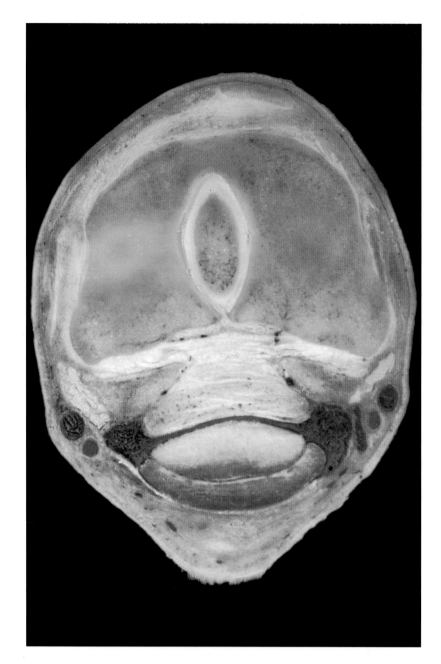

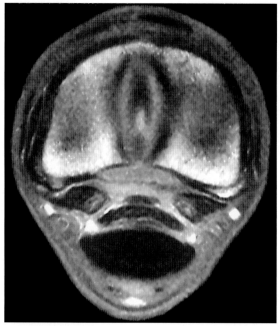

Transverse MRI scan of the fetlock after injection of latex into the arteries and fat material into the veins.

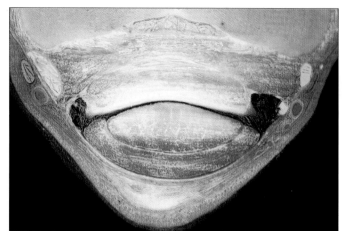

Transverse section of the fetlock after injection of coloured latex into the synovial cavities and vessels.

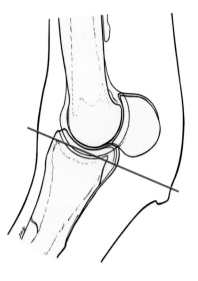

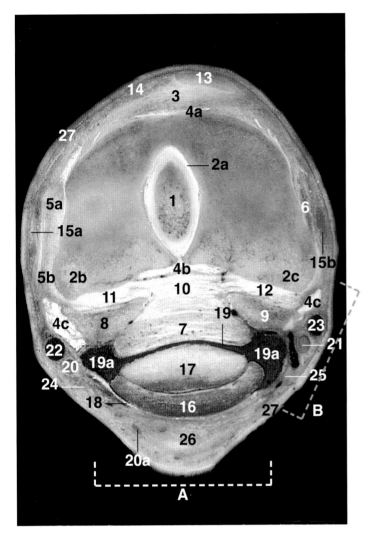

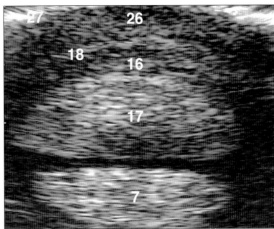

A Transverse ultrasound scan of the fetlock, palmar approach (see dotted area in illustration at left).

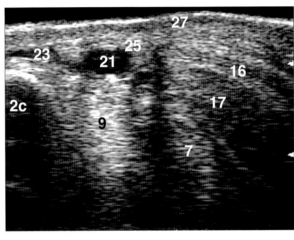

B Transverse ultrasound scan of the fetlock, palmaromedial approach (see dotted area in illustration at left).

1 Metacarpal condyle (sagittal ridge)
2 Proximal phalanx
  2a Sagittal groove
  2b Lateral palmar eminence
  2c Medial palmar eminence
3 Dorsal capsule of the metacarpophalangeal joint
4 Synovial cavity
  4a Distodorsal recess
  4b Distopalmar recess
  4c Collateral recess
5 Lateral collateral ligament
  5a Superficial part
  5b Deep part
6 Medial collateral ligament
7 Straight sesamoidean ligament
8 Lateral oblique sesamoidean ligament
9 Medial oblique sesamoidean ligament
10 Cruciate sesamoidean ligaments
11 Lateral short sesamoidean ligament

12 Medial short sesamoidean ligament
13 Dorsal digital extensor tendon
14 Lateral digital extensor tendon
15 Third interosseus muscle
  15a Lateral extensor branch
  15b Medial extensor branch
16 Superficial digital flexor tendon
17 Deep digital flexor tendon
18 Palmar annular ligament
19 Digital sheath cavity
  19a Collateral recess
20 Lateral proper palmar digital artery
  20a Ergot ramus
21 Medial proper palmar digital artery
22 Lateral proper palmar digital vein
23 Medial proper palmar digital vein
24 Lateral proper palmar digital nerve
25 Medial proper palmar digital nerve
26 Ergot cushion
27 Skin

T17: Transverse Section of the Metacarpophalangeal Joint

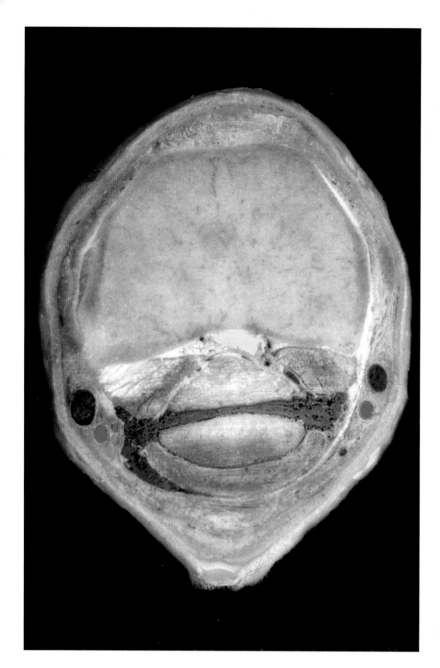

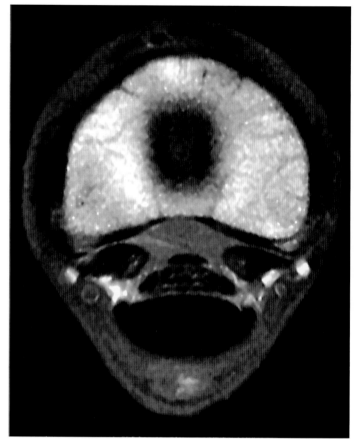

Transverse MRI scan of the fetlock after injection of latex into the arteries and fat material into the veins.

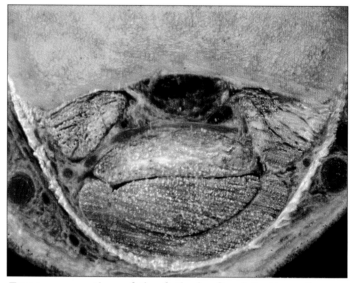

Transverse section of the fetlock after injection of coloured latex into the vessels.

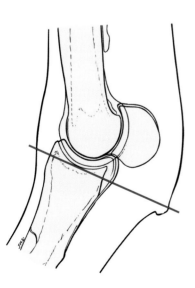

1 Proximal phalanx
  1a Lateral palmar eminence
  1b Medial palmar eminence
2 Dorsal capsule of the metacarpophalangeal (MP) joint
3 Distopalmar recess of the MP joint
4 Lateral collateral ligament (superficial part)
5 Medial collateral ligament (superficial part)
6 Straight sesamoidean ligament
7 Lateral oblique sesamoidean ligament
8 Medial oblique sesamoidean ligament
9 Cruciate sesamoidean ligament
10 Dorsal digital extensor tendon
11 Third interosseus muscle
  11a Lateral extensor branch
  11b Medial extensor branch
12 Superficial digital flexor tendon
13 Deep digital flexor tendon
14 Proximal digital annular ligament
15 Digital sheath cavity
  15a Collateral recess
16 Lateral proper palmar digital artery
  16a Ergot ramus
17 Medial proper palmar digital artery
18 Lateral proper palmar digital vein
19 Medial proper palmar digital vein
20 Lateral proper palmar digital nerve
21 Medial proper palmar digital nerve
22 Ergot
  22a Ergot cushion
23 Skin

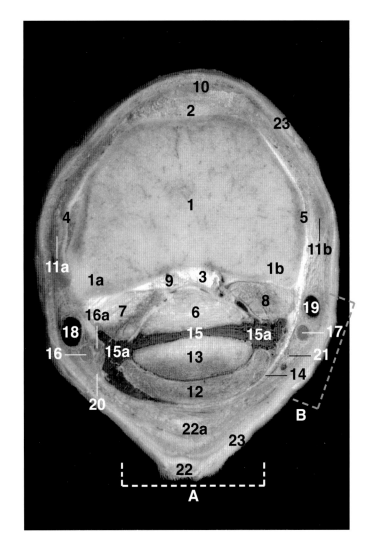

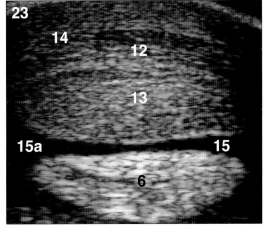

A Transverse ultrasound scan of the fetlock, palmar approach (see dotted area in illustration above, right).

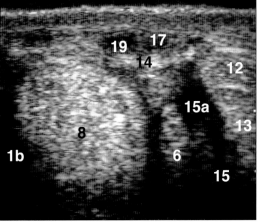

B Transverse ultrasound scan of the fetlock, palmaromedial approach (see dotted area in illustration above).

Frontal Sections of the Equine Fetlock

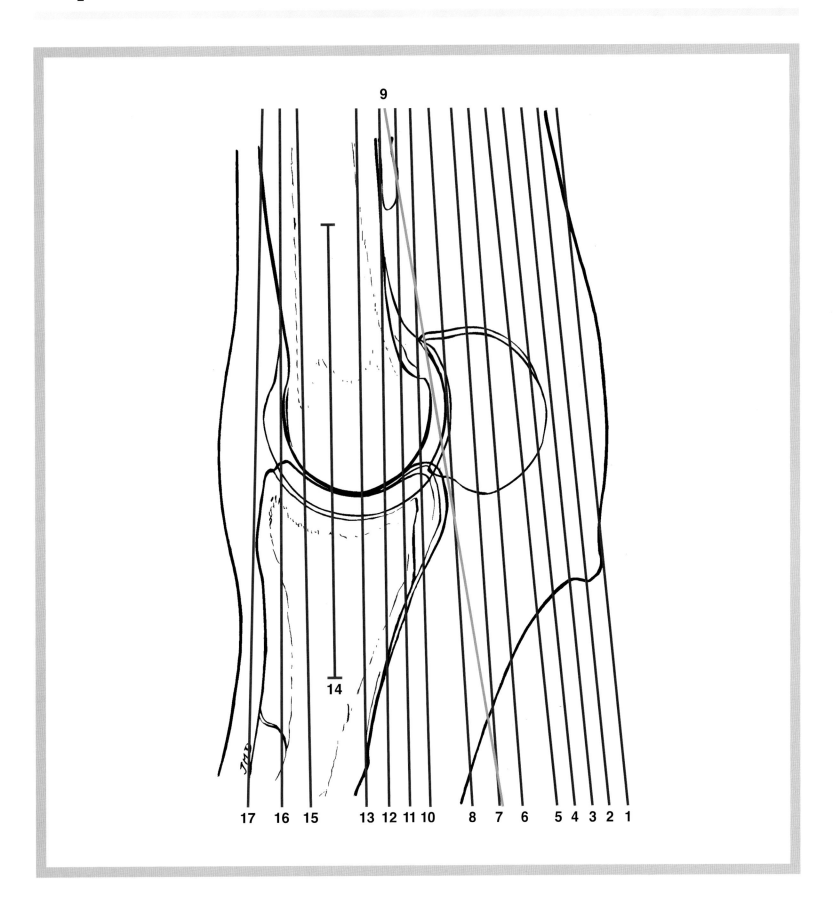

F1: Frontal Section of the Fetlock

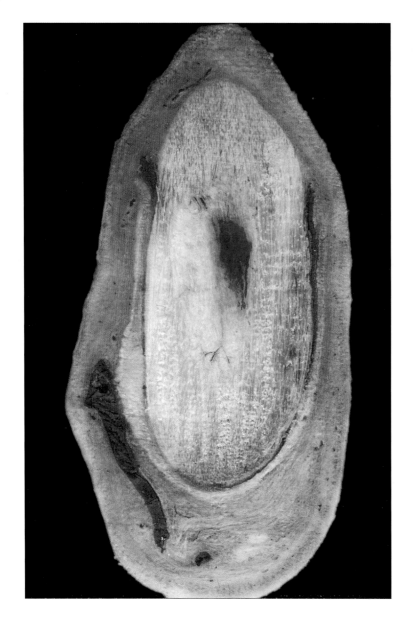

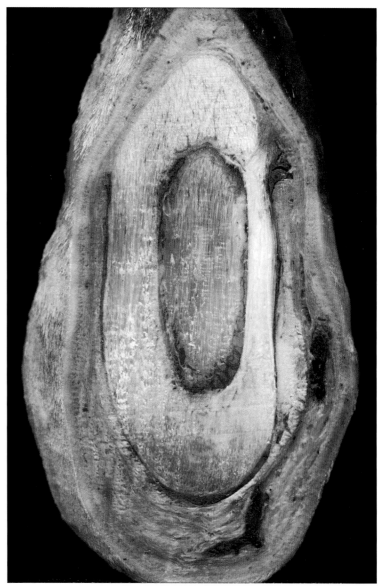

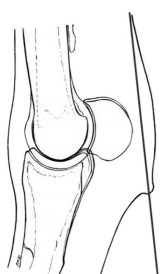

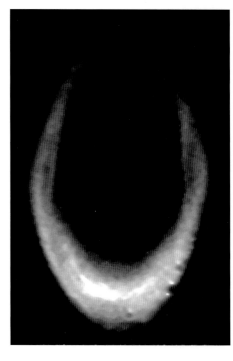

Frontal MRI scan of the fetlock after injection of latex into the arteries and fat material into the veins.

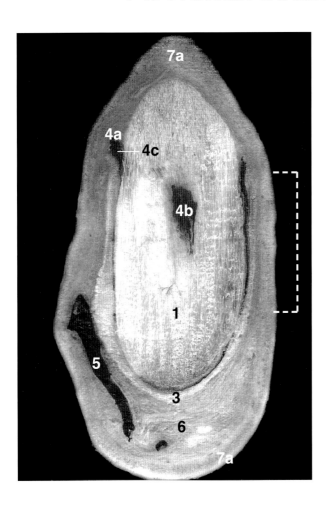

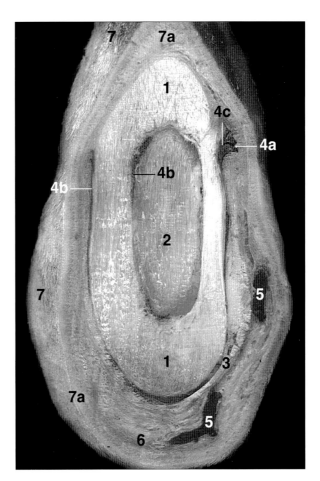

1 Superficial digital flexor
   tendon
2 Deep digital flexor tendon
3 Palmar annular ligament
4 Digital sheath
   4a Synovial membrane
   4b Synovial cavity
   4c Proximal recess
5 Ergot ramus of the proper
   palmar digital vein
6 Ergot cushion
7 Skin
   7a Skin section

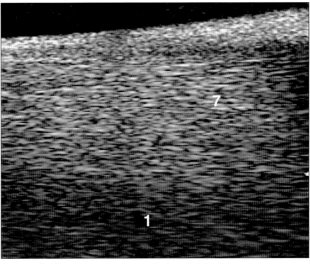

Frontal ultrasound scan of the fetlock area,
lateral approach (see dotted area in illustration
above, left).

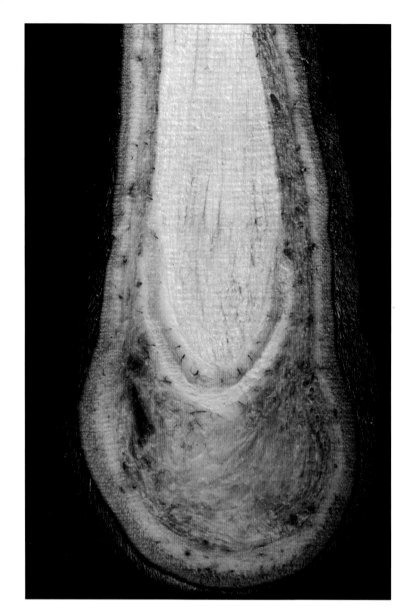

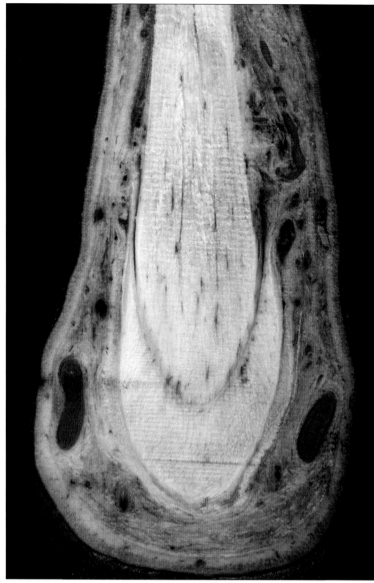

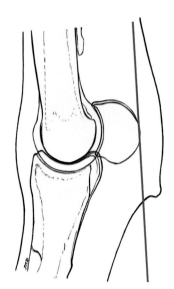

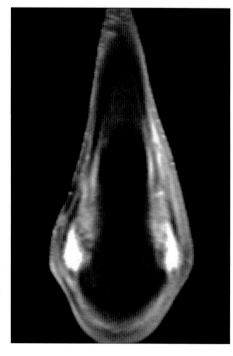

Frontal MRI scan of the fetlock after injection of latex into the arteries and fat material into the veins.

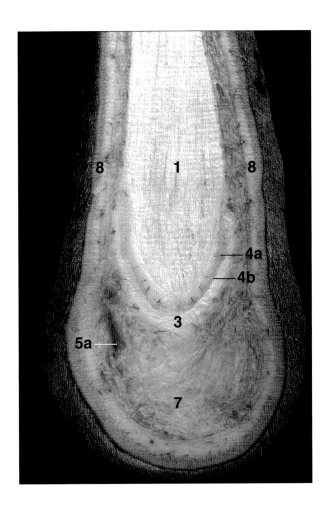

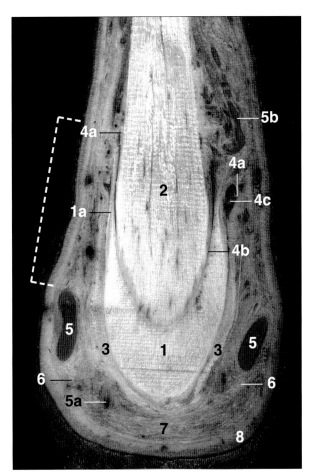

1 Superficial digital flexor tendon
  1a Manica flexoria
2 Deep digital flexor tendon
3 Palmar annular ligament
4 Digital sheath
  4a Synovial membrane
  4b Synovial cavity
  4c Proximal recess
5 Proper palmar digital artery
  5a Ergot ramus
  5b Rami for the flexor tendons
6 Proper palmar digital nerve
7 Ergot cushion
8 Skin

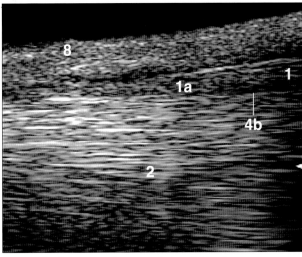

Frontal ultrasound scan of the fetlock area, lateral approach (see dotted area on illustration above).

F4: Frontal Section of the Fetlock

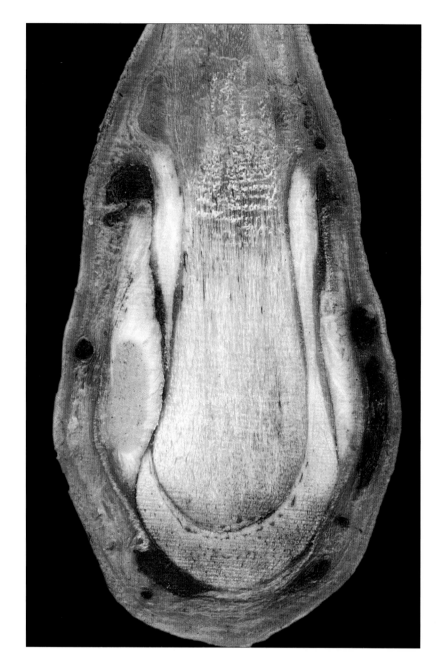

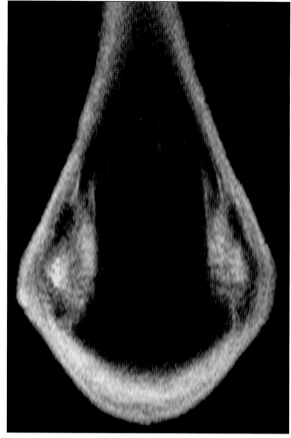

Frontal MRI scan of the fetlock.

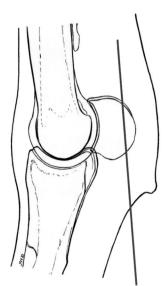

Frontal section of the fetlock
after injection of coloured
latex into the vessels.

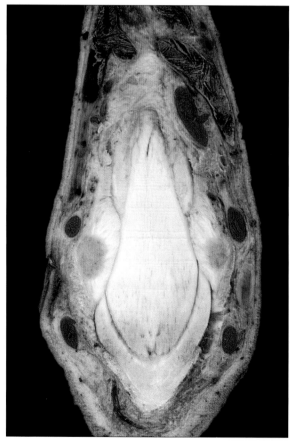

1 Lateral proximal sesamoid bone (palmar border)
2 Palmar (intersesamoidean) ligament
3 Superficial digital flexor tendon
    3a Manica flexoria
4 Deep digital flexor tendon
5 Palmar annular ligament
6 Digital sheath cavity
    6a Synovial membrane
    6b Collateral recess
    6c Proximal recess (uncompletly filled)
7 Ramus of the lateral proper palmar digital vein
8 Ramus of the medial proper palmar digital vein
9 Ergot rami (artery and vein)
10 Ergot cushion
11 Skin

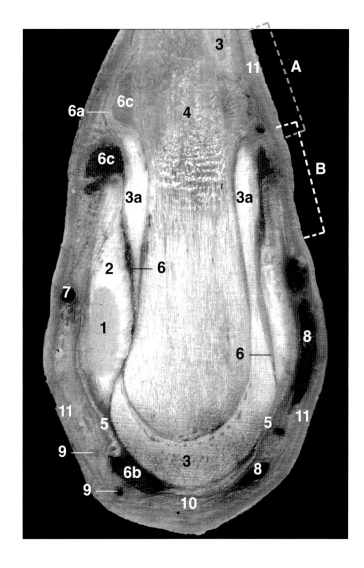

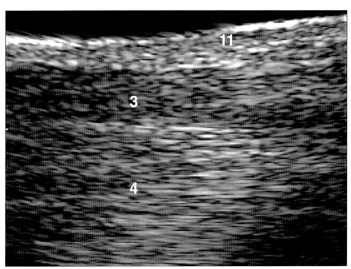

A Frontal ultrasound scan of the fetlock area, medial approach (see dotted area in illustration above, right).

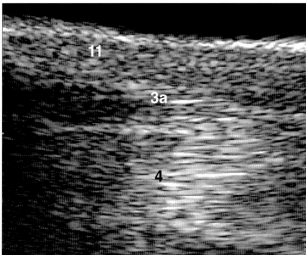

B Frontal ultrasound scan of the fetlock area, medial approach (see dotted area in illustration above).

F5: Frontal Section of the Fetlock

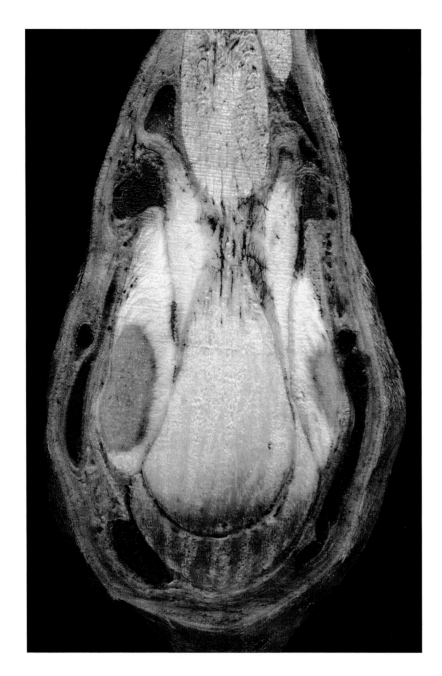

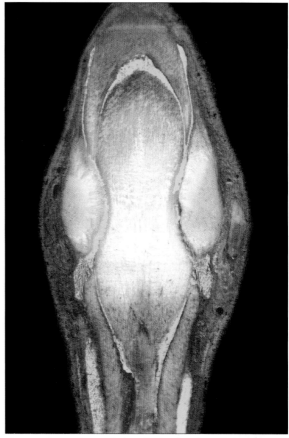

Frontal section of the fetlock after injection of coloured latex into the synovial cavities and vessels.

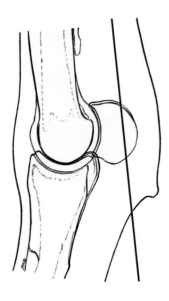

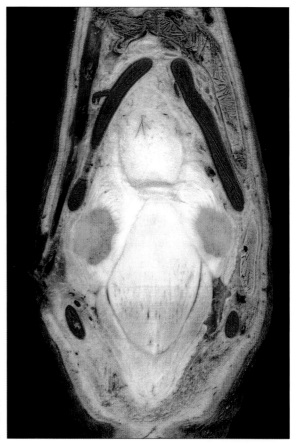

Frontal section of the fetlock after injection of coloured latex into the vessels.

F5: Frontal Section of the Fetlock

1 Lateral proximal sesamoid bone (palmar border)
2 Medial proximal sesamoid bone (palmar border)
3 Palmar (intersesamoidean) ligament
4 Superficial digital flexor tendon
   4a Manica flexoria
5 Deep digital flexor tendon
6 Palmar annular ligament
7 Proximal digital annular ligament
8 Digital sheath
   8a Synovial membrane
   8b Proximal recess (incompletely filled)
   8c Collateral recess
9 Lateral proper palmar digital artery
   9a Ergot ramus
10 Ramus of the lateral proper palmar digital vein
11 Ramus of the medial proper palmar digital vein
12 Lateral proper palmar digital nerve
13 Skin
   13a Skin section

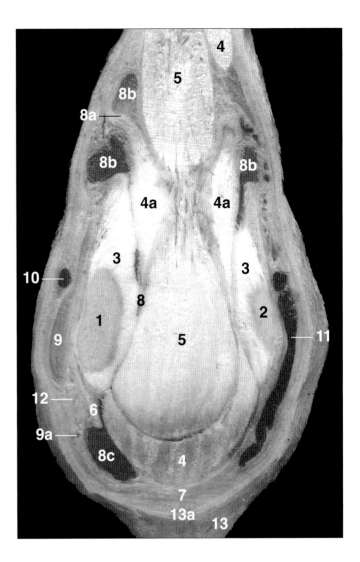

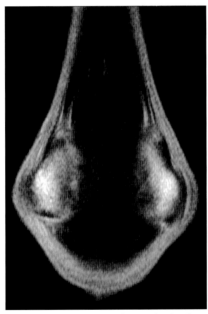

Frontal MRI scan of the fetlock.

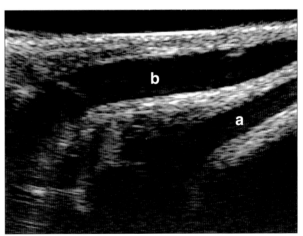

Frontal ultrasound scan of the fetlock area demonstrating the proper palmar digital artery (**a**) and vein (**b**).

F6: Frontal Section of the Fetlock

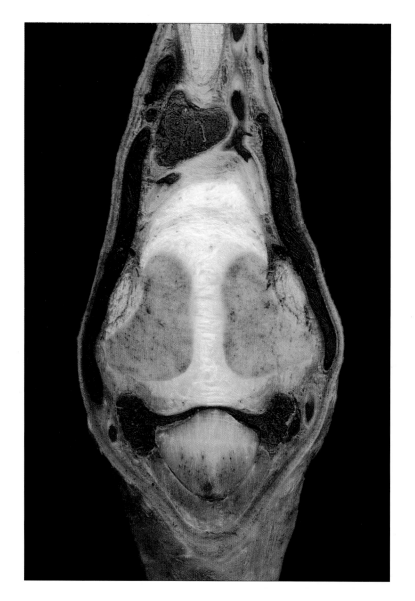

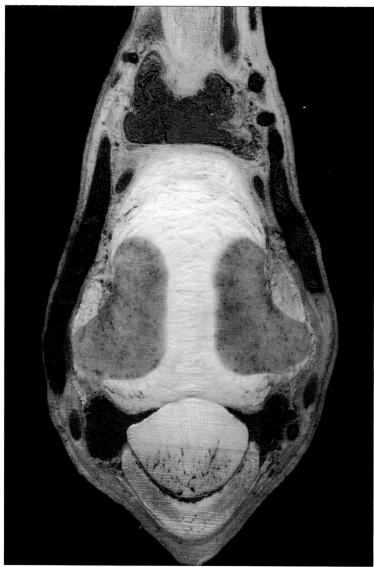

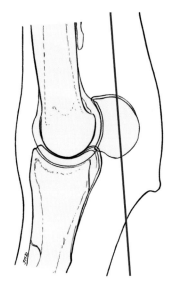

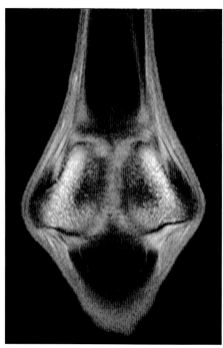

1 Lateral proximal sesamoid bone
   1a Apex
   1b Base
   1c Interosseus face
   1d Flexor surface
2 Medial proximal sesamoid bone
3 Palmar (intersesamoidean) ligament
4 Straight sesamoidean ligament
5 Third interosseus muscle (distal branch insertion)
6 Superficial digital flexor tendon

Frontal MRI scan of the fetlock.

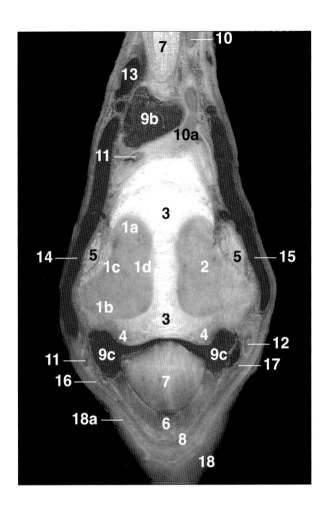

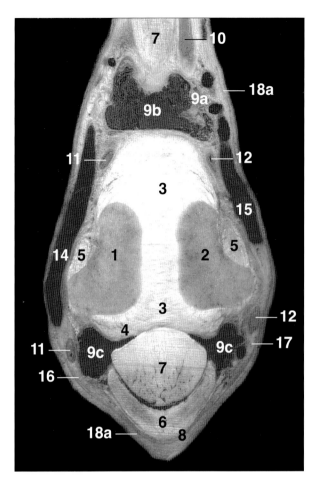

7 Deep digital flexor tendon
8 Proximal digital annular ligament
9 Digital sheath
    9a Synovial membrane
    9b Proximal recess
    9c Collateral recess
10 Medial common palmar digital artery
    10a Bifurcation
11 Lateral proper palmar digital artery
12 Medial proper palmar digital artery
13 Lateral common palmar digital vein
14 Lateral proper palmar digital vein
15 Medial proper palmar digital vein
16 Lateral proper palmar digital nerve
17 Medial proper palmar digital nerve
18 Skin
    18a Skin section

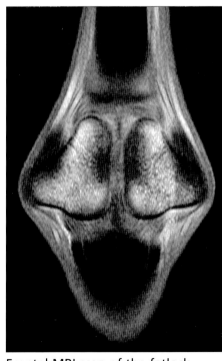

Frontal MRI scan of the fetlock.

F7: Frontal Section of the Fetlock

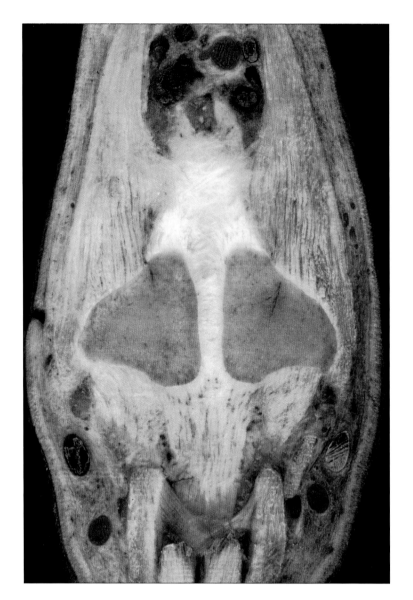

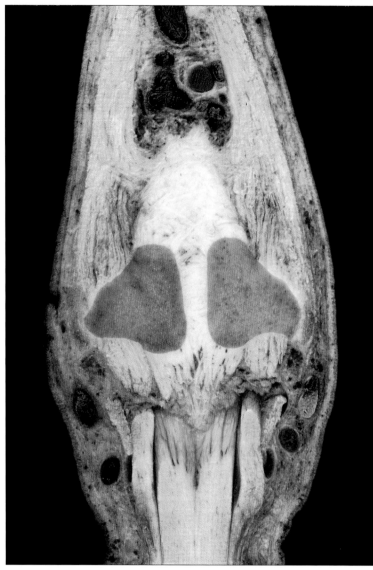

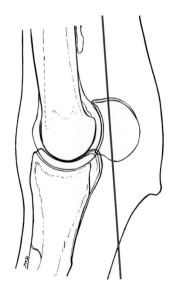

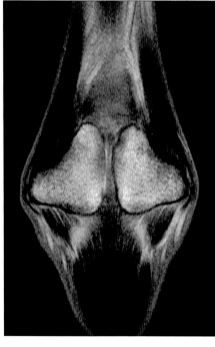

Frontal MRI scan of the fetlock.

1 Lateral proximal sesamoid bone
  1a Apex
  1b Base
  1c Interosseus face
  1d Flexor surface
2 Medial proximal sesamoid bone
3 Proximopalmar recess of the metacarpophalangeal joint
4 Palmar (intersesamoidean) ligament
5 Straight sesamoidean ligament
6 Lateral oblique sesamoidean ligament
7 Medial oblique sesamoidean ligament
8 Third interosseus muscle
  8a Lateral branch
  8b Medial branch

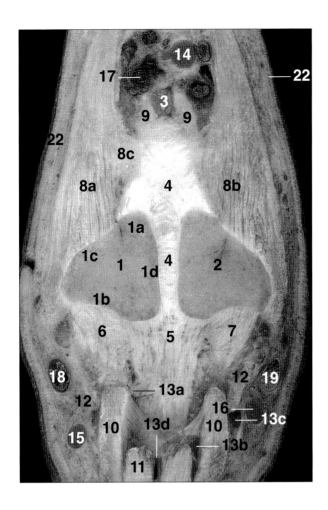

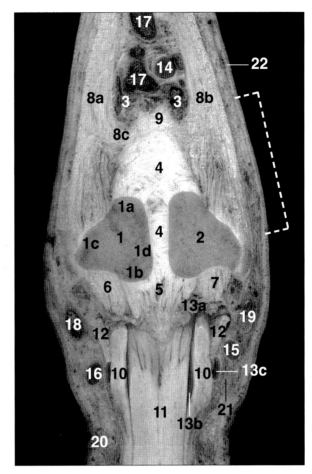

8c Attachment to palmar ligament
9 Metacarpointersesamoidean ligament
10 Superficial digital flexor tendon
11 Deep digital flexor tendon
12 Proximal attachment of the proximal
digital annular ligament
13 Digital sheath
    13a Synovial membrane
    13b Synovial cavity
    13c Collateral recess
    13d Synovial fold
14 Anastomosis between the common
palmar digital and metacarpal arteries
15 Lateral proper palmar digital artery
16 Medial proper palmar digital artery
17 Anastomosis between the common
palmar digital and metacarpal veins
18 Lateral proper palmar digital vein
19 Medial proper palmar digital vein
20 Lateral proper palmar digital nerve
21 Medial proper digital nerve
22 Skin

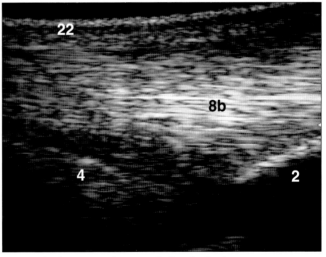

Frontal ultrasound scan of the fetlock area,
medial approach (see dotted area in illustration
above).

F8: Frontal Section of the Fetlock

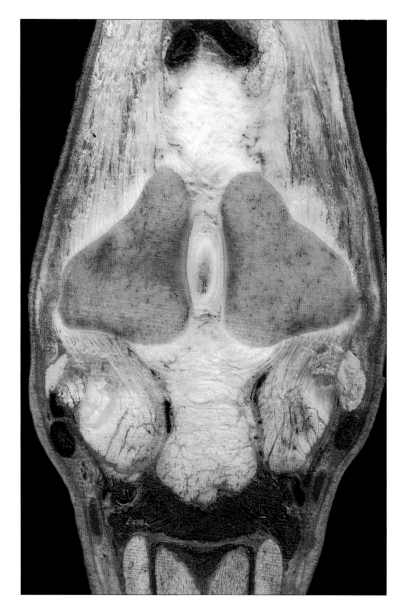

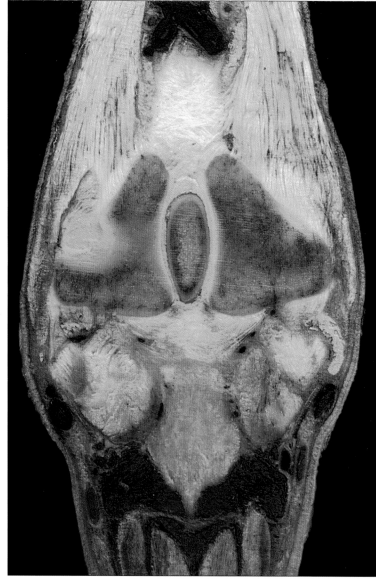

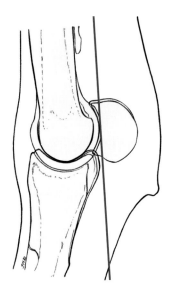

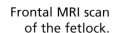

Frontal MRI scan
of the fetlock.

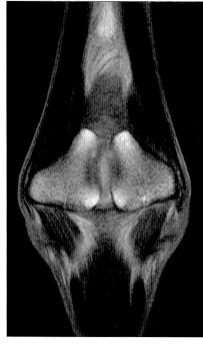

1 Metacarpal condyle (sagittal ridge)
2 Lateral proximal sesamoid bone
   2a Apex
   2b Base
   2c Interosseus face
   2d Articular surface
3 Medial proximal sesamoid bone
4 Recesses of the metacarpophalangeal joint
   4a Proximopalmar recess
   4b Distocollateral recess
5 Palmar (intersesamoidean) ligament
6 Metacarpointersesamoidean ligament
7 Straight sesamoidean ligament
8 Lateral oblique sesamoidean ligament

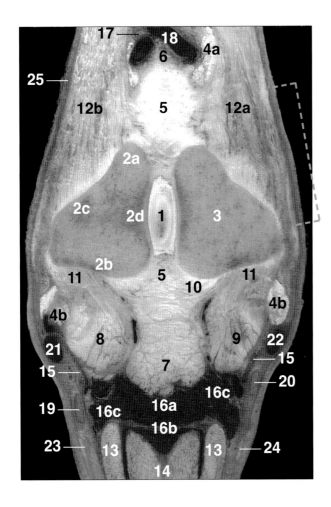

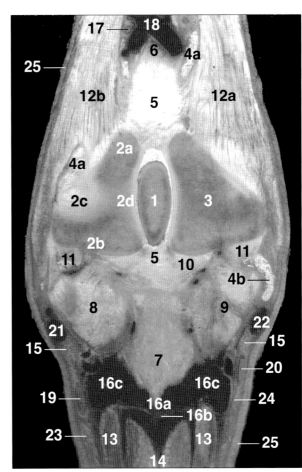

9 Medial oblique sesamoidean ligament
10 Cruciate sesamoidean ligament
11 Short sesamoidean ligament
12 Third interosseus muscle
    12a Medial branch
    12b Lateral branch
13 Superficial digital flexor tendon
14 Deep digital flexor tendon
15 Proximal digital annular ligament
    (proximal attachment)
16 Digital sheath
    16a Synovial cavity
    16b Synovial fold
    16c Collateral recess
17 Palmar metacarpal arteries
18 Palmar metacarpal veins
19 Lateral proper palmar digital artery
20 Medial proper palmar digital artery
21 Lateral proper palmar digital vein
22 Medial proper palmar digital vein
23 Lateral proper palmar digital nerve
24 Medial proper palmar digital nerve
25 Skin

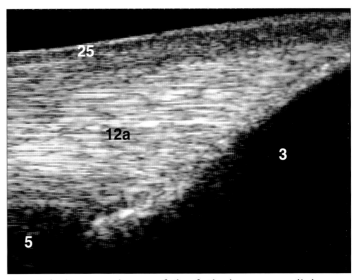

Frontal ultrasound scan of the fetlock area, medial
approach (see dotted area in illustration above, left).

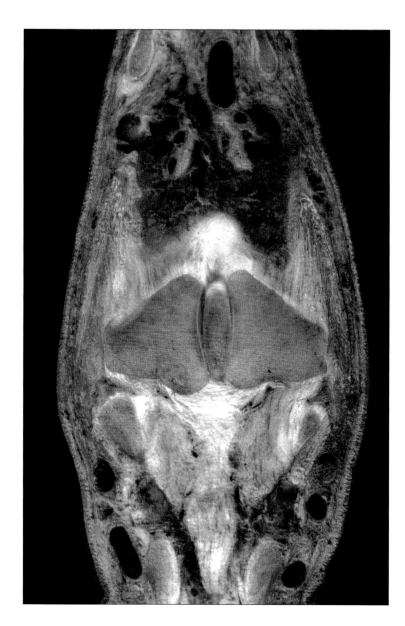

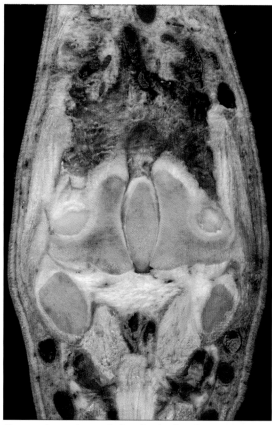

Frontal section of the fetlock after injection of coloured latex into the vessels.

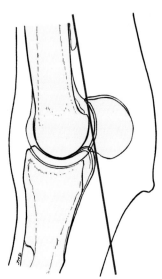

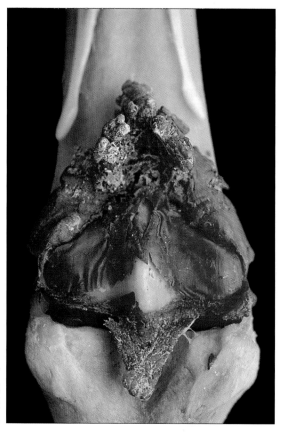

Dissected specimen after injection of coloured latex into the metacarpophalangeal joint cavity.

1 Metacarpal condyle (sagittal ridge)
2 Second metacarpal bone
3 Fourth metacarpal bone
4 Proximal phalanx
    4a Lateral palmar eminence
    4b Medial palmar eminence
5 Lateral proximal sesamoid bone
    5a Apex
    5b Base
    5c Articular surface
    5d Interosseus face
6 Medial proximal sesamoid bone
7 Synovial cavity of the metacarpophalangeal joint
    7a Proximopalmar recess
    7b Synovial villi
8 Palmar (intersesamoidean) ligament
9 Lateral collateral sesamoidean ligament
10 Medial collateral sesamoidean ligament
11 Metacarpointersesamoidean ligament
12 Straight sesamoidean ligament
13 Medial oblique sesamoidean ligament
14 Lateral oblique sesamoidean ligament
15 Cruciate sesamoidean ligament
16 Short sesamoidean ligament
17 Third interosseus muscle
    17a Lateral branch
    17b Medial branch
    17c Lateral extensor branch
    17d Medial extensor branch
18 Superficial digital flexor tendon
    18a Lateral branch
    18b Medial branch
19 Proximal digital annular ligament (proximal attachment)
20 Digital sheath (collateral recess)
21 Medial common palmar digital artery
22 Palmar metacarpal artery
23 Lateral proper palmar digital artery
24 Medial proper palmar digital artery
25 Palmar metacarpal vein
26 Lateral proper palmar digital vein
27 Medial proper palmar digital vein
28 Skin

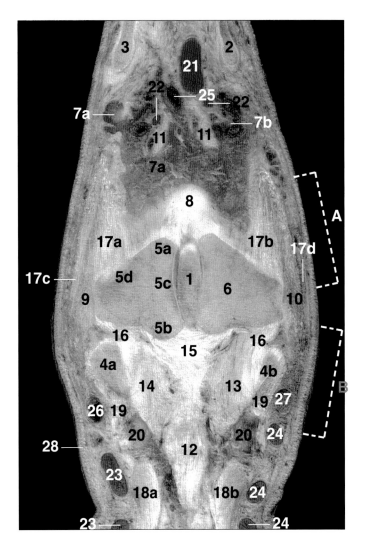

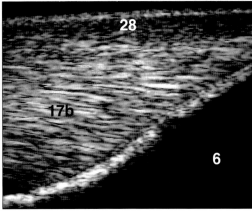

A Frontal ultrasound scan of the fetlock area, palmaromedial approach (see dotted area in illustration above).

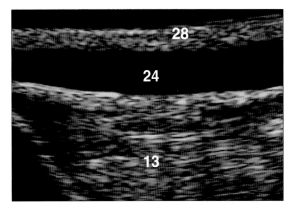

B Frontal ultrasound scan of the fetlock area, palmaromedial approach (see dotted area in illustration at top).

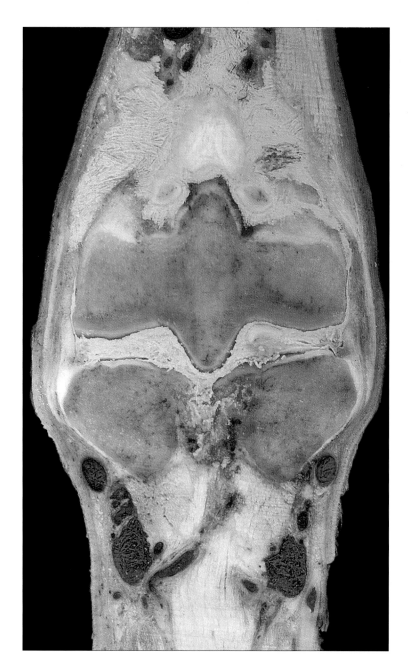

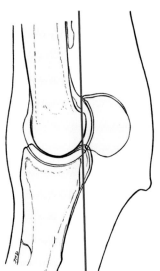

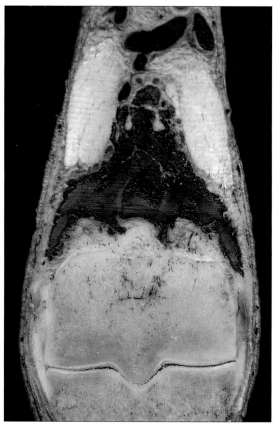

Frontal section of the fetlock after injection of coloured latex into the synovial cavities and vessels.

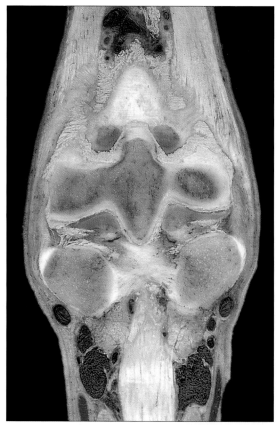

Frontal section of the fetlock after injection of coloured latex into the synovial cavities and vessels.

1 Metacarpal condyle
  1a Sagittal ridge
  1b Lateral part
  1c Medial part
2 Proximal phalanx (P1)
  2a Lateral palmar eminence
  2b Medial palmar eminence
3 Lateral proximal sesamoid bone (apex)
4 Medial proximal sesamoid bone
  4a Apex
  4b Base
5 Synovial cavity of the metacarpophalangeal joint
  5a Proximopalmar recess
  5b Distopalmar recess
6 Palmar (intersesamoidean) ligament
7 Straight sesamoidean ligament
8 Lateral oblique sesamoidean ligament
9 Medial oblique sesamoidean ligament
10 Lateral collateral sesamoidean ligament
11 Medial collateral sesamoidean ligament
12 Lateral collateral ligament (deep part)
13 Medial collateral ligament (deep part)
14 Third interosseus muscle
  14a Lateral branch
  14b Medial branch
  14c Lateral extensor branch
  14d Medial extensor branch
15 Proximal digital annular ligament (proximal attachment)
16 Digital sheath (collateral recess)
17 Palmar metacarpal artery
18 Palmar metacarpal vein
19 Ramus (artery) of P1
20 Lateral proper palmar digital vein
  20a Ramus (artery and vein) of P1
21 Medial proper palmar digital vein
  21a Ramus (artery and vein) of P1
22 Skin

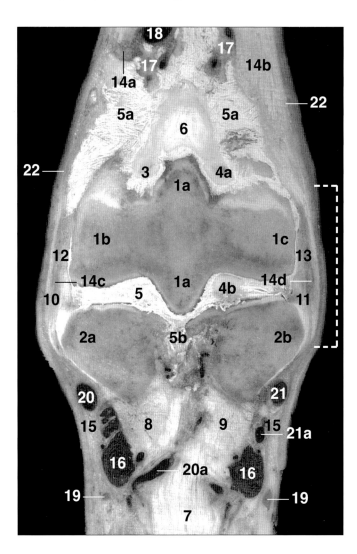

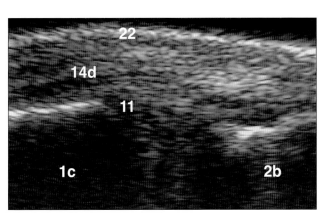

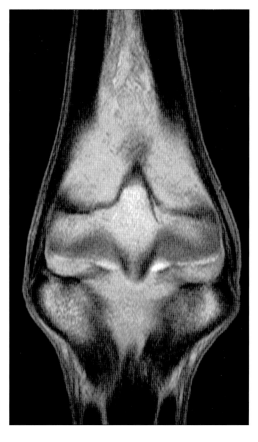

Frontal ultrasound scan of the fetlock, medial approach (see dotted area in picture above).

Frontal MRI scan of the fetlock.

F11: Frontal Section of the Metacarpophalangeal Joint

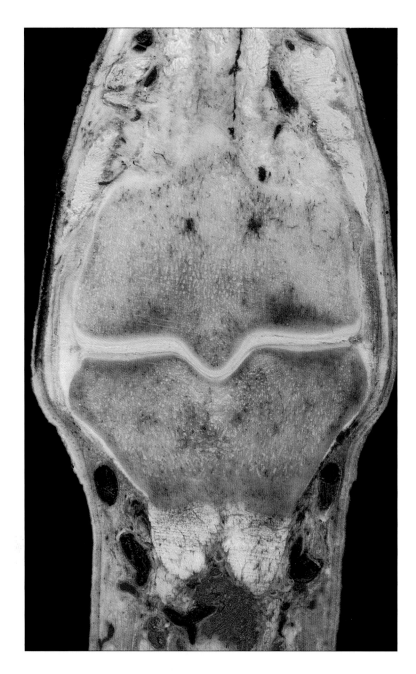

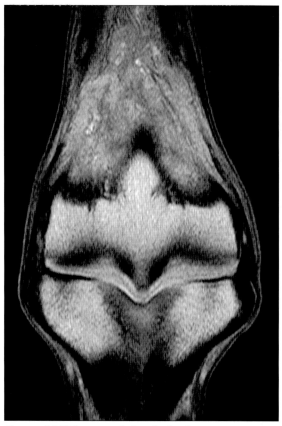

Frontal MRI scan of the fetlock.

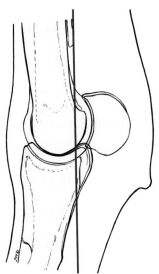

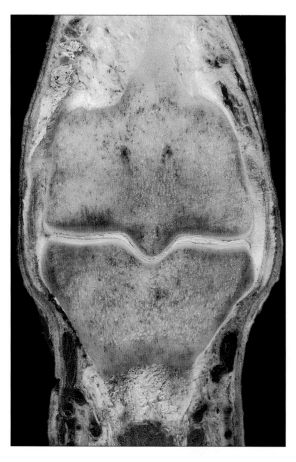

Frontal section of the
fetlock after injection of
latex into the synovial
cavities and vessels.

1 Third metacarpal bone
2 Metacarpal condyle
   2a Lateral part (lateral condyle)
   2b Medial part (medial condyle)
   2c Sagittal ridge
3 Proximal phalanx (P1)
   3a Lateral glenoid cavity
   3b Medial glenoid cavity
   3c Sagittal groove
4 Synovial membrane of the
   metacarpophalangeal (MP) joint
   4a Synovial fold
5 Synovial cavity of the MP joint
   5a Proximopalmar recess
6 Lateral collateral ligament (deep part)
7 Medial collateral ligament (deep part)
8 Lateral collateral sesamoidean ligament
9 Medial collateral sesamoidean ligament
10 Lateral oblique sesamoidean ligament
11 Medial oblique sesamoidean ligament
12 Lateral third interosseus extensor branch
13 Medial third interosseus extensor branch
14 Palmar metacarpal artery
15 Palmar metacarpal vein
16 Ramus (artery) of P1
17 Lateral proper palmar digital vein
   17a Palmar ramus of P1
18 Medial proper palmar digital vein
19 Palmar recess of the proximal
   interphalangeal joint
20 Skin

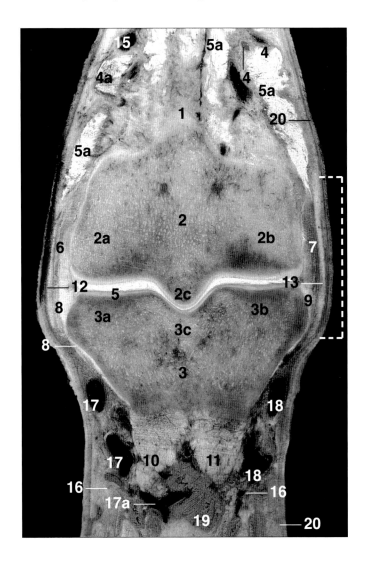

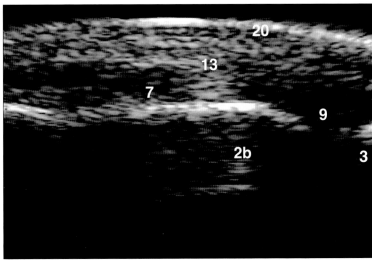

Frontal ultrasound scan of the fetlock, medial approach
(see dotted area in illustration above, right).

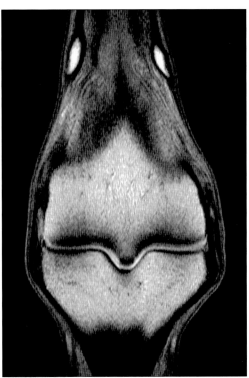

Frontal MRI scan of the fetlock.

F12: Frontal Section of the Metacarpophalangeal Joint

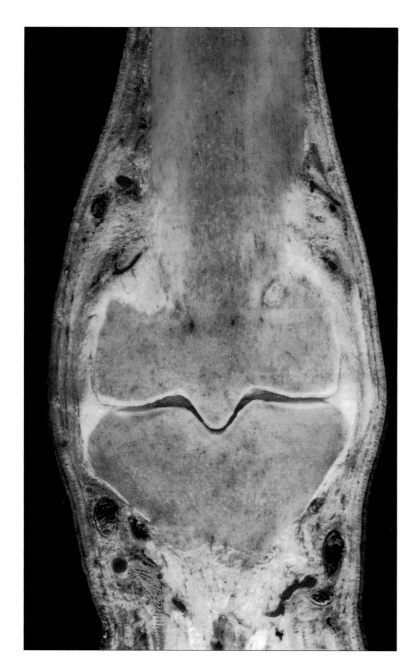

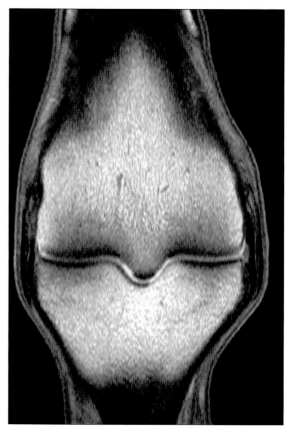

Frontal MRI scan of the fetlock.

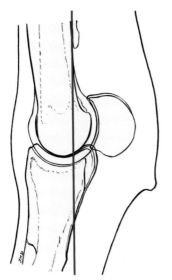

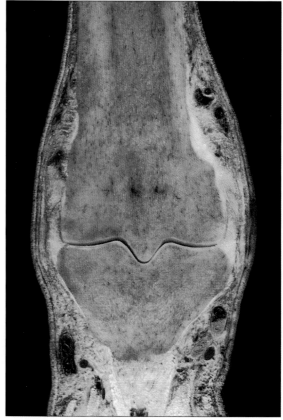

Frontal section of the fetlock after injection of coloured latex into the vessels.

1 Third metacarpal bone
2 Metacarpal condyle
    2a Lateral part (lateral condyle)
    2b Medial part (medial condyle)
    2c Sagittal ridge
3 Proximal phalanx (P1)
    3a Lateral glenoid cavity
    3b Medial glenoid cavity
    3c Sagittal groove
4 Synovial membrane of the metacarpophalangeal (MP) joint
    4a Metacarpophalangeal synovial fold
5 Synovial cavity of the MP joint
6 Lateral collateral ligament (deep part)
7 Medial collateral ligament (deep part)
8 Lateral collateral sesamoidean ligament
9 Medial collateral sesamoidean ligament
10 Lateral oblique sesamoidean ligament
11 Medial oblique sesamoidean ligament
12 Lateral third interosseus muscle extensor branch
13 Medial third interosseus muscle extensor branch
14 Proximal digital annular ligament
15 Palmar metacarpal artery
16 Palmar metacarpal vein
17 Palmar ramus of P1
18 Lateral proper palmar digital vein
19 Medial proper palmar digital vein
20 Palmar ramus of P1
21 Skin

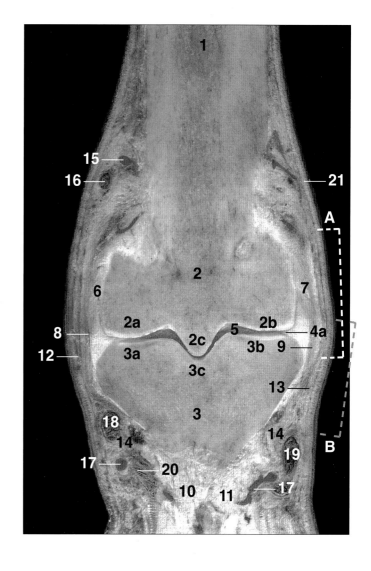

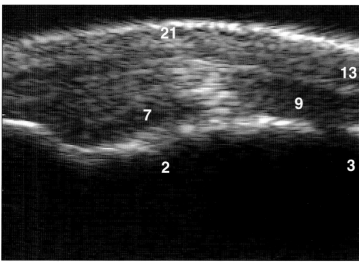

A Frontal ultrasound scan of the fetlock, medial approach (see dotted area in illustration above, right).

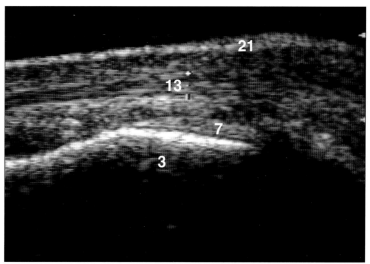

B Frontal ultrasound scan of the fetlock, medial approach (see dotted area in illustration above).

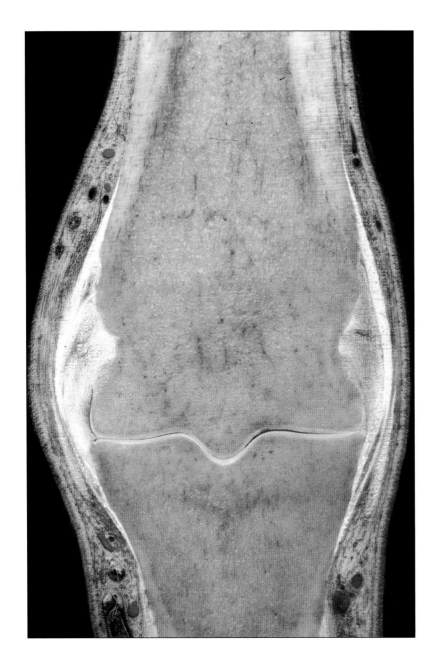

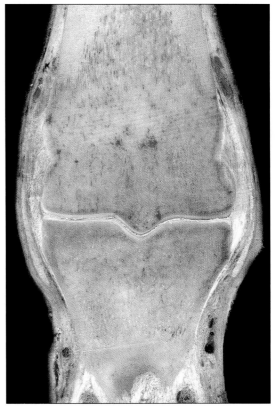

Frontal section of the fetlock after injection of coloured latex into the synovial cavities and vessels.

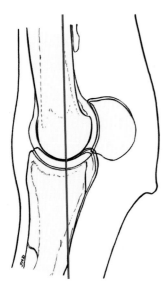

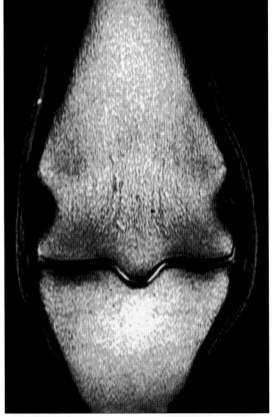

Frontal MRI scan of the fetlock.

1 Third metacarpal bone
   1a Lateral cortex
   1b Medial cortex
2 Metacarpal condyle
   2a Lateral part (lateral condyle)
   2b Medial part (medial condyle)
   2c Sagittal ridge
   2d Lateral collateral fossa
   2e Medial collateral fossa
3 Proximal phalanx (P1)
   3a Lateral glenoid cavity
   3b Medial glenoid cavity
   3c Sagittal groove
4 Synovial membrane of the metacarpophalangeal (MP) joint
   4a Metacarpophalangeal synovial fold
5 Synovial cavity of the MP joint
6 Lateral collateral ligament
   6a Superficial part
   6b Deep part
7 Medial collateral ligament
   7a Superficial part
   7b Deep part
8 Lateral collateral sesamoidean ligament
9 Medial collateral sesamoidean ligament
10 Third interosseus muscle
   10a Lateral extensor branch
   10b Medial extensor branch
11 Vascular network of the MP joint
12 Lateral dorsal ramus of P1
13 Medial dorsal rami (artery and vein) of P1
14 Lateral proper palmar digital vein
15 Dorsal metacarpal fascia
16 Skin

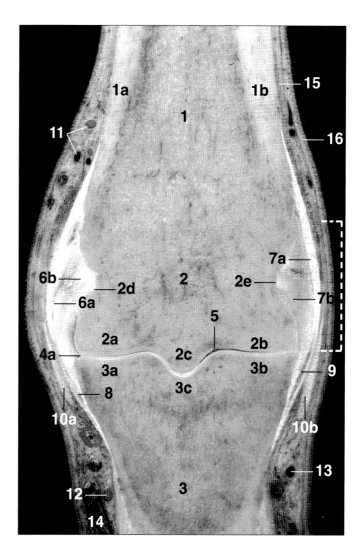

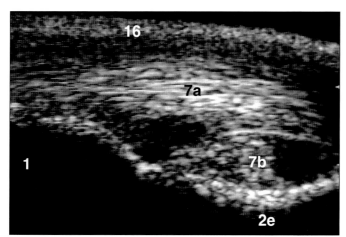

Frontal ultrasound scan of the fetlock, medial approach (see dotted area in illustration above, right).

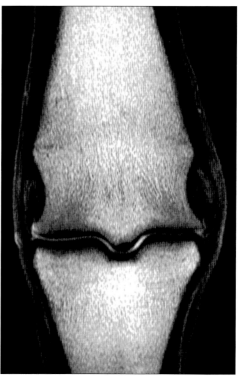

Frontal MRI scan of the fetlock.

F14: Frontal Section of the Metacarpophalangeal Joint

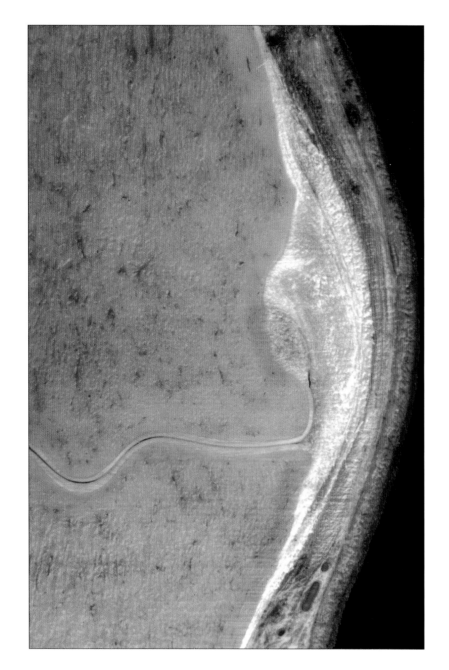

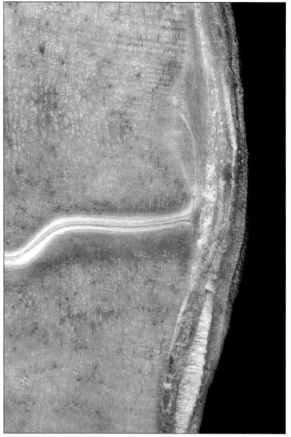

Frontal section of the fetlock after injection of coloured latex into the synovial cavities and vessels.

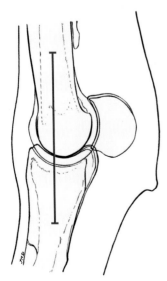

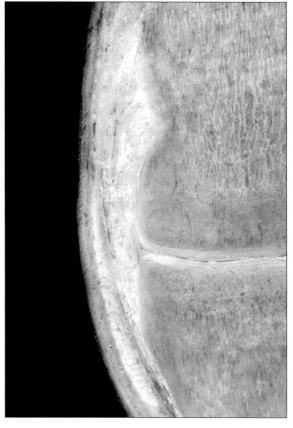

Frontal section of the fetlock after injection of coloured latex into the synovial cavities and vessels.

F14: Frontal Section of the Metacarpophalangeal Joint

367

1 Third metacarpal bone
2 Metacarpal condyle
  2a Medial part (medial condyle)
  2b Sagittal ridge
  2c Medial collateral fossa
3 Proximal phalanx (P1)
  3a Medial glenoid cavity
  3b Sagittal groove
4 Synovial membrane of the metacarpophalangeal (MP) joint
  4a Metacarpophalangeal synovial fold
5 Synovial cavity of the MP joint
6 Medial collateral ligament
  6a Superficial part
  6b Deep part
7 Dorsal capsule of the MP joint
8 Medial collateral sesamoidean ligament
9 Medial extensor branch of the third interosseus muscle
10 Dorsal ramus (artery) of P1
11 Dorsal metacarpophalangeal fascia
12 Skin

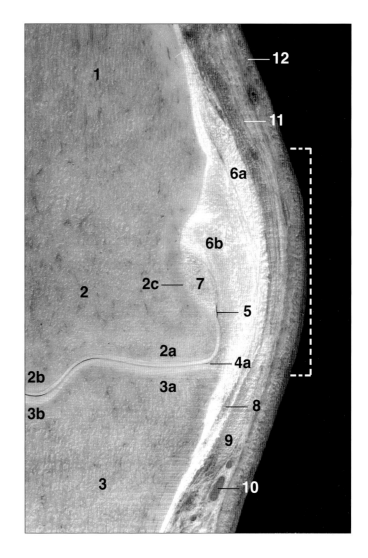

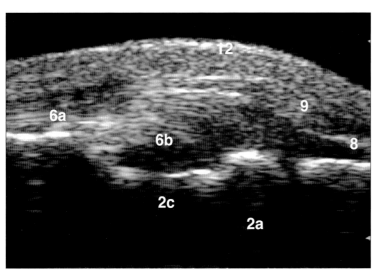

Frontal ultrasound scan of the fetlock, medial approach (see dotted area in illustration above, right).

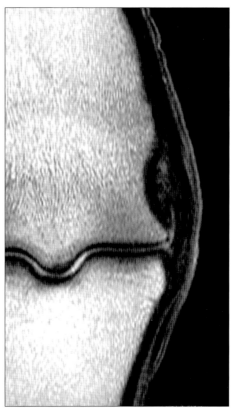

Frontal MRI scan of the fetlock.

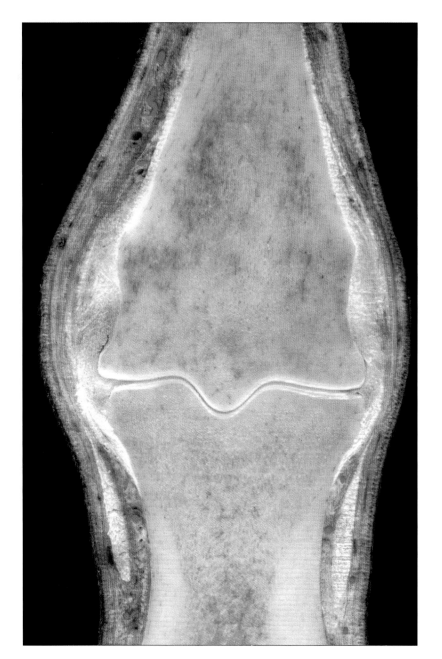

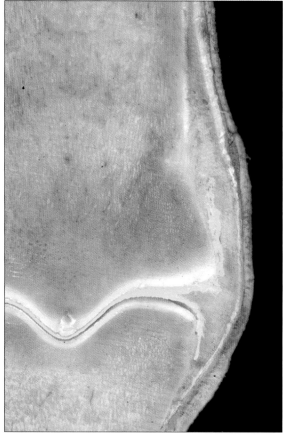

Frontal section of the fetlock after injection of coloured latex into the synovial cavities and vessels.

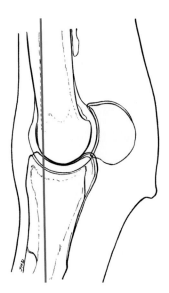

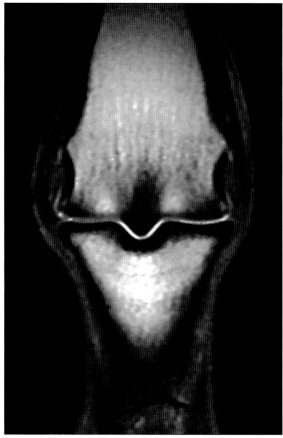

Frontal MRI scan of the fetlock after injection of latex into the arteries and fat material into the veins.

1 Third metacarpal bone
2 Metacarpal condyle
   2a Lateral part (lateral condyle)
   2b Medial part (medial condyle)
   2c Sagittal ridge
   2d Lateral collateral fossa
   2e Medial collateral fossa
3 Proximal phalanx (P1)
   3a Lateral glenoid cavity
   3b Medial glenoid cavity
   3c Sagittal groove
4 Synovial membrane and capsule of the metacarpophalangeal (MP) joint
   4a Metacarpophalangeal synovial fold
5 Synovial cavity of the MP joint
6 Lateral collateral ligament
   6a Superficial part
   6b Deep part
7 Medial collateral ligament
   7a Superficial part
   7b Deep part
8 Third interosseus muscle
   8a Lateral extensor branch
   8b Medial extensor branch
9 Vascular network of the MP joint
10 Dorsal ramus (artery) of P1
11 Dorsal metacarpophalangeal fascia
12 Skin

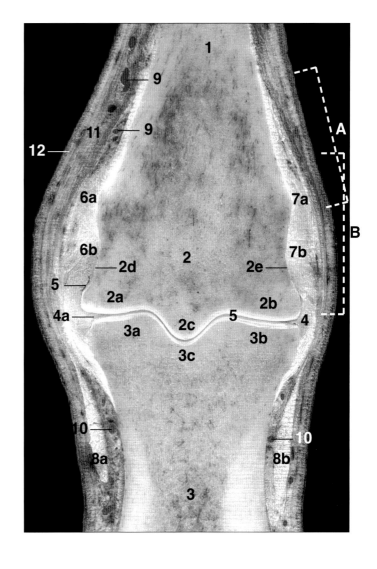

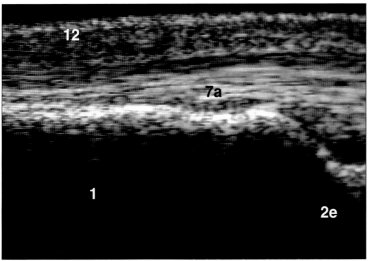

A Frontal ultrasound scan of the fetlock, medial approach (see dotted area in illustration above, right).

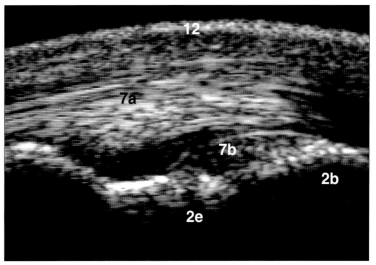

B Frontal ultrasound scan of the fetlock, medial approach (see dotted area in illustration above).

F16: Frontal Section of the Metacarpophalangeal Joint

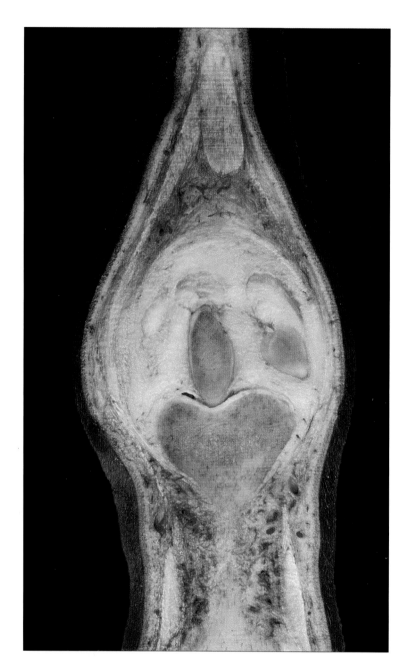

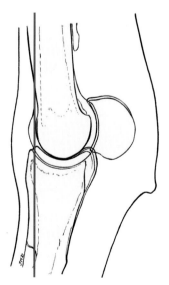

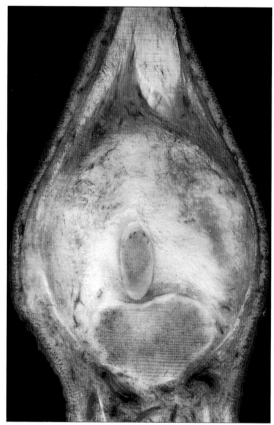

Frontal section of the fetlock after injection of coloured latex into the vessels.

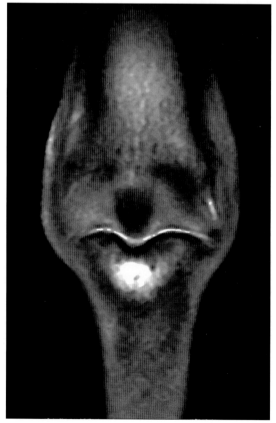

Frontal MRI scan of the fetlock after injection of latex into the arteries and fat material into the veins.

F16: Frontal Section of the Metacarpophalangeal Joint

371

1 Metacarpal condyle
  1a Medial part (medial condyle)
  1b Sagittal ridge
2 Proximal phalanx
  2a Sagittal groove
  2b Proximodorsal articular margin
3 Dorsal capsule of the metacarpophalangeal (MP) joint
4 Synovial membrane of the MP joint
  4a Proximodorsal synovial fold
  4b Metacarpophalangeal synovial fold
5 Synovial cavity of the MP joint
6 Dorsal digital extensor tendon
7 Lateral digital extensor tendon
8 Subtendinous bursa
9 Third interosseus muscle
  9a Lateral extensor branch
  9b Medial extensor branch
10 Dorsal metacarpophalangeal fascia
11 Skin
  11a Skin section

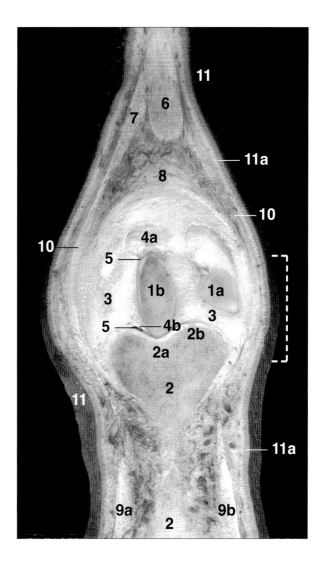

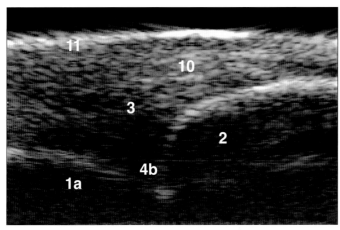

Frontal ultrasound scan of the fetlock, medial approach (see dotted area in illustration above, right).

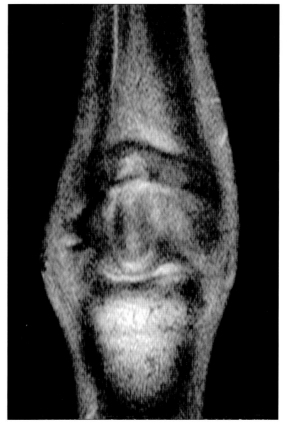

Frontal MRI scan of the fetlock.

F17: Frontal Section of the Metacarpophalangeal Joint

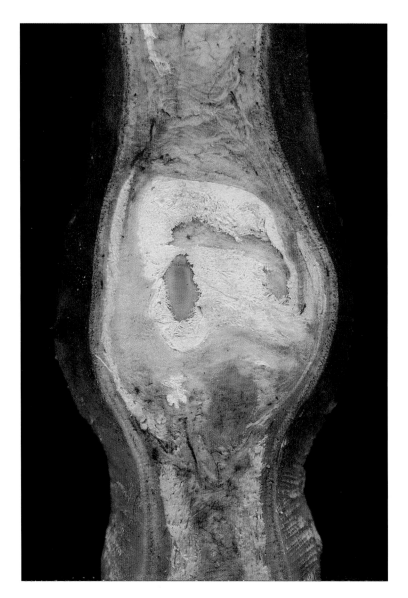

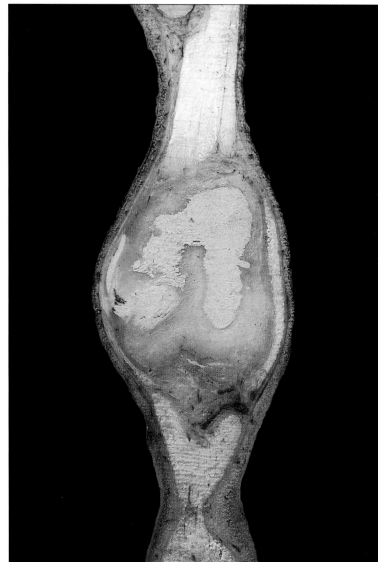

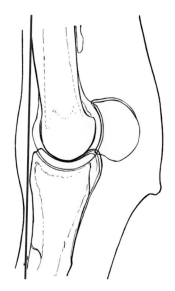

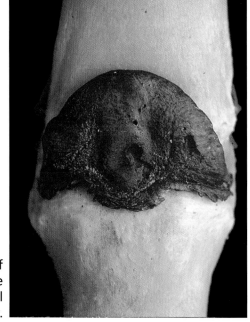

Casting preparation of the dorsal recess of the metacarpophalangeal joint, dorsal view.

F17: Frontal Section of the Metacarpophalangeal Joint

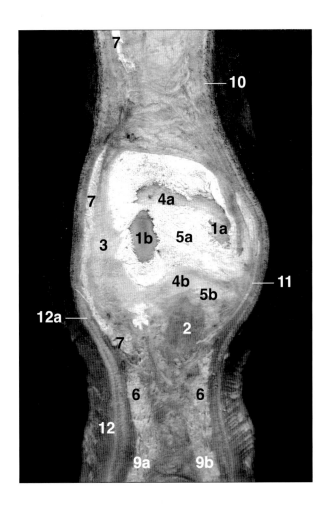

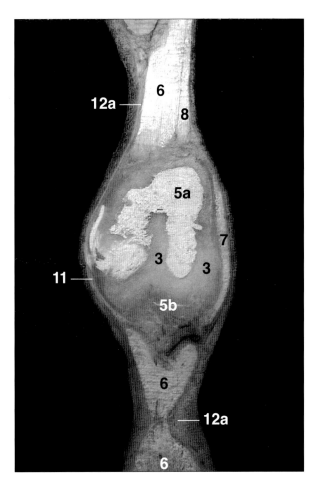

1 Metacarpal condyle
  1a Medial part (medial condyle)
  1b Sagittal ridge
2 Proximal phalanx
3 Dorsal capsule of the
  metacarpophalangeal (MP) joint
4 Synovial membrane of the MP joint
  4a Proximodorsal synovial fold
  4b Metacarpophalangeal synovial fold
5 Synovial cavity of the MP joint
  5a Dorsal recess
  5b Distodorsal recess
6 Dorsal digital extensor tendon
7 Lateral digital extensor tendon
8 Accessory digital extensor tendon
9 Third interosseus muscle
  9a Lateral extensor branch
  9b Medial extensor branch
10 Dorsal metacarpal fascia
11 Dorsal metacarpophalangeal fascia
12 Skin
  12a Skin section

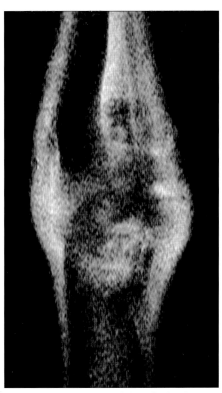

Frontal MRI scan of the fetlock.

Glossary of English and Latin Equivalents

Note: not every English name has a Latin equivalent; asterisks indicate names that are used only rarely to identify structures of the equine distal limb.

English	Latin
REGIONS	**REGIONES**
Metacarpophalangeal region (fetlock)	Regio metacarpophalangea
Pastern region	Regio compedis
Coronal region (coronet)	Regio coronalis
Foot	
BONES	**OSSA**
Cortical bone	Substantia corticalis
Compact bone	Substantia compacta
Spongious (cancellous) bone	Substantia spongiosa
Metacarpal bones II, III, IV	**Os metacarpalia II, III, IV**
Body	Corpus
Dorsal surface	Facies dorsalis
Palmar surface	Facies palmaris
Medial border	Margo medialis
Lateral border	Margo lateralis
Head (metacarpal condyle)	**Caput**
Sagittal ridge	
Lateral part (lateral condyle)	
Medial part (medial condyle)	
Dorsal margin	
Palmar margin	
Proximal phalanx	**Phalanx proximalis (os compedale)**
Base of the proximal phalanx (proximal end)	Basis phalangis proximalis
Articular fossa	Fovea articularis
Proximal sagittal groove	
Medial glenoid cavity	
Lateral glenoid cavity	
Dorsal margin	
Palmar margin	
Medial palmar eminence	Eminentia palmaris medialis
Lateral palmar eminence	Eminentia palmaris lateralis
Body of the proximal phalanx	Corpus phalangis proximalis
Trigone of the proximal phalanx	Trigonum phalangis proximalis
Head of the proximal phalanx (distal condyle)	Caput phalangis proximalis
Distal sagittal (intercondylar) groove	
Medial distal condyle	
Lateral distal condyle	
Middle phalanx	**Phalanx media (os coronale)**
Base of the middle phalanx (proximal end)	Basis phalangis mediae
Articular fossa	Fovea articularis
Medial glenoid cavity	
Lateral glenoid cavity	
Extensor process	Processus extensorius
Flexor tuberosity	Tuberositas flexoria
Body of the middle phalanx	Corpus phalangis mediae
Head of the middle phalanx (distal condyle)	Caput phalangis mediae

Distal phalanx
Spongious bone*
Subchondral bone*
Distopalmar compact bone*
Insertion fossa for the collateral ligament*
Articular surface
Sesamoidean articular surface
Parietal surface
Medial part
Medial parietal sulcus (groove)
Medial palmar process
Foramen of the medial palmar process
Incisura (notch) of the medial palmar process
Dorsal part
Lateral part
Lateral parietal sulcus (groove)
Lateral palmar process
Foramen of the lateral palmar process
Incisura (notch) of the lateral palmar process
Solar surface
Flexor surface
Semilunar line
Planum cutaneum
Medial solar sulcus
Lateral solar sulcus
Medial solar foramen
Lateral solar foramen
Solar canal
Coronal (coronary) border
Extensor process
Solar (distal) border
(Crena marginis solearis)

Medial ungular cartilage

Lateral ungular cartilage

Proximal sesamoid bone
Articular surface
Flexor surface
Interosseus face
Apex
Body
Base
Palmar border

Distal sesamoid bone
Spongious bone*
Compact bone*
Flexor surface
Sagittal ridge
Articular surface
Proximal border
Distal border
Lateral angle
Medial angle

JOINTS
Articular cartilage
Synovial fossa
Articular (joint) cavity
Articular (joint) margin

Phalanx distalis (os ungulare)

Facies articularis
Facies articularis sesamoidea
Facies parietalis
Pars medialis
Sulcus parietalis medialis
Processus palmaris medialis
Foramen processus palmaris medialis
Incisura processus palmaris medialis
Pars dorsalis
Pars lateralis
Sulcus parietalis lateralis
Processus palmaris lateralis
Foramen processus palmaris lateralis
Incisura processus palmaris lateralis
Facies solearis
Facies flexoria
Linea semilunaris
Planum cutaneum
Sulcus solearis medialis
Sulcus solearis lateralis
Foramen soleare mediale
Foramen soleare laterale
Canalis solearis
Margo coronalis
Processus extensorius
Margo solearis
(Crena marginis solearis)

Cartilago ungularis medialis

Cartilago ungularis lateralis

Ossa sesamoidea proximalia
Facies articularis
Facies flexoria
Facies musculus interossei

Os sesamoideum distale

Facies flexoria

Facies articularis
Margo proximalis
Margo distalis

ARTICULATIONES
Cartilago articularis
Fossae synoviales
Cavum articulare
Labrum articulare

Glossary of English and Latin Equivalents

Articular (joint) capsule	Capsula articularis
Fibrous layer	Stratum fibrosum
Synovial layer (synovial membrane)	Stratum synoviale
Synovial plica (fold)	Plica synovialis
Synovial villi	Villi synoviales
Synovial fluid	Synovia
Ligament	Ligamenta

Metacarpophalangeal joint — **Articulatio metacarpophalangea**

Joint (articular) capsule (dorsal capsule)	Capsula articularis
Dorsal recess (pouch)	Recessus dorsales
Proximodorsal synovial fold*	
Distodorsal recess*	
Distodorsal (metacarpophalangeal) synovial fold*	
Palmar recess (pouch)	Recessus palmares
Proximopalmar recess	
Distopalmar recess	
Collateral recess	
Distocollateral recess*	
Collateral ligament	Ligamentum collateralia
Palmar (intersesamoidean) ligament	Ligamentum palmaria
Collateral sesamoidean ligament	Ligamentum sesamoidea collateralia
Metacarpointersesamoidean ligament	Ligamentum metacarpointersesamoideum
Straight sesamoidean ligament	Ligamentum sesamoideum rectum
Oblique sesamoidean ligament	Ligamentum sesamoidea obliqua
Sagittal part*	
Short sesamoidean ligament	Ligamentum sesamoidea brevia
Cruciate sesamoidean ligament	Ligamentum sesamoidea cruciata

Proximal interphalangeal joint — **Articulatio interphalangea proximalis manus**

Articular (joint) capsule	Capsula articularis
Dorsal recess (pouch)	Recessus dorsales
Distodorsocollateral recess*	
Palmar recess (pouch)	Recessus palmares
Sagittal palmar recess*	
Collateral palmar recess*	
Collateral ligament	Ligamentum collateralia
Palmar ligament	Ligamentum palmaria
Axial palmar ligament*	
Abaxial palmar ligament*	

Distal interphalangeal joint — **Articulatio interphalangea distalis manus**

Articular (joint) capsule	Capsula articularis
Dorsal recess	Recessus dorsales
Palmar recess	Recessus palmares
Proximopalmar recess	
Distopalmar recess	
Collateral recess	
Collateral ligament	Ligamentum collateralia
Collateral sesamoidean ligament	Ligamentum sesamoidea collateralia
(Impar) distal sesamoidean ligament	Ligamentum sesamoideum distale impar
Chondrocompedal ligament	Ligamentum chondrocompedalia
Chondrocoronal ligament	Ligamentum chondrocoronalia
Chondrosesamoidean ligament	Ligamentum chondrosesamoidea
Collateral chondroungular ligament	Ligamentum chondroungularia collateralia
Cruciate chondroungular ligament	Ligamentum chondroungularia cruciata

MUSCLES — **MUSCULI**

Superficial digital flexor muscle — **Musculus flexor digitalis superficialis**

Manica flexoria — Manica flexoria

Deep digital flexor muscle
   Metacarpophalangeal fibrocartilaginous part*
   Phalangeal fibrocartilaginous part*
Dorsal digital extensor muscle
Lateral digital extensor muscle
Accessory digital extensor tendon*

Third interosseus muscle
   Distal branch
   Extensor branch
Dorsal fascia of the manus
   Dorsal metacarpal fascia*
   Dorsal metacarpophalangeal fascia*
Palmar fascia
   Palmar metacarpal fascia*
Digital fascia
   Dorsal digital fascia*
Palmar annular ligament

Digital sheath fibrous wall

Proximal digital annular ligament
   (2 pars anulares + 1 pars cruciformis)
   Proximal attachment*
   Distal attachment*
Distal digital annular ligament
   (1 pars anularis + 1 pars cruciformis)
   Proximal attachment*
   Distal attachment*
Proximal scutum
Middle scutum
Distal scutum

Digital synovial tendon sheath
   Dorsal proximal recess*
   Palmar proximal recess*
   Collateral metacarpal recess*
   Palmar middle recess*
   Collateral digital recess*
   Palmar distal recess*
   Dorsal distal recess*
Tendon vincula
   Loose connective mesotendon*
Subtendinous bursa of the third interosseus muscle
Podotrochlear bursa
   Proximal recess
   Distal recess
   Collateral recess*

ARTERIES
Palmar metacarpal arteries II and III
Lateral common palmar digital artery III
Medial common palmar digital artery II

Medial (proper palmar) digital artery
Ergot ramus*
Palmar ramus of the proximal phalanx
Dorsal ramus of the proximal phalanx
Palmar ramus of the middle phalanx
Dorsal ramus of the middle phalanx

Musculus flexor digitalis profundus

Musculus extensor digitalis communis
Musculus extensor digitalis lateralis

Musculus interosseus III

Fascia dorsalis manus

Fascia palmaris

Fascia digiti

Ligamentum metacarpeum transversum superficiale (ligamentum anulare palmare)

Vaginae fibrosae digitorum manus
Pars anularis vaginae fibrosae (ligamentum anulare digiti)
Pars cruciformis vaginae fibrosae

Scutum proximale
Scutum medium
Scutum distale

Vagina synovialis tendinum digitorum manus

Vincula tendinum

Bursa subtendinea musculus interosseus III
Bursa podotrochlearis manus

ARTERIAE
Arteriae metacarpeae palmares II et III
Arteria digitalis palmaris communis III
Arteria digitalis palmaris communis II

Arteria digitalis (palmaris propria III) medialis

Ramus palmaris phalangis proximalis
Ramus dorsalis phalangis proximalis
Ramus palmaris phalangis mediae
Ramus dorsalis phalangis mediae

Ramus of the digital torus	Ramus tori digitalis
Coronal artery	Arteria coronalis
Dorsal ramus of the distal phalanx	Ramus dorsalis phalangis distalis
Terminal arch	Arcus terminalis
Solar marginal artery (circonflex artery)	Arteria marginis solearis

Lateral (proper palmar) digital artery — **Arteria digitalis (palmaris propria III) lateralis**

Palmar ramus of the proximal phalanx	Ramus palmaris phalangis proximalis
Dorsal ramus of the proximal phalanx	Ramus dorsalis phalangis proximalis
Intermediate ramus*	
Palmar ramus of the middle phalanx	Ramus palmaris phalangis mediae
Dorsal ramus of the middle phalanx	Ramus dorsalis phalangis mediae
Ramus of the digital torus	Ramus tori digitalis
Coronal artery	Arteria coronalis
Dorsal ramus of the distal phalanx	Ramus dorsalis phalangis distalis

VEINS — VENAE

Lateral common palmar digital vein	Vena digitalis palmaris communis III

Lateral (proper palmar) digital vein — **Vena digitalis (palmaris propria III) lateralis**

Coronal vein	Vena coronalis
Terminal arch	Arcus terminalis
Palmar metacarpal veins II and III	Venae metacarpeae palmares II et III
Distal deep palmar anastomosis	Arcus palmaris profundus distalis
Medial common palmar digital vein	Vena digitalis palmaris communis II

Medial (proper palmar) digital vein — **Vena digitalis (palmaris propria III) medialis**

Coronal vein	Vena coronalis
Ungular plexus	Plexus ungularis
Superficial ungular plexus*	
Deep ungular plexus*	
Lateromedial palmar anastomosis*	

NERVES — NERVI

Medial common palmar digital nerve	Nervus palmaris medialis (nervus digitalis palmaris communis II)

Medial (proper palmar) digital nerve — **Nervus digitalis palmaris (proprius) medialis**

Dorsal ramus	Ramus dorsalis
Intermediate ramus*	
Lateral common palmar digital nerve	Nervus palmaris lateralis (nervus digitalis palmaris communis III)
Medial palmar metacarpal nerve	Nervus metacarpeus palmaris medialis
Lateral palmar metacarpal nerve	Nervus metacarpeus palmaris lateralis

Lateral (proper palmar) digital nerve — **Nervus digitalis palmaris (proprius) lateralis**

Dorsal ramus	Ramus dorsalis
Intermediate ramus*	

INTEGUMENT — INTEGUMENTUM COMMUNE

Ergot	Calcar metacarpeum
Ergot cushion*	
Ergot ligament*	

CORIUM HOOF AND PAD — UNGULA

Limbus — **Limbus**

Periople (stratum externum of the hoof wall)	Epidermis limbi (perioplum)
Horn (epidermal) tubules	Tubuli epidermales
Limbic (perioplic) dermis (limbic corium)	Dermis (corium) limbi
Dermal (corial) papillae	Papillae dermales (coriales)
Limbic cushion	Tela subcutanea limbi (pulvinus limbi)

Glossary of English and Latin Equivalents

Corona / **Corona**
- Coronal (coronary) epidermis — Epidermis coronae
  - Horn (epidermal) tubules — Tubuli epidermales
- Coronal (coronary) dermis — Dermis (corium) coronae
  - Dermal (corial) papillae — Papillae dermales (coriales)
- Coronal cushion — Tela subcutanea coronae (pulvinus coronae)

Paries (hoof wall) / **Paries**
- Parietal epidermis (stratum internum of the hoof wall) — Epidermis parietis
  - Epidermal lamellae — Lamellae epidermales
- Parietal dermis (parietal corium) — Dermis (corium) parietis
  - Dermal (corial) lamellae — Lamellae dermales (coriales)
- Horny wall — Paries corneus (lamina)
  - Limbic (perioplic) horn — Stratum externum
  - Coronal (coronary) horn — Stratum medium
  - Parietal horn — Stratum internum
  - White zone — Zona alba
  - Collateral (lateral) part (quarter) — Pars lateralis
  - Collateral (medial) part (quarter) — Pars medialis
  - Dorsal part (toe) — Pars dorsalis
  - Lateral inflex part (lateral bar) — Pars inflexa lateralis
  - Medial inflex part (medial bar) — Pars inflexa medialis
  - Lateral palmar border (lateral heel) — Margo palmaris lateralis
  - Medial palmar border (medial heel) — Margo palmaris medialis
  - Lateral palmar parietal angle — Angulus parietis palmaris lateralis
  - Medial palmar parietal angle — Angulus parietis palmaris medialis
  - Coronal (coronary) border (proximal border) — Margo coronalis
  - Solear border (distal border) — Margo solearis
  - External face — Facies externa
  - Internal face — Facies interna
  - Limbic sulcus (groove) — Sulcus limbalis
  - Coronal (coronary) sulcus (groove) — Sulcus coronalis

Sole / **Solea**
- Epidermis of the sole — Epidermis soleae
  - Horn (epidermal) tubules — Tubuli epidermales
- Dermis (corium) of the sole — Dermis (corium) soleae
  - Dermal (corial) papillae — Papillae dermales (coriales)
- Solar subcutaneous layer — Tela subcutanea soleae
- Horny sole — Solea cornea
  - Body of the sole — Corpus soleae
  - Lateral branch of the sole — Crus soleae laterale
  - Medial branch of the sole — Crus soleae mediale
  - Parietal border — Margo parietalis
  - Central border — Margo centralis
  - Lateral angle of the sole — Angulus soleae lateralis
  - Medial angle of the sole — Angulus soleae medialis
  - External face — Facies externa
  - Internal face — Facies interna

Hoof (digital) pad / **Torus ungulae**
- Epidermis of the hoof (digital) pad — Epidermis tori
  - Epidermal tubules — Tubuli epidermales
- Dermis (corium) of the hoof (digital) pad — Dermis (corium) tori
  - Dermal (corial) papillae — Papillae dermales (coriales)

Digital cushion / **Tela subcutanea tori (pulvinus digitalis)**
- Proximal attachment (suspensory ligament)*
- Toric (proximal) part of the digital cushion (bulb of the heels) — Pars torica pulvini digitalis
- Horny part of the hoof pad — Torus corneus
  - Bulb of the lateral heel — Pars lateralis
  - Bulb of the medial heel — Pars medialis
  - External face — Facies externa
  - Internal face — Facies interna

Frog
Epidermis of the frog
   Horn (epidermal) tubules
Dermis (corium) of the frog
   Dermal (corial) papillae
Cuneal (distal) part of the digital cushion
Horny frog
   Apex of the frog
   Base of the frog
   Lateral crus (branch) of the frog
   Medial crus (branch) of the frog
   External face
   Internal face
   Lateral paracuneal sulcus (groove)
   Medial paracuneal sulcus (groove)
   Central cuneal sulcus (groove)
   Spine of the frog

Cuneus ungulae
Epidermis cunei
   Tubuli epidermales
Dermis (corium) cunei
   Papillae dermales (coriales)
Tela subcutanea cunei (pars cunealis pulvini digitalis)
Cuneus corneus
   Apex cunei
   Basis cunei
   Crus cunei laterale
   Crus cunei mediale
   Facies externa
   Facies interna
   Sulcus paracunealis lateralis
   Sulcus paracunealis medialis
   Sulcus cunealis centralis
   Spina cunei

Horny hoof, hoof capsule
Solear face
   Contact face
   Fornix face
Dorsal angle
Lateral angle
Medial angle
Lateral palmar angle
Medial palmar angle

Capsula ungulae
Facies solearis
   Facies contactus
   Facies fornicis
Angulus dorsalis
Angulus lateralis
Angulus medialis
Angulus palmaris lateralis
Angulus palmaris medialis

References

International Comittee on Veterinary Gross Anatomical Nomenclature (1994) *Nomina Anatomica Veterinaria*, 4th edn. World Association of Veterinary Anatomists, Ithaca, New York.
Schaller, O. (1992) *Illustrated Veterinary Anatomical Nomenclature*. Enke, Stuttgart.

Index

Index (E–L)

Index (P)